DISORDERS OF THE RESPIRATORY SYSTEM

Volume II of
THE SCIENCE AND PRACTICE
OF CLINICAL MEDICINE

Jay P. Sanford, M.D.

Editor-in-Chief
Professor of Medicine
and Dean, School of Medicine
Uniformed Services University of the Health Sciences
Bethesda, Maryland

Disorders of the Respiratory System

Edited by
Homayoun Kazemi, M.D.

Associate Professor of Medicine
Harvard Medical School
and Physician and Chief, Pulmonary Unit
Massachusetts General Hospital
Boston, Massachusetts

GRUNE & STRATTON
A Subsidiary of Harcourt Brace Jovanovich, Publishers
New York   San Francisco   London

Library of Congress Cataloging in Publication Data
Main entry under title:
Disorders of the respiratory system.
  (The Science and practice of clinical medicine;
  v.2) Includes bibliographies and index.
  1. Respiratory organs—Diseases. 2. Lungs.
I. Kazemi, Homayoun. II. Series. [DNLM: 1. Res-
piratory tract diseases—Congresses. W1 SC679 v.2/
WF140 D612]
RC731.D57   616.2   76-5496
ISBN 0-8089-0937-1

Grune & Stratton, Inc.
111 Fifth Avenue
New York, New York 10003

Library of Congress Catalog Card Number 76-5496
International Standard Book Number 0-8089-0937-1
Printed in the United States of America

Contents

Preface

Diseases of the respiratory system are diagnosed with increasing frequency and are one of the major causes of morbidity in patients. In recent decades our understanding of the physiologic function of the lung has expanded greatly, and physiologic tools are used continuously in the diagnosis and management of patients with respiratory disorders. The biochemical functions of the lungs in terms of host defense mechanisms, homeostasis of various polypeptides in the body as a whole and in the regulation of pulmonary microcirculation and airway function are becoming better known and understood.

This book is an attempt to bring together the physiologic function and the pathophysiologic alterations in the respiratory system. It is intended primarily for the medical student, house officer, and general physician, not necessarily for the pulmonary specialist, and is the second volume of a projected textbook entitled *The Science and Practice of Clinical Medicine.* The first part of this book describes anatomy, development, and nonrespiratory functions of the lung; physiology of respiration is then presented in some detail. The subsequent chapters on respiratory diseases group together disorders that share certain common physiologic traits, and these disorders, as far as possible, are discussed in relation to their pathophysiologic alterations. These chapters are not an exhaustive compilation of all of the diseases of the respiratory system. Rather, they are reviews of the major pathophysiologic disorders that share a common pattern of physiologic alterations or comparable etiologic factors, such as occupational lung disease. In addition there are sections on diagnostic approaches—physiologic, radiologic, isotopic, and surgical—as well as a section on physical signs and symptoms in pulmonary disease.

Since this book is part of a larger work, there are certain deliberate omissions. Pulmonary infections are included in the section on infections, pulmonary emboli are discussed in the book covering disorders of the cardiovascular system, and H^+ homeostasis is presented only very briefly in this volume since it is dealt with extensively in the book on the disorders of the renal system.

This book is the result of the contributing efforts of several authors, and I am grateful to them for their help. In particular I would like to express my gratitude to my colleague Denise J. Strieder, for not only writing extensively for this book but also for helping to review and edit many of the other chapters. I would also like to thank Lilian Roberts, who supervised and typed the initial manuscript.

Homayoun Kazemi, M.D.

Contributors

Reginald Greene, M.D.
Assistant Professor of Radiology
Harvard Medical School
and Associate Radiologist
Massachusetts General Hospital
Boston, Massachusetts

Hermes C. Grillo, M.D.
Professor of Surgery
Harvard Medical School
and Chief of General Thoracic Surgery
and Visiting Surgeon
Massachusetts General Hospital
Boston, Massachusetts

Russell C. Klein, M.D.
Director of Respiratory Therapy
Charity Hospital of Louisiana at New Orleans
and Associate Clinical Professor of Medicine
Louisiana State University
School of Medicine
New Orleans, Louisiana

Barry W. Levine, M.D.
Assistant Professor of Medicine
Harvard Medical School
and Assistant in Medicine
Massachusetts General Hospital
Boston, Massachusetts

Gerald Nash, M.D.
Associate Pathologist
Cedars-Sinai Medical Center
and Clinical Associate Professor of Pathology
University of California at Los Angeles
Medical Center
Los Angeles, California

Daniel C. Shannon, M.D.
Associate Professor of Pediatrics
Harvard Medical School
and Director, Pediatric Intensive Care Unit
Massachusetts General Hospital
Boston, Massachusetts

Neil S. Shore, M.D.
Instructor in Medicine
Harvard Medical School
and Clinical Associate in Medicine
Massachusetts General Hospital
Boston, Massachusetts
and Director of Pulmonary Medicine
Salem Hospital
Salem, Massachusetts

John D. Stoeckle, M.D.
Associate Professor of Medicine
Harvard Medical School
and Attending Physician
and Chief of the Medical Clinic
Massachusetts General Hospital
Boston, Massachusetts

Denise J. Strieder, M.D.
Associate Professor of Pediatrics
Harvard Medical School
and Chief of Pulmonary Division
Children's Hospital Medical Center
and Assistant in Medicine
Massachusetts General Hospital
Boston, Massachusetts

ANATOMY OF THE LUNG

Gerald Nash

THORAX
Thoracic Skeleton

The thoracic skeleton consists of the 12 vertebrae, the sternum, and the ribs, which articulate with the vertebrae posteriorly and join the sternum anteriorly. The bony thorax is rigid, to provide protection for the thoracic organs; yet it is also pliable, to permit changes in thoracic volume during respiration. The thoracic skeleton forms a truncated cone with a small superior and large inferior opening. Anteriorly the apices of the lungs protrude about 2 in. above the superior opening; posteriorly they extend to the level of the neck of the first rib. Each thoracic vertebra has an articular facet on its superior aspect near the junction of the body and pedicle that receives the head of its corresponding rib. Thoracic vertebrae T2 through T8 also have inferior articulating facets. Each of these vertebrae articulates not only with its own rib, but also with the next lower rib. Each of the other thoracic vertebrae articulates only with its own rib. The vertebrocostal articulations are arranged in such a way that when the ribs are elevated they move outward, increasing both the anteroposterior and transverse dimensions of the thorax.

The sternum consists of three segments: manubrium, body, and xiphoid process. The manubrium receives the clavicles and the first two pairs of ribs. The body of the sternum and the manubrium has a hingelike junction, called the sternal angle, which permits changes in the anteroposterior dimensions of the thorax. The sternal body joins with the costal cartilages of ribs three through seven. The costal cartilages of ribs eight through ten join the seventh costal cartilages and thereby attach only indirectly to the sternum. The costal cartilages below the second rib ascend obliquely to join the sternum. Despite this ascent of the costal cartilages, the sternal ends of the ribs lie below the level of their vertebral connections, giving the ribs a downward inclination as they extend from the vertebrae to the sternum. The last two pairs of ribs articulate only with their vertebrae and do not join the sternum. The xiphoid process of the sternum, which receives part of the seventh costal cartilage at the xiphisternal junction, ends inferiorly in the posterior wall of the rectus sheath.

Muscles of Respiration

The principal muscles of respiration are the diaphragm and the intercostal muscles. The diaphragm is a thin muscle that separates the thoracic and abdominal cavities. It has sternal, costal, and vertebral origins and a central aponeurotic insertion called the central tendon. There are three large openings in the diaphragm through which pass the inferior vena cava, esophagus, and aorta. Each hemidiaphragm receives its motor innervation solely from the ipsilateral phrenic nerve. These motor fibers have their origins in ventral horn cells at spinal levels C3 to C5. The peripheral fringe of the diaphragm is supplied by sensory fibers from the lower intercostal nerves. The phrenic nerves provide sensory fibers to the remainder of the diaphragm. When the muscle fibers of the diaphragm contract on inspiration, the central tendon is pulled down, thereby increasing the thoracic volume. On expiration the diaphragm relaxes and returns to its resting condition. On forced expiration the abdominal muscles are brought into play, the abdominal viscera are forced upward, and the diaphragm may rise as high as the fourth intercostal space.

The intercostal muscles consist of outer and inner layers that crisscross, running in opposite directions. The fibers of each external intercostal muscle slope obliquely anteriorly and inferiorly from the inferior margin of a rib to the superior margin of the rib below. The fibers of each internal intercostal muscle run posteriorly and inferiorly from the lateral border of the sternum to the dorsal angle of the rib below. Each internal intercostal muscle is split into two layers (the internal and the innermost intercostal muscles) by the intercostal nerves and vessels. The mechanical action of the intercostal muscles has been the subject of debate. Some authorities believe that these muscles simply prevent the intercostal spaces from ballooning in and out during inspiration and expiration. Others think that the intercostal muscles play a more active role in respiration by producing movement of the ribs, notably elevation. They may also facilitate the action of other muscles on the rib cage. In addition to the diaphragm and intercostal muscles, many other muscles attached to the bony thorax may be used to augment

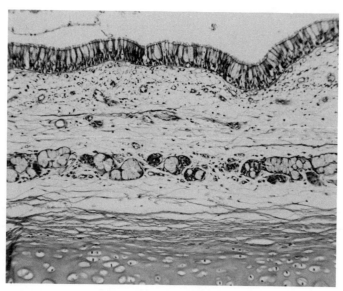

Fig. 1. Microscopic section of trachea showing pseudostratified columnar epithelium with ciliated and goblet cells, submucosal mucous and serous glands, and a portion of a cartilage plate (H&E × 130).

thoracic movements when respiratory efforts increase. These accessory muscles of respiration include the abdominal muscles, erector spinae, scalenes, sternocleidomastoids, and the serratus muscles. A familiar example of the use of accessory muscles of respiration occurs when an individual with air hunger grasps the arms of a chair to increase the force of his respiratory movements. This maneuver fixes the shoulders, enabling the anterior serratus muscles to assist in elevating the ribs.

Pleural Cavities

The pleural cavities contain the lungs and are bordered by the ribs, diaphragm, and mediastinum. The cavities are lined with parietal pleura, which consists of an inner layer of mesothelial cells lying on an outer layer of collagen and elastic fibers. The lungs are enveloped in visceral pleura, which has a structure similar to that of the parietal pleura. The visceral and parietal pleurae merge and become continuous at the root of the lung.

Lungs

The lungs are paired organs that fill most of the pleural cavities and are divided into lobes by deep fissures lined by visceral pleura. Oblique and horizontal fissures separate the right lung into three lobes, and a single oblique fissure divides the left lung into two lobes. Connective-tissue septae divide the pulmonary lobes into lobules, which are most easily recognized at the periphery of the lung, where the septae are most prominent. The bronchi, vessels, and nerves supplying the lungs enter at the pulmonary hila.

Airways

The airways include the trachea and the bronchial tree down to the level of the terminal bronchioles. They function as air conduits and do not participate in respiratory gas exchange. The trachea is a tube about 10 to 12 cm long and about 2 cm wide that begins at the cricoid cartilage. It descends through the superior mediastinum to the level of the junction of the manubrium and body of the sternum, where it bifurcates, giving rise to the main bronchi. The tracheal wall is lined by pseudostratified columnar epithelium that contains ciliated and nonciliated cells (Fig. 1). Among the latter are mucin-producing goblet cells. Against the basement membrane are small cells with oval nuclei, known as basal cells, which are thought to be able to differentiate into either ciliated or nonciliated epithelial cells. The cilia of the tracheobronchial tree have a coordinated whiplike beat that propels an overlying mucus coat upward toward the larynx, where it is either swallowed or expectorated. The mucus layer contains particulate matter from the inspired air, exfoliated epithelial cells, macrophages, and leukocytes. The mucociliary mechanism plays an important role in ridding the respiratory tract of environmental and endogenous contaminants. Beneath the basement membrane on which the tracheal epithelium lies is an elastic lamina propria. The submucosa contains mucus and serous glands whose ducts penetrate the mucosa to reach the surface. Beneath the submucosa, providing support for the wall, are a series of U-shaped cartilage plates that have their open ends facing posteriorly. A flat, transversely arranged layer of smooth-muscle fibers fills the gap between the tips of the cartilages.

The two main bronchi arise at the tracheal bifurcation and enter the lungs at the pulmonary hila. The right main bronchus is shorter than the left and deviates less from the axis of the trachea. This explains why aspirated foreign objects more often lodge in the right lung than in the left. Within the lung the main bronchi divide into lobar bronchi, one for each pulmonary lobe. The lobar bronchi give rise to segmental bronchi, ten in the right lung and eight in the left (Fig. 2). Each segmental bronchus and the portion of lung that it supplies constitute a bronchopulmonary segment. The broncho-

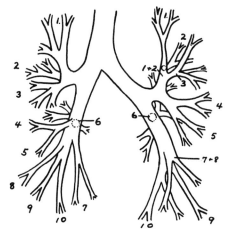

1. Apical	⎫ Upper	⎧ Apical posterior	1, 2
2. Posterior	⎬ Lobe	⎨	
3. Anterior	⎭ Bronchus	⎩ Anterior	3
4. Lateral	⎫ Middle	⎧ Superior lingular	4
5. Medial	⎭ Lobe Bronchus	⎩ Inferior lingular	5
6. Superior	⎫	⎧ Superior	6
7. Medial basal	⎪ Lower	⎨ Anteromedial basal	7, 8
8. Anterior basal	⎬ Lobe	⎪	
9. Lateral basal	⎪ Bronchus	⎨ Lateral basal	9
10. Posterior basal	⎭	⎩ Posterior basal	10

Fig. 2. Diagram of normal tracheobronchial tree showing standard numbering of segmental bronchi. (Reproduced by permission from Hinshaw HC: Diseases of the Chest. Philadelphia, WB Saunders, 1969, p 83.)

pulmonary segments are irregular and variable in size and shape, and they are separated from one another by connective-tissue septae. Knowledge of the distribution of the segmental bronchi and bronchopulmonary segments enables one to describe accurately the locations of pulmonary lesions and is important in thoracic surgery, bronchoscopy, and radiology.

The bronchi branch more or less dichotomously into successively smaller tubes, the total cross-sectional area of each generation being greater than that of the preceding one. After 6 to 25 generations the bronchial tree ends in terminal bronchioles. The large bronchi have essentially the same structure as the trachea. Medium-sized bronchi have irregularly shaped cartilage plates. The cartilage plates become smaller and more regular as the bronchi decrease in size, and they disappear at the level of the bronchioles. Bronchioles are generally less than 1 mm in diameter, are devoid of mucous glands, and have cuboidal rather than pseudostratified columnar epithelium. There are three or four orders of bronchioles, which end in terminal bronchioles. Terminal bronchioles still have ciliated epithelium, but goblet cells are few or absent. Nonciliated, heavily granulated cells known as Clara cells are also present in bronchioles. Recent studies have shown that Clara cells have ultrastructural and histochemical features characteristic of secretory cells. Although their function remains unknown it has been postulated that Clara cells are a source of the mucopolysaccharides and proteins that constitute part of

the subphase (base layer) of the alveolar surface-active layer (surfactant).

Respiratory Structures

The respiratory unit of the lung is the acinus. It is defined as the lung portion distal to a terminal bronchiole and includes respiratory bronchioles, alveolar ducts, alveolar sacs, and alveoli (Fig. 3). These are the structures that are involved in gas exchange. Respiratory bronchioles have cuboidal nonciliated epithelium and are devoid of goblet cells. Each respiratory bronchiole contains a few alveoli arising directly from its walls, and each bronchiole gives off from 2 to 11 alveolar ducts. The walls of alveolar ducts are made up entirely of alveoli and exhibit knoblike arrangements of smooth muscle surrounding the alveolar openings. The alveolar ducts terminate in either one or several alveolar sacs that are made up of a variable number of alveoli.

Alveoli are thin-walled sacs that have one open side. Alveolar walls contain a dense network of capillaries, which protrude into the alveolar spaces, as well as a supporting framework of reticulin and elastic fibers. Pores of Kohn, which are openings through the alveolar walls that measure about 7 to 9 μ in diameter, connect adjacent alveoli. These are rare or absent in children and increase in number with age. They may provide a pathway for collateral ventilation in cases of small-airway obstruction and may be involved in the spread of infection from one alveolus to another. The total alveolar surface area of the adult human lung varies between 43 and 102 m^2 de-

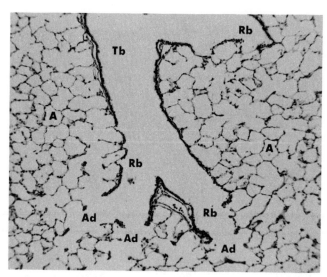

Fig. 3. Microscopic section of lung showing the respiratory structures. A terminal bronchiole (Tb) gives rise to respiratory bronchioles (Rb). The respiratory bronchioles give off alveolar ducts (Ad) that terminate in alveolar sacs made up of a variable number of alveoli (A). (H&E × 130).

pending on body length. This means that gas exchange can occur across a wide surface area and indicates that there is a great deal of reserve in the system.

The structure of the alveolar–capillary membrane was a matter of debate among histologists for many years. The controversy was resolved by the ultrastructural observations of Low and Karrer, who found that the alveolus is lined with a continuous layer of epithelium that in most areas is below the limit of resolution of the light microscope. The alveolar lining epithelium is composed primarily of two cell types (Fig. 4). Most of the alveolar surface is lined with extremely flattened cells that are similar in appearance to endothelial cells. These are membranous pneumocytes, or Type I alveolar cells. Membranous pneumocytes consist largely of thin cytoplasmic extensions that arise from a central nucleated portion. Most of the organelles, such as mitochondria and endoplasmic reticulum, are concentrated around the nucleus. The thin cytoplasmic extensions contain pinocytotic vesicles, but few other organelles. A second cell type, the granular pneumocyte or Type II cell, makes up only a small fraction of the alveolar surface. These cells are rounded and do not have cytoplasmic extensions. They bulge into the alveolar spaces or lie in niches in the alveolar wall, almost covered by adjacent Type I cells. The granular pneumocyte has microvilli on its free surface and is rich in Golgi elements, endoplasmic reticulum, and mitochondria. It also has characteristic cytoplasmic membrane-bound osmiophilic bodies. These structures, which consist largely of concentric lamellae, are called cytosomes or lamellar bodies. Lamellar bodies are rich in phospholipid, and they have been observed apparently discharging their contents onto the surface of the alveolus. These bodies may represent intracellular stores of the phospholipid portion of surfactant. In addition to their supposed contribution to the production of surfactant, the granular pneumocytes may also serve as the reserve cells of the alveolus. When the alveolar epithe-

lium has been damaged, these cells have been shown to proliferate and repopulate the alveolar surface with a cuboidal epithelium.

A rarely seen third type of alveolar epithelial cell is the Type III or alveolar brush cell. It is shaped like a truncated pyramid, with wide apical microvilli that are twice the diameter of those of the Type II cells. Its cytoplasm contains dense bundles of fine filaments. This cell is structurally similar to the chemoreceptor cell found in taste buds. Its function in the lung has yet to be ascertained.

Another cell type found in the alveoli is the alveolar macrophage. Macrophages lie free in the alveolar spaces and are not part of the epithelial lining. As phagocytes they play an important role in respiratory defense mechanisms such as inflammation and the clearing of particulate matter and bacteria from the lung. The origin of alveolar macrophages has been a subject of debate, and recent evidence supports the hypothesis that these cells are derived from marrow stem cells. It is possible that derivatives of marrow stem cells are transported via the bloodstream to the lung where, in the alveolar interstitium, they undergo division-maturation to become mature macrophages.

The endothelium of the alveolar capillaries forms an uninterrupted lining devoid of pores. Endothelial cells have an appearance similar to that of membranous pneumocytes, with central nucleated portions and thin cytoplasmic extensions containing numerous pinocytotic vesicles. Endothelial intercellular junctions permit passage of protein molecules the size of horseradish peroxidase (about 40 Å) and probably play a greater role than pinocytotic vesicles in the exchange of substances between the blood and interstitial space. In contrast, the intercellular junctions of the alveolar epithelium do not allow horseradish peroxidase to pass from the alveolar space into the interstitium.

The alveolar interstitium is the space between the

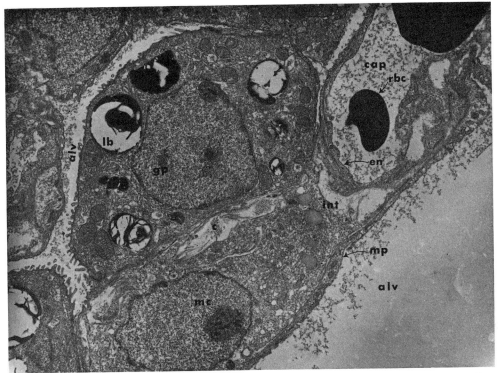

Fig. 4. Electron micrograph of alveolar-capillary membrane. Alveolus (alv) is lined with two types of epithelium: Type I membranous pneumocytes (mp) and Type II granular pneumocytes (gp) with lamellar bodies (lb). Alveolar capillary (cap) is lined with endothelium (en) and contains erythrocytes (rbc). The interstitium (int) lies between the capillary endothelium and alveolar epithelium and varies in thickness. Collagen (c) and a mesenchymal cell (mc) are present where the interstitium is widest (×7800). (Courtesy of Andrea Ceselski, Shriner's Burn Institute, Boston, Mass.)

alveolar–capillary endothelium and the alveolar epithelium. It is continuous with the interstitial space surrounding the airways and vessels. In many areas the basement membranes of the endothelium and epithelium are fused, the interstitial space is minimal, and the alveolar–capillary membrane is very thin. In other regions the endothelial and epithelial basement membranes are separated by a variable space that contains collagen and elastic fibers, fibroblasts, and other mesenchymal cells. In such regions the interstitium and the alveolar–capillary membrane are relatively wide. Thus the thickness of the alveolar–capillary membrane varies from about $0.2\,\mu$ to $10\,\mu$ with a mean of about $1.5\,\mu$.

Physiologic and biochemical evidence points to the existence of an extracellular surface-active layer overlying the alveolar epithelium. This lining layer, known as pulmonary surfactant, is believed to consist of a superficial phospholipid film lying on a subphase composed of mucopolysaccharides and protein. As mentioned previously, it is believed that the phospholipid film is produced by the granular pneumocytes of the alveolus. Ultrastructural demonstration of such an extracellular layer overlying the alveolar epithelium was not possible when standard techniques were used to prepare lung tissue for electron microscopy; however, recent studies employing new methods of lung fixation have shown a double extracellular layer lining alveoli. This layer has an ultrastructural appearance consistent with the biochemical composition of pulmonary surfactant.

Vessels and Lymphatics

Two arterial systems, pulmonary and bronchial, supply the lungs. The pulmonary arteries carry deoxygenated blood from the right ventricle to the respiratory parenchyma, accompanying the bronchial tree as far as the respiratory bronchioles. The pulmonary arterial tree is a low-resistance system, a fact reflected in the structure of the pulmonary arteries, which have a relatively thin media with more elastic tissue and less muscle than systemic arteries of comparable size. Whereas in the general circulation only the aorta and its major branches are elastic arteries, in the pulmonary circuit elastic arteries may have a diameter as small as 1 mm. Below that size the transition to muscular arteries takes place. Muscular pulmonary arteries accompany terminal and respiratory bronchioles and give rise to arterioles when they reach a diameter of approximately $70\,\mu$. Pulmonary arterioles are devoid of muscle and consist only of endothelium and a single elastic lamina surrounded by a thin layer of collagen fibers. They supply clusters of alveolar ducts. The arterioles give rise to pulmonary capillaries that form a network supplying the alveoli. The pulmonary venules drain blood from the capillaries of the pleura, alveoli, alveolar ducts, respiratory bronchioles, and bronchi, excluding the first two bronchial divisions.

These venules drain into the pulmonary veins, which run in the interlobular connective-tissue septae away from the airways and pulmonary arteries and enter the left atrium.

The bronchial arteries arise from the thoracic aorta or intercostal arteries and carry oxygenated blood to the airways. They supply the bronchial walls and provide vasa vasorum to the pulmonary arteries. Bronchial arteries are smaller in caliber and more muscular than pulmonary arteries. They lie in the peribronchial connective tissue close to the cartilage plates, supplying the bronchial tree as far as the terminal bronchioles. Much of the blood carried by the bronchial arteries enters the pulmonary veins via intrapulmonary anastamoses between bronchial and pulmonary veins. The bronchial veins primarily drain the first two or three orders of bronchi. Blood from these veins enters the azygos, the hemiazygos, or the innominate veins.

The lymphatics of the lung have three major divisions. Some lymphatics originate at the periphery of the pulmonary lobules and lie in the pleura or interlobular septa. The pleural lymphatics form polyhedral rings that outline the pulmonary lobules and drain into the interlobular lymphatics. The latter join to form the perivenous lymphatics, which also run in the interlobular septa. A second group of lymphatics have their origin around the alveolar ducts. These vessels give rise to a lymphatic network that accompanies the bronchial and pulmonary arteries. The lymphatics of the third division lie in the interlobular septa and connect the perivenous lymphatics with the bronchoarterial lymphatics. All pulmonary lymphatics drain to the hilar lymph nodes.

Innervation

Branches from the vagus nerves and the second, third, and fourth ganglia of the thoracic sympathetic chain form anterior and posterior pulmonary plexuses that supply the bronchi, arteries, and veins of the lung. The nerves supplying the bronchi are larger than those of the vessels and consist of bundles of large and small myelinated and unmyelinated fibers. The large myelinated fibers are believed to be afferent; they terminate in muscle spindles or in the bronchial epithelium. Small myelinated fibers, presumably efferent, connect with the vagal ganglion cells that are found throughout the plexus. These ganglion cells give rise to unmyelinated fibers that end in bronchial smooth-muscle and mucous glands. Ganglion cells that are probably of vagal origin have been demonstrated throughout the lung at all levels of the airways, respiratory bronchioles, alveolar ducts, and pulmonary arteries and veins.

Whereas the relatively stout nerve fibers that supply the bronchi are readily identified by the classic histologic techniques of neuroanatomy, the finer fibers that supply the pulmonary vessels have been difficult to trace and even to differentiate from reticulin fibers. In addition, the standard methods cannot distinguish between adrenergic and cholinergic fibers. The recent developments of a histochemical technique for demonstrating acetylcholinesterase and a fluorescence technique for identifying noradrenaline have enabled investigators to differentiate

cholinergic and adrenergic fibers. Studies of mammalian lung employing these methods have shown that the pulmonary arteries, bronchial musculature, and large pulmonary veins are innervated by both adrenergic and cholinergic nerve fibers. The pulmonary arterial tree has a dual vasomotor nerve supply down to the level of arterioles 40 to 70 μ in diameter. The density of innervation appears to be greatest in arterial branches just beyond the parent vessel. In the large pulmonary arteries adrenergic nerves predominate over cholinergic fibers. The bronchial arteries of most of the mammalian species tested contain adrenergic fibers only.

The existence of pulmonary stretch receptors and receptors sensitive to pressure and chemical substances has been postulated on the basis of physiologic studies. Such receptor organs have yet to be identified anatomically.

REFERENCES

Bloom W, Fawcett DW: A Textbook of Histology (ed 9). Philadelphia, WB Saunders, 1968, p 635

Bowden DH, Adamson IYR, Grantham WG, Wyatt JP: Origin of the lung macrophage. Evidence derived from radiation injury. Arch Pathol 88:540, 1969

Cutz E, Conen PE: Ultrastructure and cytochemistry of Clara cells. Am J Pathol 62:127, 1971

Hebbs C: Motor innervation of the pulmonary blood vessels of mammals, in Fishman AP, Hecht HH (eds): The Pulmonary Circulation and Interstitial Space. Chicago, University of Chicago Press, 1969, p 195

Karrer HE: The ultrastructure of capillary and alveolar walls. J Biophys Biochem Cytol 2:241, 1956

Krahl VE: Anatomy of the mammalian lung, in Fenn WO, Rahn H (eds): Handbook of Physiology, Section 3, Respiration, vol. 1. Washington, DC, American Physiological Society, 1964, p 213

Low FN: The pulmonary alveolar epithelium of laboratory mammals and man. Anat Rec 117:241, 1953

Weibel ER: Morphological basis of alveolar–capillary gas exchange. Physiol Rev 53:419, 1973

STRUCTURAL AND FUNCTIONAL DEVELOPMENT OF THE LUNG

Daniel C. Shannon

The fetal lung in utero serves no recognized useful function except for a minor role in water balance. Yet from the moment of birth the lung must immediately and continuously interact with the environment to sustain aerobic metabolism and defend against air pollutants and microorganisms. Previously untested mechanisms must first initiate and then sustain ventilation of air through a system of fluid-filled conduits and air spaces; further, a pulmonary capillary bed, accustomed to carrying 5 percent of cardiac output, must suddenly carry almost the entire output and match it in a reasonable fashion with ventilation to accomplish efficient gas exchange. Once fetal lung fluid is cleared, the alveolar surface and interstitium must be kept relatively dry and the alveoli themselves must remain inflated. Of less immediate but

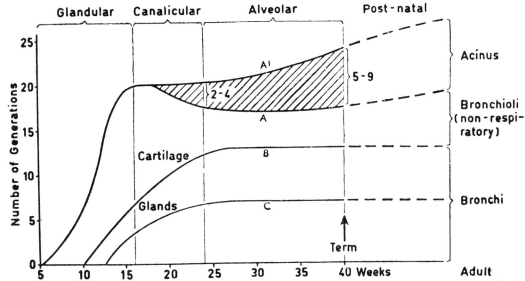

Fig. 1. The development of numbers of generations of bronchi, bronchioles, and acini in human fetuses from 5 weeks gestation to term. [Reproduced by permission from Reid L: in De Reuck AVS, Porter R (eds): Development of the Lung. Boston, Little, Brown, 1967, p 110.]

nonetheless great importance, defense mechanisms must be prepared to filter out large numbers of inhaled particles and microorganisms.

Since successful initiation and maintenance of air breathing is central to survival in man, it is no surprise that failure of development or expression of physiologic processes controlling respiration accounts for a large percentage of neonatal mortality.

BASIC STRUCTURE
Bronchial

The developing lung can be thought of as two trees arborizing toward one another, resulting in apposition of their terminal branches. The tracheobronchial tree begins as a ventral pouch of endoderm from the floor of the primitive foregut in the fourth week of gestation. Within days, precartilage appears and follows bronchial development, so that while the branching of the bronchial system proceeds to completion by the 16th week the full extent of cartilage has appeared by the 24th week (Fig. 1).

Vascular

A transitional system of perfusion of the primitive lung bud is then replaced by the definitive pulmonary vascular tree. The main pulmonary artery is derived from the right ventricle and joins the right and left pulmonary arteries, which are derived from the right and left sixth aortic arches. Branching of the system then parallels airway development and establishes functional connections with capillaries that proliferate in the glandular mesenchyme. Pulmonary venous branching occurs simultaneously and connects to buds from the left atrium, completing the pulmonary vascular system. Most of the primitive blood supply then atrophies except for a variable number of bronchial arteries that supply derivatives of the primitive lung bud down to terminal bronchioles and drain into the pulmonary veins. Origins of lymphatic capillaries, which ultimately extend peripherally to the level of respiratory bronchioles and their more central lymphatic vascular connections which accompany bronchial and arterial branches through interstitial spaces to the right lymphatic duct and the thoracic duct, are not well defined.

As a result the lung contains air spaces approximated to capillaries and appears physically capable of gas exchange by the 28th week. Although there is controversy over whether true alveoli are present even at 40 weeks of gestation, it is clear that most if not all alveoli develop postnatally, reaching their full complement of 300×10^6 at 8 years of age. Even though alveolar epithelium and capillary endothelium are closely apposed at 28 weeks gestation on the average, they will not support gas exchange unless the interstitial space between them can be kept dry by a functional lymphatic system.

Connective Tissue

Elastic tissue elements appear to arise from collagen fibers during the 25th week and are especially prominent around the entrance to alveolar ducts and between capillary and epithelial walls that will later develop into alveoli. Smooth-muscle fibers appear early in airways, and are present as a thin, often unicellular layer, down to terminal bronchioles at 40 weeks' gestation.

Cellular Differentiation: Epithelium

Knowledge of the regulation of orderly elaboration of various cell types with their specialized metabolic functions is recent and incomplete. Mesenchyme is necessary or endoderm will not differentiate into epithelial structures. Epithelium of air conduits becomes pseudostratified columnar in type, with goblet cells that produce mucus and with ciliated cells that propel it toward the trachea. The function of a third type, serous cells, is unknown. Cuboid epithelium characteristic of terminal airways of the 16-week fetus differentiates to form Type I membranous pneumocytes and Type II granular pneu-

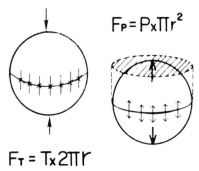

$$F_P = P \times \pi r^2$$

$$F_T = T \times 2\pi r$$

Fig. 2. Forces acting on a bubble. The force of surface tension (FT) acts at the circumference of the sphere $2\pi r$, while the force of pressure within (FP) acts on the surface of the sphere πr^2.

mocytes. While the Type I cell attenuates to provide most of the alveolar surface area, the Type II cell is responsible for production and release of a surface-active material that helps stabilize alveoli and keep them dry once air breathing begins.

Surfactant

Until Clements found that surface forces in lung extracts were directly related to surface area, it seemed perplexing that bubbles expressed from lungs did not recoil and break but were in fact extremely stable. He suggested that the ability of lung surface extracts to approach zero surface tension at low surface areas prevented atelectasis of alveoli at low lung volume, e.g., at expiration. Having observed that air-filled lungs tended to retain volume on deflation whereas saline-filled lungs did not, von Neergard postulated in 1929 that the lung must be lined by a material with low surface tension.

Physiology. The size of the alveoli at any phase in the respiratory cycle depends on a balance between pressures acting across alveolar walls. If alveoli are to remain inflated and stable when the lung is at rest, pressures acting on alveoli that tend toward inflation and surface pressures that tend toward deflation must be balanced. In very simple terms, $2\pi r \times T = \pi r^2 \times P$, or $P = 2T/r$. This is the Laplace relationship (Fig. 2) applied to the lung. P is the pressure difference across alveolar walls necessary to maintain a given size measured as the radius. This relationship predicts that larger pressure differences will be necessary as surface tension increases or alveolar size decreases. Little is known about the relative contributions of factors contributing to normal intraalveolar pressure, but the net pressure must tend toward inflation. The factors involved are interdependent and consist of the supporting effects of elastic tissue, support by the thorax at the pleural surface, intravascular pressure in both capillaries and lymphatics, alveolar interstitial fluid pressure, the geometric relationship of one alveolus to the next, and the pressure transmitted from more central airways. From current knowledge it appears that most if not all of these pressures tend to inflate alveoli; even pulmonary vascular pressure appears to exert an erectile effect (von Bosch effect) that would help inflate alveoli.

Ultimately the summation of all these forces is manifest in the alveolar interstitial pressure, which at resting lung volume (functional residual capacity) is 2–3 cm H_2O subatmospheric. Since intraalveolar pressure at rest is atmospheric, surface forces must balance interstitial pressure with an equivalent collapsing pressure. Thus any increase of alveolar surface forces or increase in interstitial pressure will promote atelectasis. There may be a margin of safety attributable to the presence of a surfactant lining whose surface tension as measured in vitro changes with surface area and approaches zero at a minimal surface area. If the primary deficit increases surface forces, however, only a greater than normal transalveolar pressure, and thus greater work, can support alveoli.

Biochemistry. Only a highly polar molecule could satisfy the requirements of low surface tension at low lung volume. Intermolecular attraction (surface tension) is minimal if polar molecules are arranged in palisade fashion at the surface. Disruption of this arrangement as surface area is increased at increasing lung volume leads to increased intermolecular forces and thus increased surface tension and greater elastic recoil, which assists passive expiration. The behavior of surface forces in a lung at various volumes can be illustrated by considering the pressure difference necessary to inflate a collapsed alveolus on the end of a respiratory bronchiole in the presence of a surfactant compared to its absence. The respiratory bronchiole of a premature infant has a radius of about 20 microns and surface tension in the presence of surfactant is about 5–10 dynes/cm compared to about 55 dynes/cm in its absence. Since one dyne equals 10^3 cm H_2O, the Laplace relationship predicts that a pressure difference of 5–10 cm H_2O will be necessary to open a collapsed alveolus when surfactant is present compared to 55 cm H_2O in its absence (Fig. 3).

Nearly all air-breathing animals share in common a surfactant lining that stabilizes terminal air spaces; it has been characterized as a phospholipid, primarily β,γ-dipalmitoyl lecithin (DPL), but is associated with other highly surface-active components. In vitro analysis has led to the conclusion that cholesterol may promote the spreading of DPL on the surface while the role of apoprotein is still disputed. The biochemical development of the surfactant system in utero has been well defined. Gluck has found that a sharp increase in lecithin, particularly in relation to sphingomyelin, occurs between 28 and 34 weeks in the human amniotic fluid, much of which arises from the lung (Fig. 4). Epstein and Farrell have demonstrated that choline incorporation via pathway I for lecithin synthesis accounts for nearly all of the DPL formed in primates and that a striking increase in activity of this pathway develops after about 85 percent of gestation.

Lamellar inclusions, observed in mitochondria of Type II alveolar lining cells, appear late in fetal life and are probably the major source of surfactant. Kikkawa has suggested that the phospholipid remains in these vessels until birth, when it is suddenly secreted onto the alveolar surface. Whatever the precise mechanism of re-

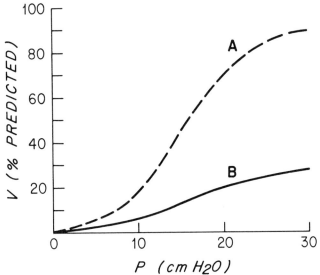

Fig. 3. The inflation limbs of the volume–pressure curves, measured in two infants: A is normal, B has severe RDS. The curves have been normalized for size to permit comparison. Curve A indicates that many alveoli open below 10 cm H₂O pressure difference. Curve B indicates that most alveoli have not yet opened at 30 cm H₂O.

lease, once on the alveolar surface it permits a five- to tenfold decrease in the pressure difference necessary to open an alveolus.

Although various inhalants and alterations in pulmonary perfusion (Table 1) can alter surface forces in the lung, their role in altering these forces in patients, outside of the premature infant, is not well defined. Certainly in a given patient with alveolar disease it is only possible to guess whether any one factor is etiologic.

Clinically, abnormality in the surfactant system is

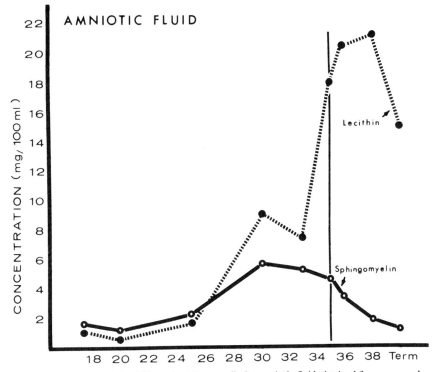

Fig. 4. The concentration of lecithin and sphingomyelin in amniotic fluid obtained from women by amniocentesis at fetal gestational age from 18 weeks to term showing a marked increase in the L/S ratio at 34 weeks. (Reproduced by permission from Gluck L, et al: Am J Obstet Gynecol 109:440, 1970.)

Table 1
Experimental Factors That Alter Surface Tension

INHALANTS		
Gases	Liquids	Perfusion Alterations
100% O_2	Water	Pulmonary artery ligation
15% CO_2	Saline	Pulmonary embolus
Oxides of nitrogen	Hydro-carbons	Cardiopulmonary bypass
Cigarette smoke		Ventilation of unperfused lung
Anesthetics		Pulmonary edema

defined in only a few circumstances (respiratory distress syndrome of the newborn, smoke inhalation, exposure to oxides of nitrogen and cigarette smoke). In a variety of other disease states abnormalities in surface forces of lung extracts have been demonstrated, but their role in the pathophysiology of those diseases remains to be defined.

REFERENCES

Dunnill MS: Postnatal growth of the lung. Thorax 17:329, 1962
Emery J: The Anatomy of the Developing Lung. London, Heinemann Medical Books, 1969
Reid L: The embryology of the lung, in De Reuck AVS, Porter R (eds): Development of the Lung. Boston, Little, Brown, 1967, p 109

NONRESPIRATORY FUNCTIONS OF THE LUNG

Barry W. Levine

In addition to its primary function as an organ of gas exchange, the lung has a significant role in host defense and is an active metabolic organ.

PULMONARY DEFENSE MECHANISMS

The lung has within it a group of defense mechanisms comprised of mechanical factors, surface fluids and epithelium, cellular reserves, immunoglobulins, and alveolar proteins and lipids, all designed to protect the host against environmental insults.

Mechanical Factors

The anatomy of the upper airway, which includes the nasopharynx, trachea, and nonrespiratory bronchi, provides a unique defense against inhaled gases or large particulate matter. The large surface area and rich vascular supply of the nasopharyngeal cavity make it an ideal absorbing surface. Both the nasal passages and tracheobronchial tree act as aerodynamic filters. The filtering property is the result of subjecting inhaled air to turbulence, which causes large particulate matter to adhere to the mucosal membranes by inertial force. Ninety percent of inhaled particles larger than 2 μ are precipitated and then cleared in this fashion.

Surface Fluids and Epithelium

The mucociliary system is composed of ciliated epithelium and a layer of viscoelastic fluid. This system extends from the nasopharynx to the terminal nonrespiratory bronchioles. The epithelium is a pseudo-stratified ciliated layer composed of 3 to 4 rows of nuclei decreasing in height peripherally into a single layer at the level of the respiratory bronchiole. Within the pseudostratified layer are goblet cells occurring singly without touching each other. There are no goblet cells within the terminal bronchioles. From the goblet cells a viscoelastic fluid emerges and rests upon the ciliated epithelium. This fluid layer is propelled upward by coordinated ciliary motion at a rate of 10–20 mm/min. Ninety percent of foreign material deposited upon this fluid layer can be cleared in 1 hr.

Cellular Reserves

Within the substance of the lung a number of different cells participate in the cleansing system. These include alveolar macrophages and Types I and II alveolar lining epithelial cells. They provide in situ detoxification independent of ciliary motion. The alveolar macrophages number about 600,000. Their phagocytic function is aided by tissue histiocytes, polymorphonuclear leukocytes, monocytes, and possibly eosinophils. Although it is a potent defense mechanism, intrapulmonary phagocytosis is very sensitive to changes in host environment. Ethanol ingestion, steroids, acute hypoxia, and hypothermia all have been shown to diminish phagocytic capability within the lung.

Alveolar Proteins and Lipids

In addition to phagocytosis occurring within the alveoli, the numerous lipids and proteins found on the epithelial lining play an important role in host defense through their physiochemical characteristics. Lipids within the alveolus act as traps by absorbing particulate matter. Protein-rich alveolar lining fluid acts as a trap by causing wetting of foreign particulate matter.

Immunoglobulins

Endobronchial secretions are known to contain various immunoblogulins whose antibody properties may play a role in pulmonary defense. The major immunoglobulin component in tracheobronchial secretions is IgA. Within these secretions IgA is 20-fold more concentrated than IgG. The form of IgA in tracheobronchial secretions differs from that in serum. A carbohydrate fragment is coupled to serum IgA, probably within the plasma cells of the bronchial submucosa, forming secretory IgA. Secretory IgA has a molecular weight of 390,000 d, of which 60,000 d is the molecular weight of the carbohydrate component.

The role of secretory IgA in pulmonary defense is not well understood. Approximately 1 of every 500 to 700 births has complete absence of serum IgA and consequently secretory IgA. However, only a third of these individuals are subject to an increased frequency of sinopulmonary disease. Furthermore, in patients with chronic bronchitis, respiratory IgA has been found in normal concentrations. Therefore the role that the presence or absence of secretory IgA plays in the pathogenesis of recurrent pulmonary infection is unclear. The recent discovery of a deficiency in IgE, the circulating antibody that mediates cutaneous anaphylaxis, may help delineate the role of antibody deficiency in pulmonary defense. In patients with combined deficiencies of serum IgA and IgE, there appears to be a predisposition to recurrent sinopulmonary infection. IgA and IgE may therefore play a role in an immunologic system that regulates the normal bacterial and viral flora of mucous membranes.

IgG, the dominant serum immunoglobulin, has a molecular weight of 160,000 d. Deficiency of IgG has multiple etiologies, but is characterized by recurrent severe infections, usually bacterial. The deficiency can be secondary to either decreased synthesis or increased catabolism. IgG deficiency may be an inherited defect or an acquired trait. Upper respiratory tract infections with sinusitis, otitis media, and recurrent pneumonia are common. Because of the long in vivo half-life of IgG, the respiratory infections in deficient individuals can be controlled with chronic parenteral γ-globulin therapy. Unfortunately the half-life of IgA in vivo is about 4 hr, and therefore parenteral therapy is of little value in this deficiency.

METABOLIC FUNCTIONS OF THE LUNG

The lung, in addition to playing a critical role in host defense, has important metabolic functions. The lung is known to store abundant amounts of histamine and serotonin; within its vascular endothelium are found potent enzymes that inactivate polypeptides and convert others to more potent forms; and finally the lung plays an important role in maintaining water and electrolyte balance.

INTRAPULMONARY STORAGE
Histamine

The lung has an abundant concentration of histamine within the pulmonary mast cells located around small pulmonary vessels. The enzymes that decarboxylate histidine and then deaminate or methylate the product to form histamine have been identified in mammalian lung tissue. Although the lung is felt to produce and store endogenous histamine, its physiologic role is yet unclear. During anaphylactic shock and tissue injury pulmonary histamine is released. This release may influence the local regulation of the pulmonary microcirculation.

Slow-reacting Substance of Anaphylaxis (SRS-A)

SRS-A is a group of chemical mediators that produce a slow, prolonged contraction of certain smooth muscles. These compounds have the biologic potential of being involved in antigen-induced bronchospasm and immunologic tissue injury due to increased capillary permeability. The release of SRS-A from the lungs when specific antigens are administered to sensitized guinea pigs seems to demonstrate this. Passive sensitization of human lung tissue with reaginic antibody has also resulted in release of SRS-A. When release occurs, there is a reduction in the number of pulmonary mast cells, suggesting that SRS-A originates or is stored in this cell type. At present SRS-A is felt to be involved in the pathogenesis of immediate hypersensitivity in man.

Serotonin

Following pulmonary emboli serotonin is released from the lung either from intrapulmonary clots (platelets) or from pulmonary mast cells. The release of serotonin from the pulmonary mast cells may cause bronchospasm or alter regional pulmonary blood flow.

INTRAPULMONARY METABOLISM
Vasoactive Polypeptides

The lung contains an abundant concentration of kininase and angiotensin-converting enzymes. These enzymes are presumably located on the pulmonary vascular endothelium. Bradykinin, which is a naturally occurring vasoactive polypeptide, is almost completely inactivated by hydrolysis during a single passage through the lung. The enzyme responsible for the inactivation is a kininase that remains potent in face of marked alterations in the physiologic function of the lung. The lung is also capable of converting the relatively inactive polypeptide angiotensin I to the more vasoactive angiotensin II. In a single passage more than 90 percent of angiotensin I is converted to angiotensin II within the pulmonary circulation. Although these are potent functions of the lung, their effects on the physiologic and biochemical homeostais of the organism are not known.

Catecholamines

Most mammalian lungs contain dopamine, norepinephrine, and epinephrine. The concentration of norepinephrine in the lung is proportional to the sympathetic innervation. There is indirect evidence that catecholamines are synthesized within the lung. Catechol-o-methyltransferase, the enzyme responsible for the breakdown of various catecholamines, is present within the lung. Therefore the lung may both produce and destroy catecholamines. It is not known what role the lung plays in the total spectrum of catecholamine metabolism.

Lipid Metabolism

The lung contains phospholipids within the interstitial space, and a phospholipid-rich layer (surfactant) coats the alveolar–tissue interface. The predominant lipid is dipalmitoyl lecithin, which is surface-active. Phospholipids are synthesized by either esterification or phosphorylation. The lung has been shown to contain the appropriate enzymes to synthesize phospholipids. The site of this synthesis is not known, although most data point to the alveolar Type II cell. The rate of lipid turnover in the lung is affected by pulmonary edema, pulmonary embolization, occlusion of a pulmonary artery, and nutritional state. Prematurity has also been associated with decreased surfactant activity, as in infant respiratory distress syndrome. It appears that maturity of alveolar cells, blood flow, and an energy source are necessary for pulmonary surfactant metabolism. When insufficient formation occurs, alveolar instability results and there is marked impairment of pulmonary mechanics and gas exchange.

WATER AND ELECTROLYTE BALANCE
Water

During respiration inspired air is conditioned by being warmed and humidified, which are dependent on air-flow dynamics, minute ventilation, and body temperature. Water loss through the lungs is also dependent on these factors. During normal ventilation 250 ml of water and 350 kcal of heat are lost per 24-hr period.

Hyperpnea increases heat transfer and water loss and acts as a homeostatic mechanism during fever. The proper conditioning of inspired air is important in maintaining the function of the ciliated epithelium. Since the nasopharynx is the major site for the appropriate exchange of water and heat, exclusion of this portion of the respiratory system (such as by a tracheostomy) will interfere with the conditioning of inspired air and the recovery of heat and water from expired air.

Solute Balance

Because of the lung's large extracellular fluid volume, it plays an important role in total-body solute balance. Water and solutes are transported across the alveolar–capillary membrane by hydrostatic forces and molecular diffusion. Between 15 and 30 osmols of carbon dioxide are excreted by the lung during a 24-hr period. The effect of various hormones on this solute balance is unknown.

REFERENCES

Green GM: The J Burns Amberson lecture in defense of the lung. Am Rev Respir Dis 102:691, 1970

Heinemann HO, Fishman AP: Non-respiratory functions of the mammalian lung. Physiol Rev 49:1, 1969

Said SI: The lung as a metabolic organ. N Engl J Med 279:1330, 1968

Tomasi TB: Human immunoglobulin A. N Engl J Med 279:1327, 1968

PHYSICAL FACTORS IN LUNG FUNCTION

Denise J. Strieder

LUNG MECHANICS

Pulmonary lobules are built on a framework made of collagen, elastic fibers, and smooth muscle. The helicoid arrangement of collagen and muscle allows for considerable volume change between collapse and full expansion. The lobules are more or less compliant, depending on whether the smooth muscle is relaxed or contracted; but at all times their volume is determined by external forces, which are needed to unfold and stretch their walls and are measured as a pressure difference.

Pressure–Volume Curve

The fundamental relationship between pressure and volume is clearly demonstrated when excised inflated lungs are allowed to deflate slowly, while the tracheal pressure and the volume of air exhaled are simultaneously recorded. The volume change for equal decrements of pressure is small at first but increases as lung volume decreases. Accordingly the pressure–volume relationship of the lung describes a curve that, as observed during deflation, is stable and reproducible (Fig. 1). The same relationship prevails whether the lungs have been inflated by positive pressure applied to the mouth or trachea or by negative pressure over the pleural surface. In both instances the forces that tend to increase lung volume are reflected in the transpulmonary pressure (P_{tp}), measured by the difference

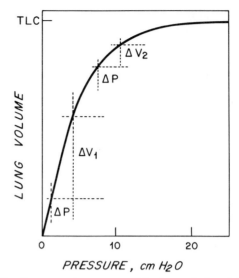

Fig. 1. Pressure–volume curve of the lungs during deflation. Compliance, which is measured by the ratio of volume increments ΔV to pressure increment ΔP decreases with increasing lung distension.

between the pressure inside the lung and the pressure at the pleural surface. When the distending pressure is removed the lungs recoil and collapse. When lung volume remains constant, distending pressure exactly balances lung recoil.

Two factors are known to contribute to lung recoil: the elastic tension within the lung tissue and the surface tension arising at the air–fluid interface. During deflation surface effects are small and lung recoil measures the elastic properties of lung tissue. During inflation the surface area of each alveolar wall increases and surface tension becomes dominant. This variability of surface forces in the lungs is due to the presence of surfactant, a surface-active material that lines the alveolar walls and permits the surface tension to vary with varying surface area from very low (10 dynes/cm) to moderately high values (40–50 dynes/cm). Surface tension is greater when surface area increases, and it falls rapidly when surface area begins to contract. In the lung, therefore, the change in surface tension that accompanies a given change of volume depends not only on the initial volume but also on the immediately preceding events (the volume history), a property known as hysteresis.

Because tension at the surface of alveolar walls is greater during inspiration than during expiration, lung recoil is greater during inspiration than during expiration. The pressure–volume relationship of the lung is best represented by a family of hysteresis loops with a common deflation curve characteristic of the elastic properties of the lung and an infinite number of inflation curves reflecting the variability of surface tension (Fig. 2).

During inhalation of a large tidal volume, transpulmonary pressure increases with increasing lung volume according to the inflation limb of the appropri-

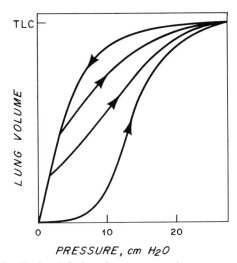

Fig. 2. During inflation the pressure–volume curve of the lungs varies with varying initial volume, describing multiple hysteresis loops. The deflation curve is the same as in Fig. 1. [Reproduced by permission from Radford EP Jr in Fenn WO (ed): Handbook of Physiology, section III, vol 1. American Physiological Society, 1964.]

ate hysteresis loop. If, then, the breath is held at any point during inflation, more surfactant molecules are recruited to the surface, and within a few seconds surface tension falls. Consequently transpulmonary pressure falls, returning to the value sufficient to balance lung recoil as given by the deflation curve. For any lung volume, therefore, the deflation curve indicates the minimal value of lung recoil that actually prevails not only during deflation but also in apnea when sufficient time is allowed for molecular rearrangement to take place at the alveolar surface and true static conditions prevail. Accordingly, the minimal lung recoil at any volume is often referred to as static recoil of the lung.

Lung Compliance

During normal breathing at rest, with good initial expansion of the lung and a small tidal volume, the hysteresis loop is quite flat. There is then no need to distinguish between inflation and deflation curves. The pressure–volume relationship over the range of one tidal volume may be represented by a single function. The ratio of volume change to pressure change ($\Delta V/\Delta P$), or compliance, approximates the slope of the deflation curve (dV/dP) at the same lung volume. To indicate the conditions of measurements and the approximation implied, it is best referred to as dynamic compliance or tidal compliance. Normal values range from 0.15 to 0.3 l/cm H_2O in adults and are smaller in children and infants, whose lung volumes are smaller.

Direct measurements of pleural pressure, which would be desirable for the determination of lung compliance as well as lung recoil, are impractical. The esophagus, however, lying deep in the mediastinum between right and left pleural reflexions, offers a suitable location for a pressure probe. A small latex balloon (8 cm in length, 1 cm in diameter) mounted at the end of a polyethylene catheter is swallowed into the lower

third of the esophagus. At this level the pressure artifacts due to cardiac activity are negligible, and in the absence of peristaltic contractions esophageal pressure reflects pleural pressure. Thus tidal or static compliance may be determined from esophageal pressure and dynamic or static volume measurements.

Changes of esophageal pressure faithfully follow the changes of pleural pressure during breathing. But absolute values of esophageal pressure also give a good approximation of the absolute value of pleural pressure, thus permitting an estimation of lung recoil. Because such estimates are most reliable at high lung volumes, lung recoil is often measured after a maximal inspiration when lung volume is equal to total lung capacity (TLC).

Respiratory System

Lung and chest wall together form the respiratory system, which is moved by the respiratory muscles as one mechanical unit. During breathing elastic tensions are developed not only in the lungs (lung recoil) but also in the chest wall. These tensions are balanced by forces that are equal in magnitude and opposite in direction and are produced by muscle activity. For example, breath-holding with an open glottis in a position of forced inspiration requires the sustained contraction of inspiratory muscles, mostly to overcome lung recoil. In a position of forced expiration it requires the sustained contraction of expiratory muscles to overcome the tensions produced in stretching costovertebral ligaments and sternocostal cartilages and the inspiratory muscles.

The magnitudes of these forces can be measured with a mechanical respirator substituting for muscle contraction. Volume changes in the respiratory system are equal to the volume of air displaced in and out of the lungs, with a maximum equal to the vital capacity (VC). Pressure differences across the respiratory system are measured between body surface and mouth (a tank respirator will produce pressures above or below atmospheric, while the mouth remains at atmospheric pressure). Muscle relaxation is obtained by voluntary inhibition or by pharmacologic means. Then the pressure–volume curve of the relaxed respiratory system can be determined. When surface forces within the lung are small (true static conditions or deflation), the pressure–volume curve of the respiratory system is S-shaped and nearly symmetric with respect to the volume axis (Fig. 3).

As a mechanical component of the respiratory system, the chest wall is taken to include all structures capable of altering lung volume—the rib cage and intercostal muscles, the diaphragm, the muscles of the abdominal wall, and even the mass of abdominal viscera. The elastic characteristics of these structures can be studied when the respiratory muscles are relaxed. Conventionally the elastic properties of the chest wall are represented on a pressure–volume curve with esophageal pressure substituted for pleural pressure on the abscissa and the volume of air in the lungs plotted on the ordinate. At high lung volumes the curve is steep, showing the chest wall to be compliant, while at low lung volumes the curve levels off, showing the chest wall to be quite

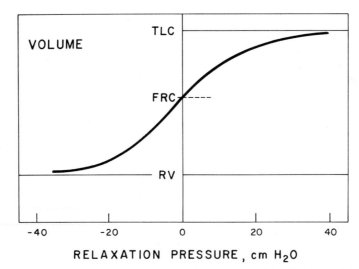

Fig. 3. Pressure–volume curve of the respiratory system (schematic). TLC is total lung capacity, FRC is functional residual capacity, and RV is residual volume of the lungs.

stiff. Thus the chest wall offers little opposition to inspiration and great resistance to compression (Fig. 4).

The increasing stiffness of the lungs with increasing lung volume determines the maximal volume of air that the lungs are able to contain, or Total Lung Capacity (TLC). The increasing stiffness of the chest wall with decreasing volume determines the end point of forced expiration and the corresponding residual volume (RV) of the lung in healthy young adults. In older individuals and in the presence of disease, other mechanisms prevail during forced expiration that lead to an increased residual volume.

The midpoint on the pressure–volume curve of the relaxed respiratory system represents a stable mechanical equilibrium whereby in the absence of muscle activity lung recoil is exactly balanced by the tendency of the relaxed chest wall to expand according to its own elastic tensions (Fig. 4). The corresponding volume is the rest-

ing Functional Residual Capacity (FRC), normally close to one-half of TLC. Should the lung become abnormally stiff, as occurs in the presence of interstitial fibrosis, the respiratory system will seek a lower resting volume, whereby greater tensions will be developed within the chest wall to balance the increased lung recoil: FRC decreases. Conversely, should the elastic recoil of lung tissue diminish. as is observed in pulmonary emphysema, the resting volume of the respiratory system moves up toward the resting volume of the chest wall, which is near 75 percent of TLC: FRC increases.

Pleural Pressure

The pleural space is normally air-free. Any air that has gained access to the pleural space disappears slowly as oxygen is taken up by tissues in the chest wall and the concentrated nitrogen diffuses out. Fluid is absorbed promptly, provided that the oncotic pressure of blood exceeds pulmonary or systemic capillary pressure, plus

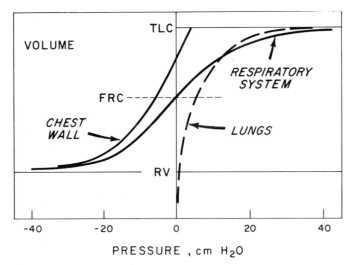

Fig. 4. Pressure–volume curves (schematic) of the chest wall (left), the respiratory system (center: same curve as in Fig. 3), and the lungs (right: same curve as in Fig. 1). At FRC the elastic forces of lung and chest wall are equal in magnitude and opposite in direction.

the oncotic pressure of the pleural fluid itself. A thin layer of fluid normally persists that is sufficient to act as a lubricant but is so thin that pleural pressure at any one point is determined by local mechanical forces.

Pleural pressure is always lower than alveolar pressure. During apnea, with the glottis open, alveolar pressure is zero (i.e., equal to atmospheric pressure); pleural pressure is equal and opposite to transpulmonary pressure $[P_{pl} = -P_{tp} \text{ (apnea)}]$ and is entirely determined by lung volume (Fig. 1). If the breath is held after a deep inspiration, pleural pressure falls to -20 or -30 cm H_2O. After a deep expiration it is -2 or -3 cm H_2O. Sustained contraction of respiratory muscles is needed to increase or maintain the elastic pull of the chest wall upon the lungs, except at FRC, where the elasticity of the chest wall exactly balances lung recoil.

Gravity also affects pleural pressure. In the erect position the weight of the lungs is partly suspended from the apex of the chest cavity and partly supported by the dome of the diaphragm. The value of pleural pressure obtained with an esophageal balloon actually prevails only at the level at which it is measured, about one-third up the height of the lungs. At FRC, for example, with an esophageal pressure of -4 cm H_2O, pleural pressure at the apex of the lungs reaches -8 cm H_2O, but at the base of the lungs it is only -2 cm H_2O. From apex to base there is a vertical gradient of pleural pressure equal to 0.25 cm H_2O per centimeter of lung height, as estimated from indirect evidence in man and direct measurements in animals. A similar gradient of pleural pressure exists in the supine position, but the vertical height of the lungs now measured from front to back is reduced. The resulting differences in pleural pressure between upper and lower regions of the lung surface are less marked.

A vertical gradient of transpulmonary pressure occurs as a mirror image of the regional changes of pleural pressure. In the apical region of the lungs where pleural pressure is the most negative, transpulmonary pressure is high and the alveoli are almost fully expanded. At the base of the lungs, where pleural pressure is near zero, transpulmonary pressure is small and the alveoli are barely open. Thus normal lungs have a vertical gradient of alveolar size determined by the pressure–volume relationship of pulmonary lobules and by the vertical gradient of pleural pressure.

Alveoli and lobules are presumed normally to have pressure–volume curves similar in shape to that of the whole lung, and identical throughout the lung. Therefore, as pleural pressure and alveolar volume vary from apex to base, so does the compliance of these air spaces. At FRC, apical alveoli are almost completely inflated. Their compliance is low, as indicated by the nearly flat slope of the pressure–volume curve of the lung in the range of high volumes; apical alveoli will respond to further increase in regional transpulmonary pressure by a small gain in volume. Basal alveoli are poorly inflated, but their compliance is high, as shown by the steep slope of the pressure–volume curve of the lung in the range of

low volumes. Therefore basal alveoli respond to the same increase in transpulmonary pressure by a substantial gain in volume. Accordingly inspired air is distributed preferentially to the base of the lung during normal tidal breathing.

The vertical gradients of pleural pressure, alveolar size, and alveolar compliance are reflected in the vertical gradient of ventilation, which characterizes the distribution of inspired air in erect man.

Alveolar Stability

Air bubbles in most fluids tend to collapse or coalesce. In contrast, 300 million alveoli with a common airway coexist in the lungs, and in any region they maintain remarkably even sizes, as is seen on histologic preparation. Both the unusual properties of pulmonary surfactant and the elastic properties of lung tissue contribute to the stability of alveolar volume.

Whenever a group of alveoli expands beyond the average volume required by the regional pleural pressure, alveolar surface tension and elastic stress immediately rise and compliance decreases; further expansion is opposed. If another group tends to collapse, surface tension and elastic stress immediately fall, and compliance increases; these alveoli tend to return to normal size. Thus the changes in recoil and compliance that accompany all changes in volume act as a mechanical feedback to correct random variations in alveolar size.

During quiet breathing, however, particularly in the supine position when lung volume is reduced, it has been shown that alveolar collapse occurs in the dependent parts of the lung and that it persists until a sigh produces increased tensions within the lung tissue sufficient to reexpand all alveolar units. Indeed, each inspiration tends to restore alveolar volume in the same way as sighing, with an effectiveness proportional to tidal volume. Shallow breathing therefore is ineffective in this respect.

The reexpansion of collapsed alveoli with increased transpulmonary pressure occurs suddenly rather than progressively, being delayed until the opening pressure required to overcome surface forces is reached. Pulmonary surfactant reduces the alveolar opening pressures well below the values of 70–100 cm H_2O that would be required by an air–water or air–plasma interface. Nevertheless relatively large pressures are still needed to open or reopen collapsed lungs. The normal newborn produces transpulmonary pressures of the order of 30 cm H_2O to draw the first breath. Similar pressures are exerted by anesthesiologists to reexpand a lobe collapsed during thoracic surgery.

When surfactant is insufficient, a significant number of alveoli collapse with each expiration. Each inspiration then requires an unusually large transpulmonary pressure to expand the alveoli. Considerable benefit may be gained by using intermittent positive pressure breathing (IPPB), with which the required work is produced by a mechanical device, or even continuous positive pressure breathing (CPPB), whereby in addition a transpulmonary pressure of 5–10 cm H_2O is maintained at the end of expiration to prevent alveolar collapse.

AIRWAY MECHANICS

Ventilation results from mechanical action of the chest upon the lungs. The chest wall, by pulling on the pleural surface, increases lung volume and produces inspiration. With the relaxation of inspiration muscles, lung recoil causes the respiratory system to return to its resting volume and produces expiration. Quantitative analysis of the underlying mechanical phenomena is needed to understand the behavior of the respiratory system under the stress of disease.

Alveolar Pressure

Alveolar pressure depends upon the elastic surface forces in the respiratory system, the action of respiratory muscles, and the resistance of the airway.

In the absence of respiratory muscle contraction and with a closed airway, alveolar pressure reflects the static pressure of the respiratory system (Fig. 4) and therefore depends on lung volume: alveolar pressure is positive at high lung volumes where lung recoil is predominant and becomes negative at low lung volumes where chest wall elasticity is predominant. One can directly experience these pressure changes by closing the mouth and nose and relaxing the respiratory muscles at the end of a forced inspiration, and then again at the end of a forced expiration. But the measurement of these relaxation pressures in the laboratory is generally omitted, because in most instances complete muscle relaxation cannot be ascertained.

During the ventilatory cycle the alveolar pressure falls with the contraction of inspiratory muscles and rises with that of expiratory muscles. Maximal inspiratory efforts made against a closed airway can lower alveolar pressure to −100 cm H_2O near residual volume but only to −10 to −20 cm H_2O near total lung capacity. Maximal expiratory efforts can raise alveolar pressure to values as high as 200 cm H_2O near total lung capacity, but only to 50 to 70 cm H_2O near residual volume.

Lung volume affects the range of possible alveolar pressures because the tensions developed in the respiratory system are volume-dependent (Fig. 4) and either help or hinder the effort of respiratory muscle. At all lung volumes the elastic recoil of the lung assists expiration but opposes inspiration. Below the resting volume of the chest wall its elastic tensions assist inspiration but resist expiration; the opposite holds above resting volume. Furthermore, the efficiency of respiratory muscles varies with muscle length and with configuration of rib cage and diaphragm; the inspiratory muscles lose mechanical advantage near TLC, and so do the expiratory muscles near RV.

The large alveolar pressure differences developed during maximal efforts against a closed airway are never reached during normal breathing. At rest only a few centimeters of H_2O are needed; a lowering of pleural pressure for inspiration is produced by contraction of the inspiratory muscles and the subsequent expiration is produced by recoil of the respiratory system. At exercise, however, the activity of both inspiratory and expiratory muscles is required to achieve the necessary flow rates. Yet alveolar pressure hardly exceeds the range of −20 to +30 cm H_2O because normal airway resistance is small.

Airway Resistance

Pressure differences between mouth and alveoli produce the flow of air in and out of the lungs. Airway resistance R_{aw} is defined as the ratio of pressure difference to rate of flow. With ambient pressure taken as a reference, mouth pressure becomes zero and airway resistance is measured by the ratio of alveolar pressure (P_A) to ventilatory flow ($\dot{V}$): $R_{aw} = P_A/\dot{V}$.

Airway resistance varies with lung volume and with the magnitude and direction of flow. However, if measurements of alveolar pressure and ventilatory flow are made with modest flow rates, with small tidal volume (as during panting), and at a specific lung volume (usually near FRC), then airway resistance may be expressed as a single result, with normal ranges of 0.5–1.5 cm H_2O/l/sec in men, 1–2.5 cm H_2O/l/sec in women, and higher values in children. The differences between airway resistance of healthy men, women, and children are due to differences in the sizes of their airways.

Actual measurement of airway resistance requires simultaneous recording of rate of flow and alveolar pressure. Inspiratory and expiratory flow rates are easily monitored by having the subject breathe through a fine screen, which acts as a linear resistor, and recording the slight pressure drop across the screen with a differential pressure transducer. The instrument is designed to assure that the pressure drop is proportional to rate of flow. Alveolar pressure, however, is accessible only to indirect determination. The method of reference makes use of a body plethysmograph, an airtight "body box" in which the subject is enclosed. With each inspiration alveolar pressure falls, alveolar air expands, and body volume increases, causing the pressure in the airtight box to rise. Conversely, with each expiration alveolar pressure rises, alveolar air is compressed, and body volume decreases, causing the pressure in the box to fall. Box pressure is monitored with a pressure transducer, and its response to changes in body volume is calibrated by introducing known aliquots of air and observing the resulting pressure rise. Independent measurement of lung volume is also needed to carry out the calculation of alveolar pressure during breathing.

With this or comparable methods, airway resistance has been shown to vary not only with body size but with rate of flow (because turbulence becomes more important with greater flow rates), with inspiration and expiration (because bronchial caliber varies through the ventilatory cycle), and with lung volume (because lung recoil also affects bronchial diameter).

Laminar and Turbulent Flow

With quiet breathing, ventilatory flow tends to be laminar. By applying Poiseuille's law the resistance of any bronchus to laminar flow may be evaluated from its length (l) and radius (r): $R = 8\eta l/r^4$, where η is the viscosity of air, which is little altered by the presence of

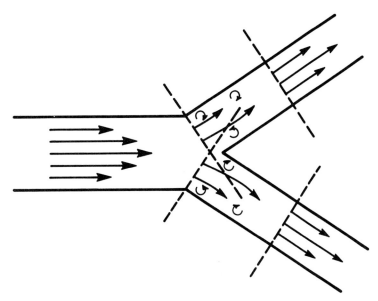

Fig. 5. Disruption of laminar flow at a bronchial bifurcation (schematic).

water vapor and a small fraction of carbon dioxide. However, fully established laminar flow is unlikely to exist in the bronchial tree, because each bronchial division disturbs the pattern of flow (Fig. 5) with an apparent increase in airway resistance.

During quiet breathing turbulence occurs near the narrows of the laryngeal passage. During exercise turbulent flow prevails in the trachea and also in the large bronchi. With turbulent flow resistance rises in proportion to the rate of flow. Resistance becomes independent of air viscosity but varies in direct proportion to specific gravity ρ and in inverse proportion to the fifth power of the bronchial radius. Yet increasing resistance with increasing rate of flow is the essential characteristic of turbulent flow: $R \sim (l\rho/\pi r^5)\dot{V}$.

The prevalence of a turbulent or laminar pattern of flow in any segment of the bronchial tree is determined by two variables: the air velocity v, which depends on the rate of flow and cross-sectional area of the bronchial segment ($v = \dot{V}/\pi r^2$), and the kinematic viscosity of the gas mixture (ratio of specific gravity to viscosity, ρ/η). The respective roles of these two factors are predicted by the Reynolds number, ($\mathbf{R} = v\rho l/\eta$); whenever air velocity is great, the Reynolds number is large and flow becomes turbulent. Such a situation prevails in the trachea and large bronchi when ventilation is large.

Table 1
Dichotomous Branching of the Bronchial Tree

Z	Name	Diameter (cm)	Cross Section (cm²)	Number 2^z	Total Cross-sectional Area (cm²)	Mean Air Velocity for $v = 1$ l/sec (cm/sec)
0	Trachea	2	3	1	3.0	330
1	Mainstem	1.3	1.35	2	2.7	370
2	Lobar	0.9	0.70	4	2.8	360
3	Segmental	0.7	0.38	8	3.0	330
4	Subsegmental	0.5	0.20	16	3.2	310
...						
12	Bronchiole	0.05	0.0021	4,096	8.6	125
13	Bronchiole	0.04	0.0012	8,192	9.8	100
...						
16	TB	0.018	0.00024	65,536	16	66
17	RB1	0.015	0.00015	131,072	20	50
18	RB2	0.012	0.00011	262,144	30	35
19	RB3	0.011	0.00010	524,288	50	20
20	AD1	0.010	0.00008	1,048,576	80	12
21	AD2	0.010	0.00008	2,097,152	160	6
22	AD3	0.010	0.00008	4,194,304	–	–
23	AS	0.005	0.00002	8,388,608	–	–

Average dimensions for human lungs inflated to three-fourths of total lung capacity; z is the generation number. (After Wiebel ER: Morphometry of the Human Lung. New York Academy Press, 1963.)

Beyond the segmental bronchi, however, the numbers of bronchi increase much more rapidly than their individual radius decreases (Table 1); thus the total cross-sectional area of the airway increases from trachea to bronchioles, slowly at first but very rapidly in the peripheral airways. Because the total volume flow is the same at a given instant at all levels of the bronchial tree, the velocity of flow varies inversely with the total cross-sectional area. Accordingly, low air velocity is the rule in the peripheral airways, the Reynolds number remains small regardless of ventilation, and flow tends to be laminar.

Central and Peripheral Airways

The branching of the bronchial tree follows a general pattern of irregular dichotomy; the daughter branches often have uneven diameters and lengths. A well-known example is offered by the tracheal bifurcation: of the two main stem bronchi, the right one is both wider and shorter than the left one. Although mathematical functions can be evolved that account for such irregularities, a simpler model of regular dichotomy (Fig. 6) gives sufficient insight into the resistive properties of the airway. Indeed, the difference between such a model and the true anatomic structures is notable mostly for the first five or six generations of bronchi.

In any dichotomous branching the number of branches doubles with each generation. With the convention that the trunk of origin (here the trachea) should be of rank 0, the nth generation comprises 2^n individual branches. The number of branchings along any single bronchial pathway varies from 10 to 25. On the average, however, bronchioles devoid of cartilage appear at or near the 12th generation, and alveolar ducts at or near the 20th. The reduction in diameter with each division is marked at first, but diminishes progressively until the alveolar ducts are reached, where division occurs with no change in size. Therefore, the summed cross-sectional area of parallel pathways increases slowly through the first 5 to 10 generations and rapidly toward the periphery (Table 1). Accordingly, most of the resistance to air flow is encountered in the central airways. In contrast, the small peripheral branches are so numerous that their total resistance is minimal. Evidence for this longitudinal partition of resistance has been provided experimentally in excised lungs by comparing alveolar pressure with the pressure measured by a transpleural catheter wedged at a branching near the 15th generation. The resistance of peripheral airways in normal adult lungs was found to be one-tenth that of the whole bronchial tree. In vivo, however, the upper airways, nose, pharynx, and larynx offer a resistance equal to that of the bronchial tree. Therefore the overall partition of resistance in healthy adults may be estimated as follows: upper airway 50 percent, central airway 45 percent, peripheral airway 5 percent. In infants, peripheral bronchi contribute a greater share to the total airway resistance.

Bronchial Diameter

Bronchi are deformable; their size and shape are partly determined by transmural pressure (equal to the difference between intrabronchial and peribronchial

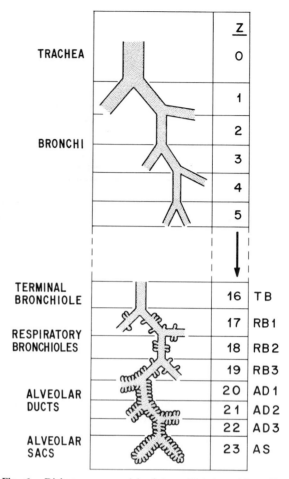

Fig. 6. Dichotomous model of bronchial branching. (Reproduced by permission from Weibel ER: Morphometry of the Human Lung, New York Academy Press, 1963.)

pressures) and by the bronchial wall compliance. Because of the presence of cartilage in their walls, bronchi have a stable volume at zero transmural pressure, and their distension in response to high transmural pressure is limited. But the membranous part of the wall determines bronchial compliance in the functional range of pressures (± 25 cm H_2O), so that bronchi stretch appreciably in length and circumference during inspiration when transmural pressure is increased. They recoil at expiration. Should transmural pressure be reversed, bronchial walls yield to compression and the cross-sectional area narrows to a slim crescent (Fig. 7).

Intrabronchial pressure varies above and below zero during the breathing cycle. At any given time it also varies along bronchial pathways, ranging from alveolar pressure to ambient pressure. During quiet breathing these variations through time and space are small, and transmural pressure is determined by peribronchial pressure.

The peribronchial space is occupied by expansions of the visceral fascia, whose laminated structure allows the bronchi to alter their spatial relations with lung tissue as required in the act of breathing. The visceral fascia in the lungs resembles the pleural space in that it

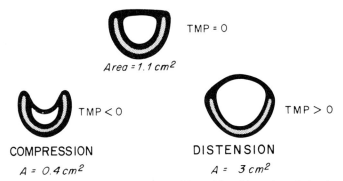

Fig. 7. Changing shape and cross-sectional area of bronchi and intrathoracic trachea with varying transmural pressure (schematic).

may be dissected by air (pneumomediastinum) or by fluid (interstitial edema). Although direct measurements of peribronchial pressure thus far have yielded discordant results, indirect but reliable evidence indicates that it is equal to or little different from pleural pressure. Bronchographic and bronchoscopic observations have shown bronchial diameter to increase with increasing lung volume. Also airway resistance falls when the lungs are expanded from residual volume to total lung capacity, all of which is consistent with a greater tethering effect on the bronchi with greater lung recoil.

The relationship of airway resistance to lung volume is hyperbolic (Fig. 8A), so that the reciprocal of airway resistance (airway conductance) is related to lung volume by a linear function (Fig. 8B). Because of this fundamental relationship, results of measurements are often expressed in terms of specific conductance, equal to the ratio of airway conductance to the lung volume at which it was measured, usually FRC. Specific conductance is independent of body size and normally averages 0.1 l/sec/cm H_2O per liter of lung volume. Because the relationship of conductance to volume is linear rather than proportional, specific conductance is not entirely independent of lung volume. Nevertheless, since airway obstruction is commonly associated with

increased FRC, specific conductance offers a more accurate index of impaired airway mechanics than does conductance alone.

Like pleural pressure peribronchial pressure probably varies from apex to base of the lung, whereas intrabronchial pressure at a given time is essentially the same in bronchi of the same rank throughout the lungs. Thus at the apex transmural pressure is higher, and bronchi of similar rank are more widely open than at the base of the lung. In normal young adults the regional differences in airway diameter and resistance have little effect on the distribution of inspired air during slow, quiet breathing. During a rapid inspiration, however, the vertical gradient of airway resistance becomes significant; apical ventilation is favored and basal ventilation reduced, which partially counteracts the effect of differences in regional compliance. Thus the distribution of inspired air in normal lungs is more even with rapid inspiration than with slow inspiration.

Small-Airway Closure

Devoid of cartilage, a bronchiole collapses whenever its transmural pressure falls below a critical value, either zero or a very small negative figure (0 to -2 cm H_2O). Since during quiet breathing transmural pressure closely approximates transpulmonary pressure, the in-

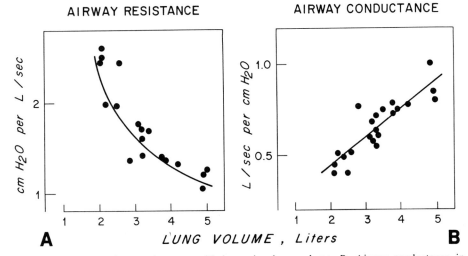

Fig. 8. A: Airway resistance decreases with increasing lung volume. B: Airway conductance increases with increasing lung volume. (Courtesy of Dr. W. Briscoe and the Journal of Clinical Investigation cumma 1958.)

cidence of small-airway closure increases with decreasing lung volume. Closure actually begins in the dependent part of the lung where transpulmonary pressure is the lowest. As lung recoil diminishes with age or with emphysema, closure affects an increasingly larger number of bronchioles at any lung volume. The lung volume at which, during a complete expiration, small airways begin to close is usually referred to as closing volume.

Only indirect methods are available to determine the closing volume in vivo. Most of these make use of the assumption that a bolus of marker gas inhaled near residual volume is distributed only to areas of the lung with open airways. Results have shown that closing volume is near residual volume in healthy young adults but approaches FRC as age increases from 20 to 60 years. In older persons closing volume is normally found in the tidal range.

Disease can affect airway closure in various ways. Loss of lung recoil, which is much more severe in emphysema than in normal aging lungs, reduces transmural pressure at all lung volumes; closing volume exceeds FRC early in the course of the disease and both FRC and residual volume increase. Because of their small diameter and radius of curvature bronchioles, like alveoli, depend on surfactant to remain open. Airway surfactant probably originates in the Clara cells, and its production is impaired by inflammatory processes affecting the bronchiolar epithelium. The presence of mucus not only interferes with the role of surfactant but also directly causes closure at positive transmural pressures. Similarly, submucosal edema encroaches on the lumen and facilitates closure. Bronchoconstriction theoretically could improve resistance to collapse by strengthening the bronchiolar wall, but since it is usually associated with submucosal edema and the presence of mucus it actually induces airway closure. Interstitial edema reduces transmural pressure because of fluid accumulation in the peribronchial space.

The physiologic consequences of airway closure are multiple, but maldistribution of inspired air is probably the single most important. Local ventilation may be absent or intermittent, and then occurring only near the end of tidal inspirations and during sighs; or it may be entirely dependent upon collateral channels (pores of Kohn, canals of Lambert) through which air spaces trapped behind closed airways receive alveolar air rather than fresh inspired air from preserved neighboring airspaces. In young children, collateral channels are poorly developed, and airway closure, when widespread in a segment of a lobe, causes atelectasis.

Dynamic Compression

During quiet breathing, expiration is driven by the recoil of the respiratory system without intervention of expiratory muscles. In the range of lung volumes normally utilized at rest, chest wall elasticity opposes lung recoil, so that pleural pressure remains negative. Similarly, pressure around the bronchi is negative, whereas in the lumen pressure is positive everywhere. Transmural pressure then remains positive, and although

bronchial caliber is smaller than at inspiration the difference is slight. In healthy young adults the airway remains well open from bronchiole to trachea; the expiratory rise in airway resistance is minimal.

During forced expiration the forces developed by expiratory muscles compress the lungs. Pleural and peribronchial pressures become positive, although everywhere less positive than alveolar pressure; the difference is precisely equal to lung recoil. Intrabronchial pressure is positive, too, but varies from terminal bronchiole (where it is close to alveolar pressure) to trachea (where it approaches zero). Therefore somewhere along every bronchial pathway there is a point where intrabronchial and peribronchial pressures are equal (Fig. 9). Peripheral to this equal-pressure point, transmural pressure is positive and the airways widely open. Central to the equal-pressure point, transmural pressure is negative and the airways are effectively compressed by the lung tissue surrounding them. The cervical trachea and upper airways, which are not exposed to peribronchial or pleural pressure, escape dynamic compression.

Lung recoil, which is responsible for the negativity of pleural and peribronchial pressures with respect to alveolar pressure, plays an essential role in protecting the intrathoracic airways from dynamic compression. Near TLC normally lung recoil is high; therefore at the beginning of a forced expiration only the lower trachea and carina are subjected to compression. As lung volume falls during forced expiration, so does lung recoil, and the equal-pressure point moves from the carina toward the periphery, reaching at least the subsegmental bronchi, with a corresponding increase in airway resistance. With loss of lung recoil as in emphysema, dynamic compression affects an abnormally large segment of the bronchial tree at all lung volumes.

Isovolume Flow–Pressure Curves

During forced expiration the intrathoracic airways are thus functionally divided into a peripheral segment upstream of the equal-pressure point, where transmural

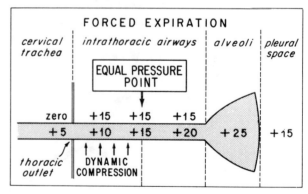

Fig. 9. Distribution of pressure during forced expiration. Pleural and peribronchial pressures are equal. Alveolar pressure is greater than pleural pressure, the difference being equal to the elastic recoil of the lung. Intrabronchial pressure as it decreases along the airway becomes equal to peribronchial pressure at the equal-pressure point.

pressure is positive and the airways fully open, and a central segment downstream, subjected to dynamic compression. Flow through the upstream segment is produced by the difference between alveolar pressure and pleural pressure, the latter prevailing at the equal-pressure point; this difference by definition equals transpulmonary pressure or lung recoil. In the downstream segment the same flow is produced by the difference between pleural pressure at the equal-pressure point and the intratracheal pressure at the level of the thoracic outlet, still positive but lower. Flow rate is actually determined by the balance between lung recoil, which initiates flow through the upstream segment, and pleural pressure, which compresses the downstream segment.

The relationship of expiratory flow rate to alveolar pressure, as plotted for various lung volumes, shows that flow increases with increasing expiratory effort until a critical pleural pressure is reached. Then flow levels off, becoming independent of effort (Fig. 10A). In raising pleural pressure, expiratory efforts develop the counterproductive effects of moving the equal-pressure point toward the periphery and increasing the force of dynamic compression.

Isovolume flow–pressure curves are of value in analyzing the mechanical events that occur during forced expiration. However, to determine a family of such curves for an individual, multiple forced expirations must be monitored for flow rate, lung volume, and alveolar or pleural pressure, to allow the plotting of data pertaining to a series of selected lung volumes. The procedure is tiring for the subject, and the data processing is rather complex. Therefore no clinical test has evolved from such investigation.

Flow–Volume Curves

In the volume range from residual volume to two-thirds or three-fourths of vital capacity a moderate expiratory effort suffices to reach maximal flow rates. Monitoring alveolar or pleural pressure then becomes unnecessary and adequate information is obtained from simultaneous measurements of lung volume and flow. Flow and volume are then instantly displayed on an X–Y recorder during a single forced expiration maneuver. Such flow–volume curves are characterized by a steep initial rise of expiratory flow rate near TLC followed by a reduction of flow rate with diminishing lung volume (Fig. 10B). In contradistinction to the rest of the flow–volume curve, the peak expiratory flow rate is effort-dependent.

Normal peak flow rates are in the range of 6–12 l/sec, implying large air velocities in the central airways, with large Reynolds numbers and turbulent flow. Accordingly, the resistance to forced expiration near TLC is found mostly in large bronchi, whose size and structure predominantly affect the peak flow. In patients a decreased peak flow rate indicates either large airway obstruction (asthmatic attack, tracheal stenosis) or a severe loss of lung recoil (emphysema).

Below TLC lung recoil falls rapidly with diminishing lung volume, and dynamic compression affects a progressively larger segment of the airway. But as flow rate diminishes turbulent flow subsides and the central airways contribute a diminishing fraction to total resistance. Maximal expiratory rates are then influenced by lung recoil and the structure of small airways upstream of the equal-pressure point. Normally the flow–volume relationship is almost linear from peak flow near TLC to zero flow at residual volume. In patients with obstructive lung disease flow decreases more rapidly than volume, and the flow–volume curve is convex toward the volume axis. To characterize such curves, maximal expiratory flow rates are measured at 25, 50, and 75 percent of vital capacity, or at FRC, all in the volume range of normal breathing. The maximal expiratory flow rate measured at 50 percent of vital capacity may fall from a normal range of 3–5 l/sec (near one-half of the peak flow rate) to below 0.5 l/sec, offering a sensitive index of small-airway disease or loss of lung recoil. But loss of lung recoil affects both peak flow rate and

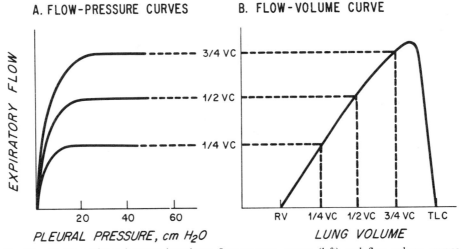

Fig. 10. Correspondence between isovolume flow–pressure curves (left) and flow–volume curves (right) (schematic).

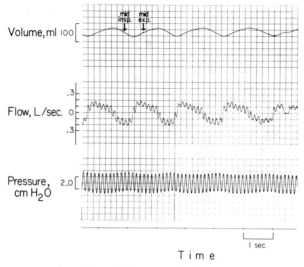

Fig. 11. Simultaneous recording of ventilation (top), air flow rate (middle), and mouth pressure (bottom). The ratio of the 8-cps modulation of pressure and flow measures the resistance of the respiratory system. (Courtesy of Dr. MEB Wohl and Pediatrics, 1970.)

maximal flow rate at low lung volume because of the increased dynamic compression in the downstream segment and the decreased driving pressure in the upstream segment.

Work of Breathing

The lungs are a passive mechanical device, acted upon by the chest wall. Energy developed by the respiratory muscles is used in the lungs to overcome lung recoil, airway resistance, and air inertia. But energy is also dissipated within the chest wall as needed to overcome recoil forces and tissue resistance and inertia. Inertial forces are comparatively small and in first approximation they may be ignored. Work is spent in proportion to the elastic recoil of the respiratory system, as measured for lungs and chest wall together, and in proportion to the resistance of the respiratory system, comprising airway and tissue resistances.

Elastic recoil is determined by the relaxed pressure–volume curve of the respiratory system (Fig. 3), which over the span of one breath may be approximated by a linear relationship with slope equal to the compliance of the respiratory system, C_{RS}. The recoil pressure during inspiration increases in inverse proportion to the compliance of the system and at the end of inspiration reaches a maximum equal to V_T/C_{RS}; the mean pressure developed to overcome elastic forces (P_{el}) is one-half of the maximum reached at the end of inspiration: $P_{el} = V_T/2C_{RS}$. The tidal volume V_T is easily measured with a spirometer or a plethysmograph or by integrating the flow signal of a pneumotachograph. Methods for determining a relaxed pressure–volume curve of the respiratory system were described in the previous section.

Resistances are determined not by volume changes but by the instantaneous rates of flow. Pneumotachographic recordings show that flow rate remains fairly constant during inspiration. Thus if inspiration occupies one-half of the duration of a respiratory cycle ($T/2$) the instantaneous inspiratory flow rate is $V_T/(T/2) = 2V_T f$, with $f = 1/T$, the respiratory frequency. The pressure required to overcome resistive forces during inspiration is proportional to the resistance, tidal volume, and frequency: $P_{res} = 2R_{RS}V_T f$. The total resistance of the respiratory system R_{RS} is normally 50 percent greater than the airway resistance alone; the difference is due to viscous friction developed within tissues in lungs and chest wall and is occasionally referred to as viscance. The method developed to measure the resistance of the respiratory system makes use of a rapid oscillation of small amplitude, as produced by a loudspeaker, superimposed over the relatively slow oscillation of spontaneous breathing; the rapid signal causes a modulation of ventilatory flow and of pressure across the respiratory system (Fig. 11). The modulation is of such small amplitude that its elastic component is negligible. The resistance of the respiratory system is then measured by the ratio of the respective amplitudes of pressure flow and modulations. Mechanical work is measured by the product force times displacement or some equivalent expression. In the case of the respiratory system the appropriate expression is the product pressure times volume, which gives a three-dimensional summation of linear forces and displacements. Pressure is the sum of elastic and resistive pressures, $P_{el} + P_{res}$, and volume is the tidal volume displaced with each breath. Thus the work performed during one inspiration is

$$W_I = V_T(P_{el} + P_{res}) = V_T(V_T/2C_{RS} + 2R_{RS}V_T f)$$

During normal breathing at rest the recoil work done at inspiration is stored in tissue elasticity and returned during expiration to perform resistive work; the expiration is said to be passive, which emphasizes the fact that respiratory muscles perform mechanical work during inspiration only. Then the power dissipated in the act of breathing is the product of inspiratory work times breathing frequency:

$$\dot{W} = fV_T(V_T/2C_{RS} + 2R_{RS}V_Tf)$$
$$= V_T^2f/2C_{RS} + 2R_{RS}V_Tf)$$

Actual values are extremely small in normal persons at rest but increase geometrically with increasing ventilation at exercise (Fig. 12). In disease states, work of breathing increases markedly as the respiratory system exhibits decreased compliance and increased resistance, while the ventilatory requirements are often abnormally high (Table 2). In asthma the increased work of breathing exceeds the estimate derived from the above equation because expiration requires active muscular work at a rate that rises with increasing severity of the attack.

PULMONARY BLOOD FLOW

Pressure in the pulmonary artery P_{PA} normally averages about 15 mm Hg; left atrial pressure P_{LA} averages 8 mm Hg. By definition the pulmonary vascular resistance (PVR) is calculated as the ratio of this arteriovenous pressure drop to the cardiac output. With an assumed cardiac output (CO) of 5 l/min, the average values quoted for mean vascular pressures yield the following results:

$$\text{PVR} = (P_{PA} - P_{LA}/(CO)$$
$$= (15 - 8)/5$$
$$= 1.4 \text{ mm Hg per l/min}$$

In contrast, the corresponding average figures for the systemic vascular resistance (SVR) yield a much higher value (with P_{Ao} and P_{RA} written for aortic and right atrial pressures, respectively):

$$\text{SVR} = (P_{Ao} - P_{RA}/(CO)$$
$$= (95 - 5)/5$$
$$= 18 \text{ mm Hg per l/min}$$

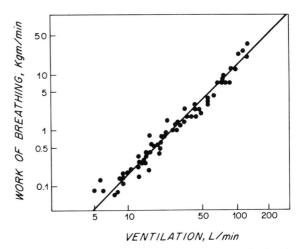

Fig. 12. Work of breathing as a function of ventilation in normal persons at rest and at exercise; the bilogarithmic plot yields a linear relationship. (Reproduced by permission of Dr. P.H. Rossier and Springer-Verlag from Physiologie and Pathophysiologie der Atmung, 1956.)

Thus the normal pulmonary circulation is characterized by a low vascular resistance, which is explained by the structure and mechanical behavior of the pulmonary vascular bed.

Pulmonary Vascular Bed

Branches of the pulmonary artery originate not only by a pattern of irregular dichotomy similar to that of the bronchial tree but also by production of supernumerary branches first appearing as occasional offshoots of subsegmental vessels but increasingly frequent toward the periphery. The conventional dichotomous arteries accompany the branches of the bronchial tree. The first 6 generations are elastic arteries; generations 7 through 10 are transition arteries, smaller than the transition vessels in the systemic circulation. Muscular arteries are found with all subsequent generations of air-

Table 2
Work of Breathing at Rest in Normal Conditions and in Asthma and Pulmonary Fibrosis.
Increased Work in Pathologic Conditions Is Due to Altered Compliance and Resistance,
and Also to Increased Ventilatory Requirements.

	Normal	Asthma	Fibrosis
Tidal volume V_T (ml)	500	700	400
Frequency f per minute	15	20	25
Compliance of respiratory system C_{RS} (ml/cm H$_2$O)	100	50*	25
Resistance of respiratory system R_{RS} (cm H$_2$O/ml/min)	0.01	2	0.1
$\dot{W}_{el} = \dfrac{1}{2C_{RS}} V_T^2 f$ (g · cm/min)	18,750	100,000	80,000
$\dot{W}_{res} = 2R_{RS} V_T^2 f^2$ (g · cm/min)	11,250	800,000	10,000
Work of breathing (g · cm/min)	30,000	900,000	90,000
Work of breathing (kgm/min)	0.3	9.0†	0.9
O$_2$ cost of breathing‡ (ml/min)	1.5	45	4.5

*Compliance is decreased because of pulmonary hyperinflation and uneven distribution.

†This value is underestimated since mechanical work performed during active expiration is not included.

‡Respiratory muscle efficiency ratio is taken equal to 10%.

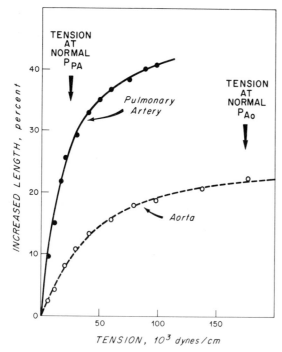

Fig. 13. Length–tension diagram of circumferential strips of normal human aorta and pulmonary artery. The arrows indicate the tension present at normal systemic and pulmonary arterial pressures. (Reproduced by permission from Harris P, Heath D: The Human Pulmonary Circulation. E&S Livingstone, 1962.)

ways down to the terminal bronchioles. Arterioles less than 7 μ in diameter and partly or totally devoid of smooth muscle first appear alongside respiratory bronchioles and are consistently found with alveolar ducts and, as branches of supernumerary arteries, at the periphery of the lobule.

The elastic pulmonary arteries exhibit marked passive dilatation with increasing pressure. When compared

to the aorta and its branches, the large pulmonary arteries are 10 times more compliant than the systemic vessels in their respective ranges of normal pressures (Fig. 13). Accordingly, any rise in pulmonary artery pressure is accompanied by a fall of resistance in large vessels.

Resistance in the pulmonary arterial bed arises from the distal branches because they have small radii (Poiseuille's law) and because their walls contain smooth muscle capable of tone and reactive constriction. Nevertheless, the thin muscular layer allows for considerable compliance to be retained and a marked fall of resistance still occurs in response to increased distending pressure.

Arterioles give off a number of precapillary vessels approximately 20 μ in diameter that supply a sheetlike capillary mesh. The capillaries, 10 μ in diameter, occupy a greater portion of the alveolar surface than the holes in the mesh (Fig. 14). They are collapsible but are thought to be nondistensible.

Venules originate from the capillary bed of respiratory bronchioles, alveolar ducts, and alveoli. Their structure is similar to that of arterioles, from which they cannot be distinguished on histologic sections. Initially they travel within the alveolar tissue to the periphery of the lobule where they pass into the interlobular septa. Larger veins are found with bronchi, arteries, and lymphatics in a common sheath of connective tissue. Pulmonary veins are devoid of valves and their smooth muscle is poorly developed.

Lymphatic capillaries originate in the pleura, in the interlobular septa and bronchovascular spaces, and in the walls of respiratory bronchioles. With successive confluents they form lymphatic trunks whose media contains well-developed bundles of longitudinal and oblique smooth-muscle fibers. Progression of lymph in these vessels results from rhythmic contractions of the smooth muscle, while lymph flow is directed toward the hilar nodes by numerous valves. Several lymphatic trunks,

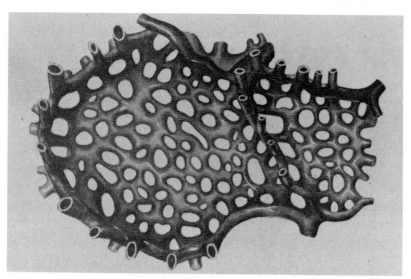

Fig. 14. Alveolar capillaries injected with india ink. (Reproduced by permission from Miller WS: The Lung. Springfield, Ill, Charles C. Thomas, 1937.)

joined by a capillary plexus, accompany each bronchus, artery, and vein.

Transmural Pressure of Pulmonary Arteries

Because of their thin walls pulmonary arteries are both collapsible and distensible. Their shape and caliber therefore vary greatly with varying transmural pressure; a circular cross section is achieved only when transmural pressure is positive, i.e., when intraarterial pressure exceeds periarterial pressure.

Intraarterial pressure is to a large extent dependent on hydrostatic forces. The arterial bed in the lungs forms a communicating system in which hydrostatic pressure develops in proportion to vertical distance. In the erect position the lungs reach about 12 cm above and below the main pulmonary arteries. Thus a hydrostatic pressure difference ranging from 0 to 12 cm H_2O (0 to 9 mm Hg) is added to the pulmonary artery pressure in the basal vessels and subtracted from it in the apical vessels. The pressure head available for lung perfusion increases linearly from apex to base with a gradient of perfusing pressure nearly equal to 1 cm H_2O per centimeter of vertical distance. Mean intraarterial pressure then shows greater variations because of hydrostatic effects (typically from 6 mm Hg at the apex to 24 mm Hg at the base of the lung in the erect position) than because of hydrodynamic pressure drop (less than 5 mm Hg from large arteries to precapillary vessels).

Periarterial pressure is variable also. The hilar vessels, enveloped in pleural reflexions, are directly exposed to pleural pressure. Their branches travel with bronchi and veins in their common sheath of connective tissue, where they are surrounded by lung parenchyma and exposed to regional lung recoil; the mechanical forces acting on these vessels differ from those affecting the alveolar capillaries, which is emphasized by the name extraalveolar vessels that is given to them. The pressure surrounding the extraalveolar arteries is not accessible to direct measurement. The evidence so far suggests that it is determined by the same mechanisms and takes the same values as pleural pressure (as explained previously). In the erect position at FRC periarterial pressure probably varies between mean values of -8 cm H_2O at the apex to -2 cm H_2O at the base. Consequently the effect of perivascular pressure on arterial caliber is negligible at the base; basal arteries are widely open because intraluminal pressure is sufficiently high. At the apex, however, the negative perivascular pressure exerts a tethering effect and supports the patency of arteries in spite of low intraluminal pressure.

The changes in pleural pressure that occur during breathing are transmitted to the heart and great vessels and cause periodic variation of pulmonary artery pressure. Since the same respiratory oscillations occur in the perivascular space, quiet breathing has no effect on transmural pressure and regional arterial resistance. However, the amplitude of the respiratory oscillations, ± 3 to 5 cm H_2O, represents an appreciable fraction of regional pulmonary arterial pressure whose effects are likely to be felt most strongly at the apex of the lung.

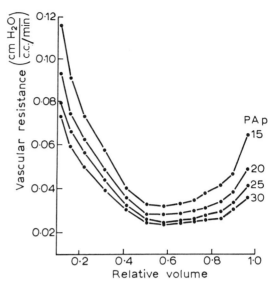

Fig. 15. Pulmonary vascular resistance at different lung volumes and pulmonary artery pressure. (Reproduced by permission of Drs. LJ Thomas Jr, A Roos, ZJ Grillo and of the American Physiological Society from J Appl Physiol, 1961.)

Certainly with full inspiration to TLC pleural pressure normally becomes so markedly negative that although systemic venous return and heart rate increase pulmonary artery pressure falls and perfusion to apical regions of the lungs ceases altogether.

Lung Volume and Vascular Resistance

In collapsed lungs the small arteries are closed and their resistance is infinite. Flow begins when pulmonary artery pressure exceeds an opening pressure that for various mammalian lungs is of the order of 7 mm Hg. With progressive lung inflation smaller opening pressures are observed, until at normal volume, near FRC, the vessels are patent and flow can be generated even with low pressure. Once flow is established, pulmonary vascular resistance decreases with increasing lung volume from the collapsed state to FRC. But above FRC, and particularly as lung volume approaches TLC, vascular resistance increases with increasing lung volume (Fig. 15).

Resistance falls at first with increasing lung volume because lung recoil increases and with it the transmural pressure and cross-sectional area of extraalveolar vessels. At high lung volume, however, these vessels are fully distended and no longer respond to further increases of transmural pressure with significant dilatation. Simultaneously the alveolar vessels, mostly the capillaries, are flattened by the increasing stretch of alveolar walls; as their resistance increases, so does the overall resistance. In addition, the resistance observed at any lung volume is greatest when flow is first established and falls rapidly if pressure and flow are raised; therefore the relationship of vascular resistance to lung volume is represented by a family of U-shaped curves, each determined for a constant perfusing pressure (Fig. 15).

In diseased lungs, changes in regional lung volume alter the distribution of blood flow. Atelectasis is accompanied by a sharp reduction of perfusion to the diseased lobe. It is likely also that extreme changes in total lung volume contribute to the pathogenesis of pulmonary hypertension in obstructive lung disease and in kyphoscoliosis.

Interstitial Pressure

Interstitial tissue envelops the alveolar and extraalveolar vessels. The alveolar interstitium is made of a thin layer of connective tissue, interplaced between alveolar and capillary basement membranes, or, in the holes of the capillary mesh, between two adjacent alveolar basement membranes. Extraalveolar connective tissue comprises the pleura, the interlobular septa, the space surrounding respiratory bronchioles, and the bronchovascular sheaths. Interstitial fluid generated in the alveolar walls is collected by lymphatic capillaries in the septa, the peribronchiolar space, and the sheaths; it is assumed that pressure differences are responsible for the progression of fluid from alveolar to extraalveolar interstitium.

Except for the interposition of alveolar epithelium and surfactant, the alveolar interstitium is exposed to alveolar pressure; during normal breathing this is equal to ambient pressure. But Laplace's law predicts that pressure differences between alveolar lumen and interstitium will arise when the air–fluid interface is curved. In normally expanded lungs, alveoli are shaped like irregular cuboids, one face of which is open for free communication with ducts and atria; the wall surface is flat except along the edge of adjacent alveoli. There three alveolar walls come into contact, with angles averaging 120 deg rounded off by a curving of the epithelium, which generates a pressure difference across the surface: $P = \gamma/r$ (from Laplace's law for a cylindric interface, with γ the surface tension and r the radius of curvature). Interstitial pressure becomes negative with respect to alveolar pressure and therefore ambient pressure. However, the pulmonary surfactant lining the alveolar epithelium reduces surface tension to 10 dynes/cm or less, so that pressure in the alveolar interstitium is negative by 1–2 cm H_2O only.

Pressure in the extraalveolar interstitium is determined by local lung recoil. Like pleural pressure, it is negative during normal breathing and lower in the uppermost regions than in the dependent regions of the lungs, with mean values ranging from -8 to -2 cm H_2O.

Thus in normal resting conditions pressure is more negative in the extraalveolar than in the alveolar interstitium and free fluid is drained toward the extraalveolar spaces where it is collected by lymphatics. The removal of fluid is in part dependent upon lung recoil and therefore less efficient in the dependent regions of the lung. This mechanism, as well as the effect of gravity upon the clearance of secretion, contributes to the pathologic changes of hypostatic pneumonia.

When the normal balance between fluid production by the blood capillaries and its removal by the lymphatics is lost, interstitial edema results. Fluid accumulates first in the extraalveolar interstitium (Fig. 16), where pressure rises. The transmural pressure available to bronchi and vessels decreases, and local ventilation and perfusion are reduced. As interstitial edema progresses, fluid backs up into the alveolar interstitium and diminishes alveolar compliance, causing further reduction of function in the dependent regions of the lungs. Should any more fluid accumulate it would break through the epithelium and flood the alveoli, giving the classic picture of pulmonary edema.

If the surfactant lining is damaged or removed, alveolar surface tension increases toward the high values observed for an air–water interface (72 dynes/cm); a strong negative pressure is developed in the alveolar interstitium, causing increased fluid leakage from the capillaries according to Starling's law. Interstitial edema can result from this mechanism as well as from elevated hydrostatic pressure within the capillaries.

Regional Distribution

Interactions between numerous mechanical factors determine vascular and perivascular pressures and therefore regional blood flow.

The local perfusing arterial pressure P_a prevalent in the small arteries in any region of the lung is set by the

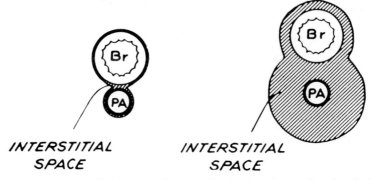

INTERSTITIAL   INTERSTITIAL
SPACE   SPACE

Fig. 16. Extraalveolar interstitial space. Left: normally the bronchovascular sheath is applied against bronchus and artery. Right: at the onset of pulmonary edema, fluid accumulation begins in the extraalveolar space. (Reproduced by permission of NC Staub and the American Physiological Society from J Appl Physiol, 1962.)

mean pulmonary artery pressure plus or minus the hydrostatic pressure gradient $\rho g h$ (with ρ the specific gravity of blood, g the acceleration due to gravity, and h the vertical distance).

The local venous pressure P_v is similarly set by the mean left atrial pressure plus or minus the hydrostatic pressure gradient.

The driving pressure, available to generate regional blood flow, is the pressure drop from regional arteries to regional veins.

The transmural pressure, which sets the regional vascular resistance, depends upon arterial and venous pressures and local perivascular pressure. The latter is close to pleural pressure for extraalveolar vessels and is close to alveolar pressure for the capillary bed.

At rest in the supine position the pressure in regional arteries and veins is positive everywhere, and the entire vascular bed is well expanded. The pressure drop ΔP across the vascular bed is constant for all lung regions: $\Delta P = (P_{PA} + \rho g h) - (P_{LA} + \rho g h) = P_{PA} - P_{LA}$. Differences in regional blood flow occur, nevertheless, because transmural pressure varies with the hydrostatic gradient. In the dependent regions vessels are more distended and have lower resistance than in the uppermost. Consequently blood flow to the dependent regions is greater than to the uppermost regions.

At rest in the erect position the same conditions still prevail in most of the lung. On the venous side, however, as pressure decreases linearly above the left atrium a point is reached where venous pressure is nil or negative. Above this level blood flow is determined by the difference between arterial pressure, which is small but still positive, and alveolar pressure, which averages zero: $\Delta P = (P_{PA} - \rho g h) - P_A = P_{PA} - \rho g h$. Thus in the resting condition flow in the upper regions decreases in direct proportion to the distance up the height of the lung.

If at rest lung volume is increased from FRC to TLC, intravascular pressures fall, while the vertical distance from main pulmonary artery to lung apex increases. As a result the arterial pressure head fails to reach the apex of the lung and there is no detectable apical blood flow.

In the presence of left ventricular failure the increased left atrial pressure creates a new situation whereby vascular pressures exceed alveolar pressure everywhere in the lung, regardless of body position or cardiac output. However, venous pressure in the dependent regions of the lung rises to the point where it exceeds the oncotic pressure of plasma proteins. Fluid transudation then exceeds the capability of the lymphatic system for fluid removal; interstitial edema sets in and regional blood flow decreases.

Thus the mechanical conditions that govern regional blood flow are determined by the relative magnitudes of arterial, alveolar, oncotic and venous pressures, whose varying relationships characterize four distinct distribution zones (Table 3). Not all four zones are found in the same lung in vivo, but the patterns of distribution actually observed with the use of radioactive gases can be understood in terms of a four-zone model.

Pressure–Flow Relationship

In the range of normal lung volumes the rise in pulmonary artery pressure required to double the pulmonary blood flow is barely measurable with the usual methods. This observation is explained by several factors, both physiologic and technical.

The recruitment of additional parallel channels permits a marked reduction of vascular resistance with increased blood flow. At rest the cardiac output goes preferentially to the dependent regions of the lungs. During exercise, when cardiac output is increased several times, the uppermost regions accommodate a fair share of the increased flow and perfusion is almost evenly distributed. Simultaneously the pulmonary capillary blood volume increases by a factor of two or more; values of 60–90 ml have been observed at rest and of 150–200 ml at exercise. Thus the maximal capacity of the capillary bed, as determined from anatomic measurements, is fully used only during exercise. In patients with chronic lung disease the impossibility of recruiting new vascular channels in response to increased flow appears to be the major mechanism for the elevation of pulmonary artery pressure during exercise.

Passive distension, which causes resistance to fall in all perfused channels, has its greatest effect during systole when a large part of the stroke volume finds its way through the arterial bed with resistance at its lowest. But even a small increase in mean pressure reduces resistance markedly in the normal range of pulmonary vascular pressures.

Kinetic energy is underestimated by the usual measurements of pulmonary artery pressure. Kinetic energy in a fluid is usually written $\rho v^2/2$, with v the linear velocity of the fluid and ρ its specific gravity, which for blood is near 1.06 g/ml. Blood leaving the right or left ventricle has the same velocity and therefore the same kinetic energy, which is negligible in the aorta where pressure is high. In the pulmonary artery where pressure is low it represents a significant fraction of total energy and is generally underestimated by catheter-tip measure-

Table 3
Factors Determining Regional Blood Flow
(P_{pp} Is the Oncotic Pressure of Plasma Proteins)

Zones	Pressure Relationships	Flow	Resistance
I	$P_{alv} > P_{art} > P_v$	$\dot{Q} = 0$	Infinite
II	$P_{art} > P_{alv} > P_v$	$\dot{Q} = \dfrac{P_{art} - P_{alv}}{R}$	Moderate
III	$P_{art} > P_v > P_{alv}$	$\dot{Q} = \dfrac{P_{art} - P_v}{R}$	Low
IV	$P_{art} > P_v > P_{pp}$	$\dot{Q} = \dfrac{P_{art} - P_v}{R}$	High

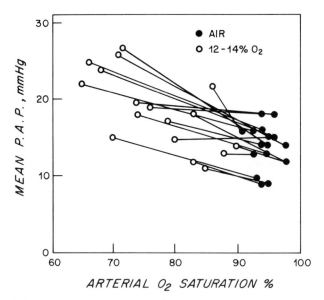

Fig. 17. Effect of alveolar hypoxia as estimated from arterial blood O_2 saturation on the pulmonary artery pressure of normal men. (Reproduced by permission of Dr. H. Fritts, Jr. Circulation 1960.)

ments of downstream pressure. The role of kinetic energy is most important when blood velocity is greatest, such as during systole and during exercise; then the kinetic error on usual measurement rises to approximately 10 percent of pulmonary artery pressure and 20 percent of the pressure drop across the lungs. Kinetic energy is transformed into pressure head in distal arteries where blood velocity decreases.

For cardiac outputs in excess of twice the normal resting values, mean pulmonary artery pressure rises significantly. Resistance, which had fallen sharply with the doubling of blood flow, decreases more slowly as flow increases further. When flow rises in response to strenuous exercise, the vascular bed accommodates fourfold to fivefold increases without fluid accumulation. When the high flow is due to a ventricular septal defect, interstitial edema occurs near a threefold increase; the different response is due to the chronicity of high blood flow and the occurrence of left ventricular overload in pathologic left-to-right shunt.

Vasomotor Control

The regulation of the pulmonary circulation is dominated by one mechanism that is unique to this vascular bed: vasoconstriction in response to hypoxia. The pulmonary hypertension induced by hypoxia is easily demonstrated in animals and in man. Breathing a gas mixture of 12 percent to 14 percent O_2 in N_2 at sea level causes a rise of pulmonary artery pressure proportional to the fall of arterial O_2 saturation (Fig. 17). Left atrial pressure and central blood volume remain unchanged but cardiac output rises, although less than pulmonary artery pressure, indicating a rise of pulmonary vascular resistance. The response is reversed by returning to normoxia.

Measurements of vascular resistance, however, fail to give an accurate picture of vasomotor activity in the pulmonary vessels because of the normal inequality of pulmonary blood flow; any increase in resistance of the better perfused regions is followed by recruitment of additional pathways, which limits the resulting change in overall resistance. This redistribution of blood flow is well demonstrated with isotopic methods in normal volunteers breathing a low-O_2 gas mixture; the upper regions of the lungs receive a greater fraction of pulmonary blood flow, so that the normal vertical gradient of regional blood flow is reduced or lost. Redistribution can be traced also during unilateral hypoxia in man or animal breathing through a divided tracheal tube. With this method the increased ventilation and cardiac output due to systemic hypoxia can be avoided by supplying one lung with pure O_2 while the other receives the low-O_2 mixture. Since both lungs are perfused with the same pulmonary arterial and left atrial pressures, blood flow is distributed in inverse proportion to the vascular resistance of each side. The finding that in these circumstances the blood flow going to the oxygenated lung is twice as great as that going to the hypoxic lung indicates that vascular resistance has nearly doubled on the hypoxic side.

Preparations of isolated lungs or lobes, perfused in situ by a pulsatile pump with blood of known gaseous composition, have yielded evidence that both alveolar and systemic hypoxia are capable of inducing pulmonary vasoconstriction and that the response is due to a dual mechanism of local regulation and neurogenic control. The response to alveolar hypoxia is often attributed to local regulation caused by direct exposure of small pulmonary arteries to hypoxic environment and medi-

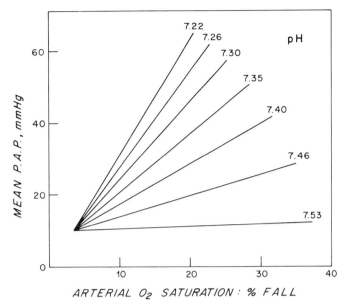

Fig. 18. Effect of hypoxia on pulmonary artery pressure at different levels of acidosis, as indicated by arterial blood pH. (Reproduced by permission of Dr. Y. Enson and the Rockefeller University Press from J Clin Invest, 1964.)

ated by local release of a chemical agent, possibly histamine. It appears likely, however, that sympathetic reflex activity contributes to the vasoconstriction of alveolar hypoxia, since resection of the stellate ganglion in the dog causes a marked reduction of the response to unilateral hypoxia.

Arterial vasoconstriction reduces the perfusion of hypoxic regions in the lungs and increases that of better oxygenated areas; therefore it limits the extent and consequences of ventilation/perfusion inequality. Whether it is active in normal persons breathing air at sea level is uncertain, although the small but definite fall of pulmonary artery pressure induced by breathing pure O_2 certainly suggests this. The beneficial role of hypoxic vasoconstriction in lung diseases is particularly well demonstrated in asthma; bronchodilating drugs cause vasodilatation as well, so that partial relief of the airway obstruction may be associated with a fall in arterial O_2 tension, unless O_2 is administered simultaneously.

With chronic alveolar and systemic hypoxia, persistent vasoconstriction results in medial hypertrophy, pulmonary hypertension, and eventually cor pulmonale. In such instances the pulmonary vasculature shows continued responsiveness to any acute worsening of hypoxia; conversely the pulmonary artery pressure decreases in response to O_2 therapy, not only acutely but also chronically when O_2 is administered over a period of weeks. Hypoxic vasoconstriction is a major factor also in the pathogenesis of high-altitude pulmonary hypertension and chronic mountain sickness. However, even in adults native to high altitude the pulmonary hypertension is reversible after prolonged residence at sea level.

Acidosis and increased CO_2 tension exaggerate the vascular response to hypoxia (Fig. 18). This effect has been well documented in patients with chronic lung disease, particularly chronic bronchitis, and contributes to the occurrence of right ventricular failure as a complication of respiratory failure. The respective roles of local regulation, neurogenic control, and effector responsiveness in this reaction have not been identified.

Other neurogenic control mechanisms can directly affect the pulmonary circulation. A rise in left atrial and pulmonary venous pressures causes reflex arterial vasoconstriction. Stimulation of the vagus nerve yields inconclusive results, but acetylcholine given by slow infusion in the pulmonary artery clearly causes dilatation of the pulmonary vessels, more marked when preliminary vasoconstriction has been induced by hypoxia.

Drugs, ions, and naturally occurring vasoactive substances also affect the pulmonary circulation. Except for histamine, which seems to be associated with hypoxic vasoconstriction, their effect is generally the same on pulmonary as on systemic vessels.

VENTILATION AND GAS EXCHANGE
Gas Laws

In the physiologic range of temperatures and pressures, not only O_2 and N_2 but also CO_2 follow the law of perfect gases: $PV = nrT$ (where P is pressure, V is volume, T is absolute temperature, n is the number of gas molecules, and r is the gas constant). This expression states that in an aliquot of gas (1) at constant temperature the product pressure times volume is constant (Boyle's law), (2) at constant pressure the volume is proportional to the absolute temperature (Charles's law), and (3) at constant volume the pressure is propor-

Table 4
Factors for Converting Gas Volumes from
ATPS Conditions to BTPS
or STPD Conditions

Temperature (deg C)	Conversion Factor ATPS to BTPS	Barometric Pressure	Conversion Factor ATPS to STPD
18	1.104	700	0.842
		720	0.867
		740	0.892
		760	0.916
		780	0.941
20	1.102	700	0.834
		720	0.858
		740	0.883
		760	0.907
		780	0.932
22	1.091	700	0.825
		720	0.849
		740	0.874
		760	0.898
		780	0.922
24	1.080	700	0.816
		720	0.840
		740	0.864
		760	0.888
		780	0.912
26	1.068	700	0.807
		720	0.831
		740	0.855
		760	0.879
		780	0.903
28	1.057	700	0.797
		720	0.821
		740	0.845
		760	0.869
		780	0.892
37	1.000	700	0.755
		720	0.777
		740	0.800
		760	0.822
		780	0.845

tional to the absolute temperature (Gay-Lussac's law). Boyle's law is applied daily in the pulmonary laboratory to determine lung volume in the body plethysmograph; so is Charles's law to calculate the effect of thermal dilatation on measurements of gas volumes. Gay-Lussac's law does not apply to phenomena taking place in the lungs where the circulation of a large blood flow assures a constant temperature. Occasionally it must be taken into account for measurements made outside the body.

Gas mixtures such as air follow the law of perfect gases: the volume imparted to each molecule in the mixture depends on pressure and temperature only, not on the nature of individual gases. This property is codified by Dalton's law: each gas in a mixture exerts a partial pressure proportional to its concentration. It follows that the partial pressures of different gases in a mixture

add up to the total pressure, equal or close to barometric pressure.

In the upper airways inspired air is warmed and humidified by contact with the fluid layer covering the respiratory mucosa. Fully saturated air contains water vapor at a partial pressure determined by temperature alone (Table 4). Room air is usually less than fully saturated but full saturation at room temperature prevails in most physiologic devices used for measuring gas volumes. The physical conditions present in the lungs are referred to by the abbreviation BTPS, for body temperature and pressure, saturated; those conditions present in collecting devices are referred to by the abbreviation ATPS, for ambient temperature and pressure, saturated. Results of ATPS measurements are readily converted to BTPS conditions by means of conversion factors calculated with Charles's and Dalton's laws (Table 4).

Measurements of gas volumes can also be converted to STPD conditions (standard temperature and pressure, dry) (0°C and 760 mm Hg) (Table 4). The result is then independent of body temperature and ambient pressure, which is advantageous when interest is attached to the mass of a gas aliquot rather than the volume it may occupy in varying conditions. Such is the case for O_2 uptake and CO_2 output.

In a saturated gas mixture the total pressure of dry gases (exclusive of water vapor) varies with varying temperature; it is equal to barometric pressure P_B minus water vapor pressure P_{H_2O}, or at sea level and normal body temperature: $760 - 47 = 713$ mm Hg. Within the dry-gas phase the fractional concentrations of the various components remain unchanged. According to Dalton's law the partial pressure of each component is given by the product of its fractional concentration and the total dry-gas pressure. Thus at sea level the partial pressures of O_2, CO_2, and N_2 in alveolar air are related to respective fractional concentrations as follows: $P_{O_2} = 713 F_{O_2}$, $P_{CO_2} = 713 F_{CO_2}$, and $P_{N_2} = 713 F_{N_2}$. The rare gases, primarily argon, which like N_2 are poorly soluble and do not participate in chemical reactions, are comprised in the N_2 fraction.

The quantitative relationships that characterize pulmonary gas exchange are expressed in the form of equations, with the use of conventional symbols listed in Table 5. In the equations quoted later in this section the conversion factors between ATPS, BTPS, and STPD conditions have been omitted.

Gas Exchange

Tidal breathing is characterized by an amplitude (the tidal volume) and a frequency (the breathing rate). The tidal ventilation, which measures the unidirectional flow of air into or out of the lungs, is equal to the product of tidal volume and respiratory rate: $\dot{V} = fV_T$.

In the lungs O_2 is taken up and CO_2 released. If CO_2 output equals O_2 uptake, inspired and expired ventilations are equal. If CO_2 output is smaller than O_2

uptake, expired ventilation is slightly smaller than inspired ventilation. The ratio of CO_2 output to O_2 uptake is the respiratory exchange ratio, distinct from the respiratory quotient that characterized cellular metabolism. The respiratory exchange ratio is equal to the respiratory quotient only when a steady state is achieved for gas exchange and the O_2 and CO_2 stores of the body remain constant.

Inspired air is normally devoid of CO_2. Therefore the CO_2 output can be calculated simply from the expired ventilation $\dot{V}_E$ and the CO_2 concentration in expired air: $\dot{V}_{CO_2} = \dot{V}_E \times F_{E_{CO_2}}$. But to determine O_2 uptake, both the inspired and expired O_2 concentrations are taken into account and a distinction is made between inspired and expired ventilations: $\dot{V}_{O_2} = (\dot{V}_I \times F_{I_{O_2}}) - (\dot{V}_E \times F_{E_{O_2}})$. Direct measurement of inspired ventilation is unnecessary, however. Since N_2 is not exchanged in the lungs, any excess of O_2 uptake over CO_2 output results in a slight increase of N_2 concentration in expired air, which is easily determined with the analysis of expired gas samples. The ratio if inspired to expired ventilation is then given by the ratio of expired to inspired N_2 concentrations: $\dot{V}_I = \dot{V}_E (F_{E_{N_2}} / F_{I_{N_2}})$. The correction introduced by the nitrogen ratio is small in the steady state when the respiratory exchange ratio remains close to unity.

Alveolar Ventilation

The continuous analysis of expired air reveals a changing composition through expiration, starting with gas from the upper airways and the bronchial tree, unchanged from inspired air (phase I), followed by rapidly changing concentrations due to the mixing of

gas coming from the airways and the alveoli (phase II), and ending with a plateau of nearly constant gas composition characteristic of alveolar air (phase III). If gas is sampled at or near the mouth, the first phase of expiration cannot be distinguished from inspiration; the continuous recording of P_{O_2} and P_{CO_2} yields a series of square waves with the gas tensions changing rapidly from a baseline of inspired concentrations to the level of alveolar plateaus. During expiration, however, the change from inspired to alveolar gas tensions is not instantaneous but rather describes an asymmetric S-shaped function that represents the mixing of airway

Table 5
Symbols in Pulmonary Physiology

Primary Symbols	Subscripts
C = compliance, concentration, or capacity	A = alveolar
D = diffusing capacity	a = arterial
F = fractional concentration	ao = airway opening
f = breathing frequency	aw = airway
G = conductance	c = capillary
P = pressure	c' = end capillary
Q = blood flow	E = expiratory or expired
R = resistance or respiratory exchange ratio	E' = end-expiratory
S = saturation	el = elastic
V = volume	I = inspiratory or inspired
$\dot{V}$ = ventilation or air flow rate	L = lung
W = work	M = membrane
	res = resistive
	RS = respiratory system
	T = tidal
	v = venous
	$\bar{v}$ = mixed venous

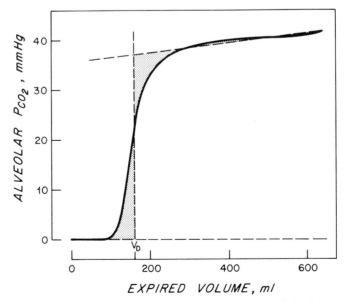

Fig. 19. P_{CO_2} in expired air as a function of expired volume: the anatomic dead space is determined by a vertical line drawn in such position as to leave the two shaded zones with equal surface areas (schematic).

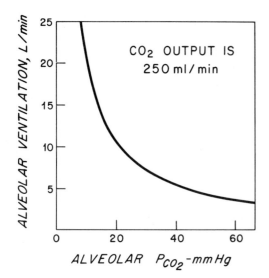

Fig. 20. For a given value of CO_2 output, alveolar ventilation is inversely proportional to alveolar P_{CO_2}.

gas and alveolar gas due to the varying length and volume of individual bronchial pathways.

The volume of inspired air remaining in the airways at the end of inspiration and first exhaled when expiration begins measures the anatomic dead space. This volume can be estimated in vivo by displaying concentration versus expired volume on an X–Y recorder and then calculating the square front equivalent to the observed S-shaped curve, according to the mean-value theorem (Fig. 19). The method of Fowler makes use of pure O_2 as inspired gas and N_2 as a marker gas, the concentration of which is monitored with a fast-responding N_2 analyzer. Reproducible results are obtained for normal subjects in whom the alveolar plateau of N_2 concentration is nearly straight and horizontal. Difficulties arise in many disease states when the alveolar plateau has significant slope and curvature.

From such data it is apparent that each expired tidal volume comprises a volume of inspired air, normally equal to the anatomic dead space, and some alveolar air sampled from all ventilated alveoli: $V_T = V_A + V_D$. Similarly, expired ventilation is equal to the sum of dead space ventilation fV_D and alveolar ventilation $\dot{V}_A$, defined as the fraction of ventilation that participates in gas exchange: $\dot{V}_E - \dot{V}_A + fV_D$. It follows that CO_2 output and O_2 uptake can be calculated in terms of alveolar ventilation and alveolar concentrations, as well as in terms of expired ventilation and expired concentrations. Here again CO_2 output is given by a simpler equation than is O_2 uptake; CO_2 output is equal to the product of alveolar ventilation and alveolar CO_2 concentration: $\dot{V}_{CO_2} = \dot{V}_A F_{A_{CO_2}}$. Rearranged, the latter relationship yields a fundamental equation $F_{A_{CO_2}} = \dot{V}_{CO_2}/\dot{V}_A$, or $P_{A_{CO_2}} = (P_B - 47)\,\dot{V}_{CO_2}/\dot{V}_A$, establishing that alveolar CO_2 concentration, or partial pressure,

is inversely proportional to alveolar ventilation (Fig. 20). The constant level of alveolar P_{CO_2} therefore depends on the exact adjustment of alveolar ventilation to the appropriate value needed for CO_2 elimination. Consequently, alveolar hypoventilation leads to high alveolar P_{CO_2} and alveolar hyperventilation to low alveolar P_{CO_2}. Should a low P_{CO_2} become desirable (as in diabetic ketoacidosis), P_{CO_2} can be reduced from a normal value of 40 mm Hg down to 20 mm Hg by doubling the alveolar ventilation. But to decrease P_{CO_2} to 10 mm Hg, alveolar ventilation should quadruple, which over a prolonged period of time represents an impossible burden. Indeed, P_{CO_2} values below 15 mm Hg are rarely observed. In addition, increased metabolic rate calls for a proportional increase of alveolar ventilation; the relationship of alveolar ventilation to CO_2 output is described by a family of curves, each one characteristic of a given P_{CO_2} (Fig. 21).

The expired P_{CO_2} is always lower than the alveolar P_{CO_2}. This difference results from the dilution of alveolar air with dead-space gas devoid of CO_2. It follows that dead-space volume can be calculated by comparing alveolar and expired P_{CO_2}, as shown by the Bohr equation:

$$V_D = V_T(P_{A_{CO_2}} - P_{E_{CO_2}})/P_{A_{CO_2}}.$$

Normal values in young adults average 150 ml, or 2.2 ml/kg of body weight, which is in good agreement with anatomic measurements. Alveolar ventilation can be determined with a similar equation:

$$\dot{V}_A = \dot{V}_E F_{E_{CO_2}}/F_{A_{CO_2}}.$$

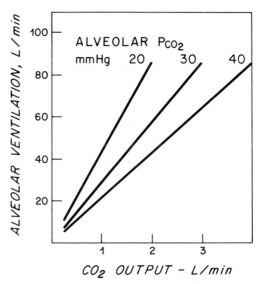

Fig. 21. For a given value of alveolar P_{CO_2} the alveolar ventilation is proportional to CO_2 output.

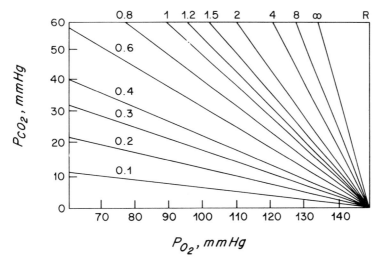

Fig. 22. P_{O_2}–P_{CO_2} diagram with a family of R lines showing how the respiratory exchange ratio is related to alveolar P_{O_2} and P_{CO_2}. (Reproduced by permission from Rahn H, Fenn WO: A Graphical Analysis of the Respiratory Gas Exchange: The O_2–CO_2 Diagram. Washington, American Physiological Society, 1955.)

Normal resting values range from 4 to 8 l/min, depending on metabolic rate and therefore on body size.

Composition of Alveolar Gas

The composition of alveolar gas differs from that of inspired air because CO_2 is exchanged for O_2. If the exchange is one-to-one, CO_2 replaces O_2 without change in the common volume or pressure of the two gases; the sum of alveolar P_{O_2} and P_{CO_2} is then equal to inspired P_{O_2}, which is known. Then a measurement of alveolar P_{CO_2} is sufficient to calculate alveolar P_{O_2}. For example, at sea level P_{O_2} in inspired air at 37°C equals 149 mm Hg; if the respiratory exchange ratio is 1 and alveolar P_{CO_2} is 40 mm Hg, then alveolar P_{O_2} is given by the difference 149 − 40 = 109 mm Hg.

If the respiratory exchange ratio is less than 1, the sum of alveolar P_{O_2} and P_{CO_2} is smaller than inspired P_{O_2}. A good approximation of alveolar P_{O_2} is then given by the equation $P_{A_{O_2}} = P_{I_{O_2}} - (P_{A_{CO_2}}/R)$. At sea level with a normal respiratory exchange ratio of 0.84 and a normal P_{CO_2}, this equation yields $P_{A_{O_2}} = 150 - (40/0.84) = 102$ mm Hg. The interdependence between the inspired P_{O_2}, the alveolar P_{O_2} and P_{CO_2}, and the respiratory exchange ratio is illustrated by the O_2–CO_2 diagram (Fig. 22), which predicts the effect of a change in any of these variables upon the composition of alveolar gas.

Oxygen uptake and CO_2 output and the respiratory exchange ratio depend on alveolar ventilation and perfusion and therefore may vary widely among individual alveoli. Where ventilation is high relatively to perfusion, P_{CO_2} falls and CO_2 output increases as more CO_2 is extracted from each unit of blood flow; the local P_{O_2} rises.

However, once hemoglobin is saturated the O_2 uptake per unit of blood flow reaches a maximum, so that the total uptake is determined by blood flow and is relatively independent of ventilation. Thus gas exchange in the presence of a high ventilation/perfusion ratio is characterized by a CO_2 output greater than O_2 uptake and a respiratory exchange ratio greater than 1, with a low P_{CO_2} and a high P_{O_2}. Where ventilation is low relatively to perfusion, P_{CO_2} rises only slightly because its maximal value is the P_{CO_2} of mixed venous blood, normally 45–48 mm Hg; but P_{O_2} falls rapidly. Because the O_2 and CO_2 dissociation curves of blood are different, local hypoventilation reduces CO_2 output more than O_2 uptake and the local respiratory exchange ratio is diminished.

For any value of the ventilation/perfusion ratio the composition of alveolar air can be calculated if the blood O_2 and CO_2 dissociation curves and the mixed venous blood gases are known. The possible alveolar air compositions range from that of inspired air where blood flow is nil to mixed venous P_{O_2} and P_{CO_2}, where ventilation is nil. A spectrum between these extremes is defined by one curve on the O_2–CO_2 diagram (Fig. 23), which represents the locus of possible respiratory exchange ratios as determined by varying ventilation/perfusion ratios.

In normal lungs in the erect position, apical alveoli may receive three times more ventilation than perfusion; if so, their P_{O_2} is 132 mm Hg, their P_{CO_2} 28 mm Hg, and exchange ratio 2.0 (Fig. 23). Halfway up the lungs ventilation and perfusion are nearly equal; P_{O_2} is 102 mm Hg, P_{CO_2} is 40 mm Hg, and the exchange ratio is 0.85. At the base of the lungs the ventilation/perfusion ratio is

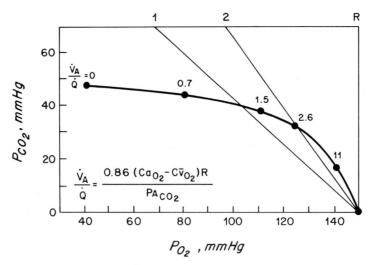

Fig. 23. P_{O_2}–P_{CO_2} diagram with the $\dot{V}/\dot{Q}$ curve, locus of all possible alveolar P_{O_2} and P_{CO_2}, for inspired air at sea level and normal mixed venous gas tensions. Two R lines are also indicated. (Reproduced by permission from Rahn H, Fenn WO: A Graphical Analysis of the Respiratory Gas Exchange: The O_2–CO_2 Diagram. Washington, American Physiological Society, 1955.)

low; where it reaches 0.63, P_{O_2} is 89 mm Hg, P_{CO_2} is 42 mm Hg, and the exchange ratio is 0.65 (Fig. 23). Thus mechanical factors responsible for the normal vertical gradients of ventilation and perfusion ultimately affect regional gas exchange; the result is a vertical gradient of alveolar P_{O_2} and P_{CO_2}.

In diseased lungs extreme variations in local ventilation and perfusion are caused by local changes in airways, alveolar walls, and vessels. Consequently the ventilation/perfusion ratio of individual alveoli may vary from zero where there is no ventilation to infinity where there is no blood flow. Complex methods have been developed to determine the statistics of gas composition in the individual alveoli of diseased lungs. A simplified approach consists of assessing the end result of uneven distribution of ventilation/perfusion ratios in terms of physiologic dead space and alveolar–arterial P_{O_2} difference.

Physiologic Dead Space

In all circumstances P_{CO_2} is the same in blood leaving an alveolus as that in the alveolar air. Therefore the same P_{CO_2} ought to be found in end-tidal air as in arterial blood, provided each alveolus contributes equal fractions of total ventilation and blood flow; this condition, however, is met only when the distribution of ventilation/perfusion ratios is uniform. Such is the case in healthy young persons studied in the supine position, when the effect of gravity upon distribution is small and is similar for ventilation and perfusion. Then the end-tidal and arterial P_{CO_2} are equal.

Whenever the distributions of ventilation and perfusion differ markedly, the contributions of individual alveoli to the end-tidal air and to the arterial blood are different. Overventilated alveoli, which have a low P_{CO_2}, contribute a greater share to expired air than to arterial blood. Underventilated alveoli, which have a low P_{CO_2}, contribute a greater share to expired air than to arterial blood. Underventilated alveoli, which have a slightly increased P_{CO_2} (less than or equal to mixed venous P_{CO_2}), contribute a smaller share to end-tidal air than to arterial blood. Thus the end-tidal air represents a mixed air sample weighted in favor of overventilated alveoli and arterial blood represents a mixed blood sample weighted in favor of underventilated alveoli. The result is a measurable difference between arterial and mean alveolar P_{CO_2}. Arterial P_{CO_2} remains normal only if the overall ventilation is increased to a value appreciably higher than would be needed with an even distribution (Fig. 24). The difference between the alveolar ventilations required for the same CO_2 output in ideal lungs with homogenous distribution and in actual lungs with uneven distribution is considered wasted ventilation, just as the ventilation of the anatomic dead space is wasted with respect to gas exchange. The term alveolar dead space is also used with the same analogy in mind.

In the presence of uneven distribution it is customary to include alveolar dead space in the estimate of physiologic dead space. This is done by assuming that expired air is a mixture of dead space ventilation and "ideal" alveolar ventilation, the latter characterized by a P_{CO_2} equal to arterial P_{CO_2}. Physiologic dead space is then calculated with a modified Bohr equation in which arterial P_{CO_2} is substituted for alveolar P_{CO_2}:

$$V_D = V_T(P_{a_{CO_2}} - P_{E_{CO_2}})/P_{a_{CO_2}}$$

In clinical settings the term physiologic dead space is used in reference to the value calculated with the arterial rather than the alveolar P_{CO_2}. The ratio of physiologic dead space to tidal volume, or V_D/V_T ratio, is often preferred to assess the impaired efficiency of CO_2

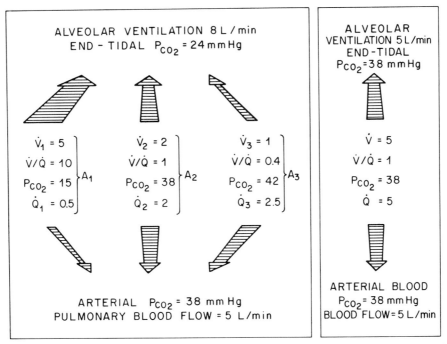

Fig. 24. Uneven distribution of ventilation/perfusion ratios generates a significant arterial–alveolar P_{CO_2} difference and requires increased alveolar ventilation (left). Compare with the efficiency of gas exchange in the presence of an even distribution of ventilation/perfusion ratios (right).

elimination; it is usually expressed as a percentage, which in normal persons at rest ranges from 20 percent to 35 percent, but rises in the presence of maldistribution. As V_D/V_T increases, P_{CO_2} can be maintained at a normal level only at the price of increasing tidal ventilation. Values in excess of 70 percent are usually associated with CO_2 retention, illustrating once more the impossibility of maintaining a gross elevation of tidal ventilation in a chronic fashion.

Alveolar–Arterial P_{O_2} Difference

Arterial P_{O_2} is always lower than alveolar P_{O_2}. For normal adults breathing air at sea level this alveolar–arterial P_{O_2} difference averages 10–15 mm Hg, with an upper limit of normal of 25 mm Hg. It arises from two normal mechanisms. First, a small fraction of cardiac output (normally less than 5 percent) bypasses the alveoli. Blood coming through this anatomic shunt has a gaseous composition characteristic of systemic venous blood and reaches the left ventricle from bronchial veins draining into pulmonary veins and from Thebesian veins draining directly into the ventricle. Second, a sizable fraction of pulmonary venous blood comes from areas of low ventilation/perfusion ratios and shows a deficit in O_2 content, which because of the shape of the hemoglobin O_2 dissociation curve cannot be compensated by subsequent mixing with blood coming from areas of high ventilation/perfusion ratios. By analogy with the anatomic shunt, this distribution component of the alveolar–arterial P_{O_2} difference is sometimes referred to as physiologic shunt.

The anatomic component of the alveolar–arterial

P_{O_2} difference increases whenever disease causes hypertrophy of bronchial vessels (as observed in chronic bronchitis, bronchiectasis and cystic fibrosis) or the perfusion of nonventilated areas in the lungs (as with lobar pneumonia or a pulmonary arteriovenous fistula). The distribution component increases with all lung and airway diseases, as alveolar compliance, airway resistance, and vascular resistance are diversely affected in individual lobules. In addition, diseases that damage the interstitial or vascular structures of the lungs may prevent complete diffusion equilibrium of capillary blood with alveolar air, which adds a diffusion component to the alveolar–arterial P_{O_2} difference. Specific tests of varying complexity have been devised to distinguish between these different physiologic mechanisms. But the alveolar–arterial P_{O_2} difference as measured during air breathing still gives the best estimate of overall performance of the lungs with respect to O_2 transfer.

In practice the determination requires a measurement of arterial P_{O_2} and an estimate of alveolar P_{O_2}, the latter being most often calculated with the alveolar air equation in which arterial P_{CO_2} is substituted for alveolar P_{CO_2}. It is assumed that the effect of anatomic shunt on arterial P_{CO_2} is negligible, a valid assumption at rest and in the presence of normal cardiac output when the normal arteriovenous P_{CO_2} difference is in the range of 4 to 8 mm Hg. With a representative value of 6 mm Hg for the arteriovenous P_{CO_2} difference the rise in arterial P_{CO_2} caused by a 10 percent shunt (shunt fraction = 0.10) is only $6 \times 0.10 = 0.6$ mm Hg. When the arterial P_{CO_2} is used in the alveolar air equation, the same error in absolute value is made on the calculated alveolar P_{O_2}, which in most instances represents less than 1 percent in relative value. In some laboratories the directly measured end-tidal P_{O_2} is used to assess the alveolar–arterial O_2 difference.

The contributions of shunt, maldistribution, and diffusion impairment to the alveolar–arterial P_{O_2} difference are diversely affected by varying the inspired P_{O_2}. If the inspired P_{O_2} is lowered, either by breathing a low O_2 concentration at sea level or by exposure to high altitude, the contributions of maldistributions and shunt become small as compared to that of diffuse limitation. If the inspired P_{O_2} is raised by breathing a high O_2 concentration at sea level or by exposure to hyperbaric environment, diffusion is not a limiting factor any more, and the contribution of maldistribution is reduced. During pure O_2 breathing the alveolar–arterial P_{O_2} difference is determined by shunt alone.

DIFFUSION

The alveoli are small diffusion chambers with one face open for gas exchange with air from the alveolar ducts and the remaining wall surface occupied by alveolar epithelium and capillaries for gas exchange with blood. Diffusion is an important factor for gas exchange at the alveolar–ductal interface. It is the only mechanism effective at the alveolar–capillary interface.

Diffusion within the Gas Phase

Alveolar ventilation is defined as the volume of inspired air that is exchanged for alveolar air per unit of time. According to this definition the lungs are considered as a black box whose input and output can be directly measured in terms of bulk flow and gas composition. Similarly individual pulmonary lobules, each connected to the common airway by a terminal bronchiole, have an input and an output. Here, however, regional inhomogeneity must be taken into account. Because of vertical gradients of pleural pressure and regional compliance, basal lobules receive about twice as much ventilation as apical lobules. It is now recognized that inhomogeneity also prevails within individual lobules because of local differences in diffusive advantage. These differences are exemplified by comparing the conditions of gas exchange for the alveoli scattered in the wall of respiratory bronchioles, for those lining the first and second order ducts, and for the end alveoli of the alveolar sacs.

Respiratory bronchioles are part of the conducting system of the lungs. Inspired air flows through these units, first bringing dead-space gas that must be re-inhaled at the beginning of inspiration and then fresh inspired air that is continually renewed until the end of inspiration. Thus as inspiration proceeds, the alveoli of the respiratory bronchioles receive most of their ventilation as fresh air. There the role of diffusion is limited to mixing the inspired aliquot with the preexisting alveolar gas, which is achieved instantaneously because of the small dimensions of the alveoli and the stirring effect of volume change.

Not all alveoli receive a share of fresh inspired air in this fashion. Along the first- and second-order ducts alveoli may or may not receive an aliquot toward the end of inspiration, depending on the size of the tidal volume. A 1-liter inspiration displaces air from all bronchi and from the respiratory bronchioles and reaches halfway down the first-order ducts. A 2-liter inspiration, which reaches the second-order ducts, still leaves two-thirds of all alveoli dependent on diffusion for gas exchange.

Diffusion within the gas phase is helped by the short axial distances along the terminal units of the lungs and by their large total cross-sectional area, which leads to low velocity of bulk motion. In addition, cardiac activity and tidal breathing itself result in an appreciable stirring effect. Thus diffusion exchange on the whole is quite effective, and considerable understanding of alveolar gas exchange can be reached with the simplifying assumption that diffusion mixing within the lobule is complete, at least for normal lungs and during quiet breathing. It is now appreciated, however, that intralobular mixing is dependent upon axial gradients of P_{O_2} and P_{CO_2}. In each lobule the proximal alveoli have higher P_{O_2} and lower P_{CO_2} than distal alveoli, a type of uneven distribution that is referred to as stratified inequality.

The magnitude of stratified gradients of alveolar gas composition is not known, and only indirect evidence of their existence has been secured as yet. The study of geometric models with dimensions comparable to those of pulmonary lobules yields numerical solutions of the diffusion equation. Results indicate that 1 sec after an interface between fresh inspired air and alveolar air has been established in the first- or second-order ducts, the axial gradients of partial pressures will still represent 5–15 percent of the initial diffusion gradients. These values are likely to be underestimated because they overlook the partitioning of lobular volume into ducts and alveoli and because they assume an end-inspiratory pause that is not observed in normal breathing.

Breath-holding at the end of inspiration is known to alter the shape of the alveolar plateau of gas concentration as recorded during the following expiration. The single-breath O_2 test permits the establishment of an O_2–N_2 interface in the pulmonary lobule and shows that the expired N_2 concentration decreases when a breath-holding period of increasing duration takes place between inspiration and expiration. Most of the change occurs from 0 to 5 sec of breath-holding, and a residual slope is constantly observed that is thought to reflect regional inhomogeneity, whether due to gravity or lung disease. Because O_2 and N_2 concentrations in the lungs are affected by respiratory gas exchange, a better estimate of diffusion mixing within the gas phase can be achieved with the use of an insoluble marker gas, such as neon or argon, or a pair of markers with widely different diffusion constants, such as He and SF_6; the concentration ratio of these two gases in expired air

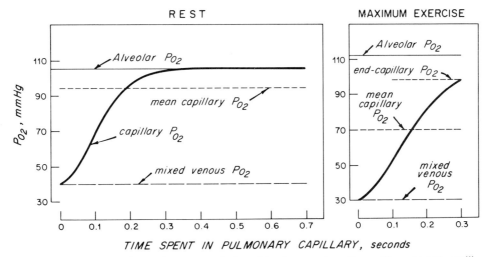

Fig. 25. Capillary blood P_{O_2} rises progressively as blood passes along the capillary. At rest, equilibration within 0.3 sec or half of the contact time. During heavy exercise the contact time is shortened, and O_2 uptake is markedly increased: capillary blood P_{O_2} fails to reach complete equilibration. Note, however, that the mean alveolar–capillary P_{O_2} difference is larger at exercise than at rest.

ought to vary only as a result of different diffusion pathways in the terminal lung units. This and similar tests permit the demonstration of stratified inhomogeneity in normal lungs and of its worsening in diseased lungs, when the structure of the terminal lung units is distorted as in emphysema.

The consequences of stratified inequality with respect to respiratory gas exchange in the lungs are similar to those of regional inequality, namely increased physiologic dead space and alveolar–arterial P_{O_2} difference. However, the quantitative partitioning of distribution inequality into its regional and stratified components has not yet been achieved.

Pulmonary Diffusing Capacity

Alveolar–capillary gas exchange is driven by differences in partial pressures between air and blood and is dependent on the diffusion coefficient of the alveolar membrane for O_2 or CO_2, itself proportional to the solubility of each gas in tissues. The driving pressure gradient is several times greater for O_2 than for CO_2, although the difference varies from rest to exercise and with varying inspired O_2 tension. But the solubility of CO_2 in tissues is 20 times greater than that of O_2. The balance is in favor of CO_2, so that diffusion limitation, when present, affects the transfer of O_2 earlier and more severely than that of CO_2. Accordingly measurements of pulmonary diffusing capacity are aimed at assessing the characteristics of the air–blood barrier with respect to O_2 transfer.

Oxygen uptake by blood in the alveolar wall capillaries is proportional to the P_{O_2} difference between alveolar air and capillary blood and to the surface area of the alveolar membrane available for gas exchange (A) and inversely proportional to the thickness of the membrane (X). These relationships are expressed by the following equation, derived from Fick's first law of diffusion: $V_{O_2} = d(A/X)(P_{A_{O_2}} - P_{c_{O_2}})$, where d is the diffusion coefficient of the alveolar membrane for O_2. However, the surface area and thickness of the membrane are inaccessible to measurement. To obviate this difficulty, the diffusing capacity of the lung is defined as $d(A/X)$ and is therefore taken as equal to the ratio of gas transfer to pressure gradient: $D_L = V_{O_2}/(P_{A_{O_2}} - P_{c_{O_2}})$. The O_2 uptake is easily calculated from analyses of inspired and expired air and the measurement of ventilation. But the partial pressure of O_2 in alveolar air varies in space and time because of regional and stratified inequality of ventilation/perfusion ratios and because of the tidal character of ventilation whereby alveolar P_{O_2} is highest at the end of inspiration and lowest at the end of expiration. P_{O_2} in the blood also varies during capillary transit and as a reflection of local alveolar air composition. Therefore the pulmonary diffusing capacity is estimated as a function of mean alveolar O_2 tension $P_{\bar{A}_{O_2}}$ and mean O_2 tension in the pulmonary capillary blood $P_{\bar{c}_{O_2}}$, so that the exact equation is written $D_{L_{O_2}} = \dot{V}_{O_2}/(P_{\bar{A}_{O_2}} - P_{\bar{c}_{O_2}})$. The mean alveolar P_{O_2} can be readily calculated with the alveolar air equation or measured in a sample of end-tidal air; but the mean capillary P_{O_2} can be estimated only by a complex procedure.

Blood entering the capillaries of the lungs has a uniform composition—that of mixed venous blood, which at rest is normally characterized by a P_{O_2} near 40 mm Hg and O_2 saturation near 75 percent. In the capillaries the blood is exposed to alveolar air with a mean P_{O_2} of 100 mm Hg and O_2 transfer begins at a rapid instantaneous rate. The O_2 content of blood begins to rise, as well as its O_2 tension. The alveolar–capillary gradient decreases and the instantaneous rate of O_2 transfer decreases accordingly. The O_2 tension and saturation in the blood progressing along the capillaries continue to rise, but at a slower rate. If O_2 content and P_{O_2} were mutually

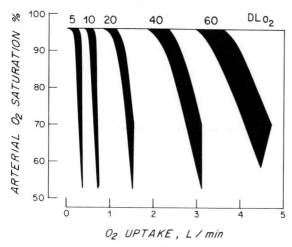

Fig. 26. Diffusing capacity as a factor limiting exercise tolerance at sea level, in the presence of lung disease. For each value of the O_2 diffusing capacity there is a narrow range of O_2 uptake that causes hypoxemia because of diffusion limitation. (Reproduced by permission of RH Shepard and the American Physiological Society from J Appl Physiol 1958.)

proportional, the rate of change of blood P_{O_2} during the capillary transit time should be exponential. The actual function relating capillary blood P_{O_2} to transit time is significantly different from an exponential and is actually sigmoid in shape because of the nonlinearity of the hemoglobin dissociation curve (Fig. 25).

The average capillary transit time in normal persons at rest is close to 0.7 sec, about twice the time needed for the blood to reach equilibrium and alveolar P_{O_2} during air breathing at sea level. It follows that the mean capillary P_{O_2} is very close to the alveolar P_{O_2} and that even a small error on the capillary P_{O_2} results in a large error on the mean alveolar–capillary P_{O_2} gradient and therefore on the estimate of the diffusing capacity. More favorable conditions for the determination of alveolar–capillary gradient and diffusing capacity are created by alveolar hypoxia caused either by breathing air at high altitude or by breathing a low O_2 concentration at sea level. With hypoxia the alveolar P_{O_2} falls faster than the mixed venous P_{O_2}. Therefore the initial alveolar capillary P_{O_2} gradient is small, O_2 transfer proceeds at slower rates from beginning to end of the capillaries, and all the capillary transit time is used for O_2 transfer. Nevertheless with marked alveolar hypoxia (12–14 percent O_2 inspired at sea level) the capillary blood P_{O_2} fails to reach an equilibrium with alveolar air and a significant alveolar–capillary P_{O_2} difference persists at the venous end of the capillaries, which is the hallmark of diffusion limitation to gas exchange (Fig. 26). In these conditions the precise course of the P_{O_2} transit-time relationship is less critical and with suitable approximations the function can be numerically integrated and its mean value determined by the trial-and-error method of Riley and

Cournand. Normal values for the mean alveolar–capillary gradient, for air breathing at sea level, are of the order of 6–10 mm Hg and for O_2 diffusing capacity 25–40 ml/min/mm Hg at rest.

Direct determination of the O_2 diffusing capacity finds few applications in clinical physiology because of the complexity of the method and the uncertain validity of some necessary simplifying hypotheses, particularly in the presence of lung disease. Instead the pulmonary diffusing capacity is usually determined with the use of a marker gas, carbon monoxide.

Carbon Monoxide Diffusing Capacity

The solubility of CO in tissues is comparable to that of O_2 and CO also combines with hemoglobin. In the range of P_{CO} values used for testing purposes the carboxy–hemoglobin dissociation curve is extremely steep, so that appreciable amounts of CO are taken up with very little change in blood P_{CO}; alveolar air and capillary blood P_{CO} do not reach equilibrium during a single capillary passage. Therefore CO uptake is limited by the rapidity with which CO passes across the alveolar membrane, i.e., by the diffusing capacity of the lungs for CO. Furthermore, because the carboxy–hemoglobin dissociation curve is steep and because presumably there is no CO in blood before the test, the capillary P_{CO} remains very small and in first approximation can be taken as negligible. Accordingly the diffusing capacity of the lungs is calculated as the ratio of CO uptake to alveolar CO tension: $D_{L_{co}} = \dot{V}_{CO}/P_{A_{co}}$.

Measurements are made with any one of three methods. The steady-state diffusing capacity is determined during tidal breathing with 0.1 percent CO in inspired air for several minutes; mean alveolar P_{CO}, which ranges from 0.1 to 0.8 mm Hg, is calculated with a variant of the alveolar air equation or is measured in a sample of end-tidal air. Normal values for the steady-state CO diffusing capacity range from 20 to 30 ml/min/mm Hg. The single-breath diffusing capacity is calculated from the rate of disappearance of CO from alveolar air after inhalation of one breath of 0.3 percent to 0.5 percent CO in air. The normal values with this method range from 30 to 50 ml/min per mm Hg. The rebreathing diffusing capacity is derived from the rate of disappearance of CO from a closed system formed by the lungs and a rebreathing bag; the normal values are similar to that of the steady-state method. These tests are most markedly affected in the presence of interstitial lung disease, such as sarcoidosis, chronic interstitial pneumonitis, and the pneumoconioses. Lowest values in ambulatory patients reach 2–5 ml/min/mm Hg for either method.

Diffusing Capacity of Alveolar Membrane

Whereas measurements of the pulmonary diffusing capacity for CO are clinically useful, the analysis of physiologic events during the determination reveals that several of the underlying assumptions are not strictly valid. Factors that are not included in the definition of the pulmonary diffusing capacity and should not affect its measurement actually cause large changes in the results. Thus the measured CO diffusing capacity decreases by more than 50 percent when capillary blood P_{O_2} is raised by increasing alveolar P_{O_2} from 100 mm Hg (room air breathing) to 600 mm Hg (pure O_2 breathing). This observation establishes the fact that despite the great affinity of hemoglobin for CO chemical competition for hemoglobin between O_2 and CO affects the uptake of CO by capillary blood in the presence of low P_{CO}. Furthermore the measured diffusing capacity is dependent upon chemical factors, in this instance the mass-action law as applied to the reaction: $Hb + CO \rightarrow HbCO$. In this reaction the velocity of combination of CO with hemoglobin depends on the concentration of dissolved CO (equal to $\alpha_{CO} P_{c_{CO}}$, with α_{CO} the solubility coefficient of CO in blood), the concentration of dissolved O_2 (equal to $\alpha_{O_2} P_{c_{O_2}}$, with α_{O_2} the solubility coefficient of O_2 in blood) and the concentration of hemoglobin. All three terms appear in the equation giving the reaction velocity: $v = m(\alpha_{CO} P_{cCO}/\alpha_{O_2} P_{c_{O_2}})Hb$, where m is a parameter whose values are determined by the blood O_2 saturation. This expression simplifies into $v = \theta_{CO} P_{c_{CO}}$, where θ_{CO} is a nonlinear function of hemoglobin concentration and P_{O_2} in the capillary blood. The reciprocal of θ_{CO}, however, proves to be a linear function of P_{O_2}, approximated by the expression $1/\theta_{CO} = 0.73 + 0.0053(P_{A_{O_2}} - 5)(15/Hb) = 0.73 + 5.3 \ 10^{-3}(15/Hb) \cdot (P_{A_{O_2}} - 5)$, where 15 g/100 ml stands for the normal blood hemoglobin concentration and 5 mm Hg for the mean alveolar–capillary P_{O_2} difference (the latter assumption in this instance is not critical); 0.73 and 5.8×10^{-3} are experimental constants.

For the combination of CO with hemoglobin to proceed, $P_{c_{CO}}$ must be significantly different from zero. Indeed, the rising blood P_{CO} during CO transfer limits the diffusion of the gas across the alveolar membrane until an equilibrium is reached whereby CO transfer from alveolar air to plasma equals CO transfer from plasma to hemoglobin. Transfer across the membrane is given by the product of the diffusing capacity of the membrane for CO ($D_{M_{CO}}$) and the CO pressure difference between alveolar air and capillary blood: $\dot{V}_{CO} = D_{M_{CO}}(P_{A_{CO}} - P_{c_{CO}})$. Transfer within the capillary blood (from simple solution in plasma to chemical binding with hemoglobin inside the red blood cell) is given by the product of the reaction velocity ($\theta_{CO} P_{c_{CO}}$) and total capillary blood volume (V_c) available for the reaction: $\dot{V}_{CO} = P_{c_{CO}} \theta_{CO} V_c$. This equation yields the value $P_{c_{CO}} = \dot{V}_{CO}/(\theta_{CO} V_c)$, to be substituted into the membrane transfer equation: $\dot{V}_{CO} = D_{M_{CO}}\{P_{A_{CO}} - [\dot{V}_{CO}/(\theta_{CO} V_c)]\}$. Dividing both sides of this equation by $\dot{V}_{CO}$ and $D_{M_{CO}}$ yields $1/D_{M_{CO}} = (P_{A_{CO}}/\dot{V}_{CO}) - (1/\theta_{CO} V_c)$. The term $P_{A_{CO}}/\dot{V}_{CO}$ can be identified as the reciprocal of the conventional diffusing capacity, so that the equation is then rewritten $1/D_{L_{CO}} = 1/D_{M_{CO}} + (1/\theta_{CO} V_c)$.

Thus the analysis of CO transfer yields evidence

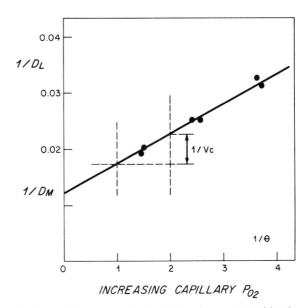

Fig. 27. Diffusing capacity for CO has been measured by the single-breath method at varying alveolar and mean capillary blood P_{O_2}. The reciprocal of D_L is then plotted against $1/\theta$ (see text for definition and unit). On the resulting regression line, the Y intercept equals the reciprocal of the diffusing capacity of the membrane D_M and the slope equals the reciprocal of the capillary blood volume V_c.

that the diffusing capacity of the alveolar membrane D_M is significantly different from the conventional diffusing capacity of the lungs D_L. Its determination requires that the conventional measurement be repeated several times at varying O_2 tensions. Then the linear relationship between the reciprocal of the diffusing capacity and the reciprocal of θ_{CO} can be identified by calculating a least-square regression equation and plotting the data to check the goodness of fit (Fig. 27). The y intercept of the regression line is equal to the reciprocal of the diffusing capacity of the membrane for CO, and the slope is equal to the reciprocal of the capillary blood volume. Normal results show that the diffusing capacity of the membrane for CO is twice as great as the conventional diffusing capacity, ranging from 60 to 100 ml/ min per mm Hg for the steady-state or rebreathing techniques. The method also provides a means for in vivo determination of the capillary blood volume, with results ranging normally from 50 to 90 ml at rest. The average value of 70 ml for the capillary blood volume, divided by a normal value for cardiac output of 6 l/min or 100 ml/ sec, gives the normal mean capillary transit time $t = 70/100 = 0.7$ sec, as previously mentioned.

These data are directly applicable to the transfer of O_2, for which one can write: $1/D_{L_{O_2}} = (1/D_{M_{O_2}}) + [1/\theta_{O_2} V_c]$. The blood volume evidently is unchanged. The diffusing capacity of the membrane for O_2 is related to that for CO by the ratio of the square roots of CO and O_2 molecular weights (Graham's law): $D_{M_{O_2}} = (32/28)D_{M_{CO}} = 1.23 \ D_{M_{CO}}$. In vitro measurements of

θ_{O_2} have shown this parameter to vary from 2.8 ml/min per mm Hg and ml of blood at a P_{O_2} of 40 mm Hg or less to 0.5 ml/min per mm Hg and ml of blood at a P_{O_2} of 98 mm Hg. However, the general equation cannot be solved for O_2 transfer in the same fashion as for CO transfer, because the conventional O_2 diffusing capacity is unaffected by altering alveolar air composition within a safe range.

The CO method and the trial-and-error O_2 method are in general agreement in showing that normally the diffusing capacity of the alveolar membrane for O_2 is greater and the capillary transit time longer than needed for gas exchange at rest during air breathing at sea level. Otherwise various discrepancies between the two methods have been identified by detailed analysis of individual examples, which is to be expected in view of the many simplifying assumptions underlying both methods.

Diffusing Capacity and Hypoxemia

The conventional CO diffusing capacity is a sensitive and reliable index for the evaluation of pulmonary gas exchange in interstitial lung diseases. Early in the course of these diseases the diffusing capacity is often found to be significantly reduced (80 percent to 50 percent of predicted) when the resting arterial P_{O_2} is still in normal range. Such observations are consistent with the fact that normal diffusing capacity is greater than needed for gas exchange at rest at sea level. In instances when effective treatment is available, improvement of the diffusing capacity documents clinical progress and repeated measurements are helpful in following the course of the disease and in guiding therapy.

However, even when observed in the presence of moderately impaired diffusing capacity, resting hypoxemia is normally attributable to another mechanism, namely uneven distribution of ventilation/perfusion ratios because of associated airway disease or the uneven distribution of interstitial pathology. With advanced interstitial disease the diffusing capacity is low and hypoxemia is the rule. Even then the respective roles of diffusion impairment and maldistribution in causing the hypoxemia cannot be identified with certainty by a single measurement at rest.

Exercise tests are of the greatest value to evaluate diffusion impairment because exercise raises the demand on pulmonary gas exchange, shortens the capillary transit time and leaves maldistribution of ventilation/perfusion ratios unchanged or improved. In normal persons diffusion is not a limiting factor to gas exchange at sea level. With exercise cardiac output rises by a factor of 3 to 5 while diffusing capacity and capillary blood volume increase by a factor of 2 to 2.5. The capillary transit time is shortened to one-half or one-third of normal, which is still compatible with complete equilibration of blood P_{O_2} with alveolar P_{O_2}. In patients with interstitial lung disease, diffusing capacity and capillary blood volume show some rise with exercise, but more important they remain far below the normal range.

Capillary transit time, which was short but possibly adequate at rest, becomes insufficient for blood P_{O_2} to reach equilibration. Typically, a critical level of exercise can be identified at which arterial P_{O_2} falls precipitously. Beyond this point diffusion limitation is responsible for the hypoxemia.

REFERENCES

Avery ME, Said S: Surface phenomena in lungs in health and disease. Medicine 44:503–526, 1965

Blout SG Jr, Vogel JHK: Altitude and the pulmonary circulation. Adv Intern Med 13:11–32, 1967

Campbell EJM, Agostoni E, Newsom Davis J: The Respiratory Muscles: Mechanics and Neural Control. Baltimore, WB Saunders, 1970

Farhi LE: Ventilation–perfusion relationship and its role in alveolar gas exchange, in CG Caro (ed): Advances in Respiratory Physiology. Baltimore, Williams & Wilkins, 1966, pp 148–197

Fishman AP, Hecht H: The Pulmonary Circulation and Interstitial Space. Chicago, University of Chicago Press, 1969

Forster RE: Exchange of gases between alveolar air and pulmonary capillary blood: Pulmonary diffusing capacity. Physiol Rev 37:391, 1957

Harris P, Heath D: The Human Pulmonary Circulation. Edinburgh, Livingstone, 1962

Macklem PT: Airway obstruction and collateral ventilation. Physiol Rev 51:368, 1971

Mead J: Mechanical properties of the lungs. Physiol Rev 41: 281, 1961

Mead J, Turner JM, Macklem P, Little JB: Significance of the relationship between lung recoil and maximum expiratory flow. J Appl Physiol 22:95, 1967

West JB: Causes of carbon dioxide retention in lung disease. N Engl J Med 284:1232–1236, 1971

OXYGEN AND CARBON DIOXIDE TRANSPORT

Homayoun Kazemi

OXYGEN TRANSPORT

Partial Pressure of O_2 in Air and Blood

Oxygen is transferred from the atmosphere to the alveolar air where it crosses the alveolar–capillary membrane into blood, reacts with hemoglobin there, is carried to the tissues by blood flow, dissociates from hemoglobin, crosses the tissue membranes, and is utilized within the cells. In this process oxygen must diffuse across a number of membranes. To cross a membrane a pressure gradient is required, i.e., the partial pressure of O_2 has to be higher on one side than on the other for oxygen to cross the membrane.

At sea level the partial pressure of oxygen in the inspired air $P_{I_{O_2}}$ is 149 mm Hg. $P_{I_{O_2}}$ = atmospheric pressure (760) minus partial pressure of water vapor at 37°C (47) times oxygen content of ambient air (20.9 percent). This is the head of pressure available to the system as air enters the nasopharynx. The partial pressure of O_2 in the alveolar air, $P_{A_{O_2}}$, is close to 105 mm Hg. There is a

PARTIAL PRESSURE OF OXYGEN
(Ambient air at 1 atmosphere)

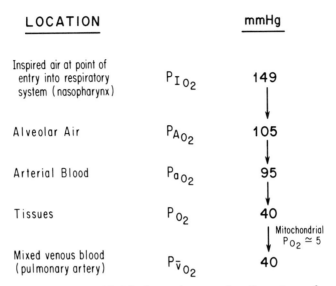

Fig. 1. Partial pressure of oxygen (P_{O_2}) in the respiratory and cardiac systems—from the nasopharynx to the mixed venous blood.

large pressure gradient (65 mm Hg) for transfer of O_2 from alveolar air to the mixed venous blood returning to the lungs at a P_{O_2} of about 40 mm Hg (Fig. 1). The arterial oxygen tension $P_{a_{O_2}}$ of 95 mm Hg is less than alveolar P_{O_2}, and this alveolar–arterial O_2 gradient (A–aD_{O_2}) is due to the normally occurring ventilation/perfusion inequality and venous admixture. The $P_{a_{O_2}}$ is well above the mean tissue P_{O_2} of 40 mm Hg (Fig. 1), so that again a large O_2 gradient is available for transfer of oxygen from arterial blood into tissues. The mitochondrial P_{O_2} of about 5 mm Hg is much less than that in the mixed venous blood of 40 mm Hg; so a protective pressure gradient for O_2 is available to the mitochondria. The mixed venous blood returns to the pulmonary capillary bed at a P_{O_2} of 40 mm Hg, and rapid equilibration between oxygen in the alveolar air and pulmonary capillary blood takes place. On the average, with normal cardiac output, the red blood cell's transit time in the pulmonary capillary bed is 0.7 sec. Complete equilibration between alveolar P_{O_2} and pulmonary capillary blood P_{O_2} takes place in 0.2–0.3 sec, so that sufficient time is available for complete equilibration of oxygen between blood and air.

Oxygen Transport in Blood

Once oxygen crosses the alveolar–capillary membrane it is transported in blood in two forms, one as physically dissolved O_2 and the other in combination with hemoglobin. The quantity of oxygen carried in both forms depends on the partial pressure of oxygen. However, of the two forms by far the major quantity of O_2 is transported bound to hemoglobin.

Physically Dissolved Oxygen

Oxygen, like any gas, goes into physical solution in a liquid medium. The quantity that enters into solution depends on the partial pressure of the gas and its solubility coefficient α in that liquid. The oxygen solubility coefficient is relatively low in blood, 0.0031 cc/100 cc blood per millimeter of P_{O_2} at 38°C. Thus with a partial pressure of 95 mm Hg in the arterial blood, 95×0.0031 (or 0.29) cc of O_2 is carried per 100 cc of blood, a value that is also expressed as 0.29 volumes percent.

Oxygen Transport by Hemoglobin

Each hemoglobin molecule has four binding sites for oxygen, and when all four sites are bound to oxygen the hemoglobin molecule is fully saturated with O_2 and is termed oxyhemoglobin. Unsaturated hemoglobin is called reduced hemoglobin. When fully saturated with oxygen 1 g of hemoglobin combines with 1.34 cc of oxygen. The total amount of oxygen carried by blood, the oxygen content, depends primarily on two factors: (1) the quantity of hemoglobin and (2) the partial pressure of oxygen. If the hemoglobin content of blood is 15 g/100 ml and P_{O_2} is 100 mm Hg, so that hemoglobin is fully saturated, then the amount of oxygen carried by hemoglobin equals $15 \times 1.34 = 20.1$ cc/100 cc of blood or 20.1 volumes percent; at the same 0.31 volumes percent O_2 will be transported in dissolved form. If under the same conditions of oxygenation the hemoglobin is reduced to 10 g/100 ml, then oxygen carried by hemoglobin will be $10 \times 1.34 = 13.4$ cc/100 cc or 13.4 volumes percent and the dissolved O_2 will again be 0.31 volumes percent, indicating the significance of hemoglobin in O_2 transport. The oxygen content of normal blood with a hemoglobin of 15 g/100 ml as a function

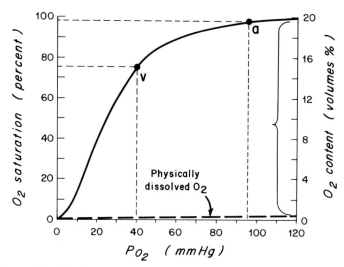

Fig. 2. Oxyhemoglobin dissociation curve. O_2 saturation is given by the vertical axis on the left and O_2 content by the vertical axis on the right. Note the S shape of the curve and the location of arterial point a on the flat part of the dissociation curve and the venous point v on the steep portion of the curve. The hemoglobin content of this blood is 15 g/100 ml, and the amount of O_2 carried in physical solution is much less than that bound to hemoglobin, as indicated by the bracket on the O_2 content axis.

of P_{O_2} is depicted in Fig. 2, where with the normal arterial P_{O_2} of 95 mm Hg 19 cc of O_2 are carried by hemoglobin and only 0.29 cc as physically dissolved O_2 per 100 cc of blood.

The degree of saturation of hemoglobin molecules is primarily a function of the partial pressure of oxygen, and the relationship is defined by the oxyhemoglobin dissociation curve (Fig. 2). It is an S-shaped curve with the top of the S being rather flat. At low P_{O_2} (less than 60 mm Hg) there are marked changes in saturation for small changes in P_{O_2}, whereas at P_{O_2} exceeding 70 mm Hg there are small changes in saturation for large changes in P_{O_2}. The S shape of the dissociation curve is of practical value in oxygen pickup by blood in the pulmonary capillary bed and in delivery of oxygen to the tissues. The normal arterial point a is on the flat part of the oxyhemoglobin dissociation curve (Fig. 2), and hemoglobin is well saturated with oxygen. The arterial P_{O_2} can fall by more than 20 mm Hg and hemoglobin will still be over 90 percent saturated and oxygen content will not be reduced significantly. This is a protective mechanism at the point of oxygen loading, since there can be significant falls in oxygen partial pressure without marked reductions in O_2 saturation or content of the arterial blood. On the other hand, at the point of oxygen unloading at the tissue level the P_{O_2} is low, as depicted by the normal mixed venous point v at 40 mm Hg on the oxyhemoglobin dissociation curve (Fig. 2). Since the venous point falls on the steep part of the dissociation curve, small falls in P_{O_2} will result in large reductions in O_2 saturation and content. This allows for ready release of oxygen from hemoglobin at the tissue level.

Shifts in Oxyhemoglobin Dissociation Curve

The relationship between hemoglobin, oxygen saturation, and oxygen partial pressure is defined by the oxyhemoglobin dissociation curve. However, the position of the dissociation curve is influenced by a number of factors, and shifts in the dissociation curve are of importance in delivery of oxygen to tissues. It has become the convention to study shifts in the oxyhemoglobin dissociation curve by measuring the P_{O_2} at which hemoglobin is 50 percent saturated, the so-called P_{50} value. For normal hemoglobin at normal pH of 7.40, normal P_{CO_2} of 40 mm Hg, and temperature, the P_{50} is 27 mm Hg (Fig. 3), i.e., hemoglobin is 50 percent saturated at a P_{O_2} of 27 mm Hg. If the dissociation curve is shifted to the right then the P_{50} value increases, and if it is shifted to the left the P_{50} value decreases.

Shifts to the right occur with increases in P_{CO_2} or falls in pH (Bohr effect), as well as elevation of temperature and increase in the erythrocyte concentration of 2,3-diphosphoglycerate (2,3-DPG) and other organic phosphates. A shift to the right of the oxyhemoglobin dissociation curve is helpful in the unloading of oxygen at the tissue level. Because the venous point is on the steep part of the dissociation curve, a shift to the right and elevation of P_{50} allows for more unloading of oxygen from hemoglobin for the same P_{O_2} (Fig. 3). Shifts to the left occur when P_{CO_2} is decreased and pH is increased (Bohr effect), or when temperature is reduced or the 2,3-DPG concentration in the erythrocyte falls. Shifts to the left impede oxygen unloading at the tissue level, because with the venous point being on the steep part of the oxyhemoglobin dissociation curve less oxy-

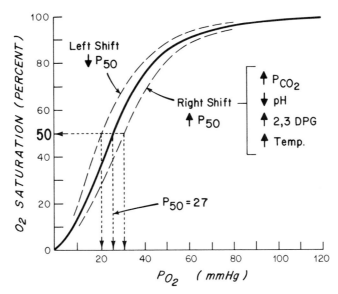

Fig. 3. Shifts in the oxyhemoglobin dissociation curve. The P_{50} value increases with a shift of the curve to the right and decreases with a shift to the left. Factors that lead to a shift to the right when changed in the opposite direction shift the curve to the left.

gen will be released from hemoglobin for the same P_{O_2} (Fig. 3).

Although shifts in the oxyhemoglobin dissociation curve can also influence oxygen loading in the pulmonary capillary bed, they are not quite as critical there because the final arterial point is on the flat part of the oxyhemoglobin dissociation curve, and changes of a few millimeters Hg in P_{O_2} do not have as significant an effect on O_2 saturation as they do at the venous point. If because of disease, however, the arterial oxygen tension falls below 60 mm Hg, so that the arterial point is then on the steep part of the dissociation curve, shifts in the oxyhemoglobin dissociation curve become quite significant; in that instance a shift to the right impedes oxygen uptake by hemoglobin and a shift to the left facilitates loading of oxygen onto the hemoglobin molecule.

Cardiac Output and O_2 Transport

Oxygen transport depends on (1) the arterial P_{O_2}, since that determines the oxygen saturation, (2) an adequate quantity of hemoglobin, since it is the primary carrier of oxygen, and (3) an adequate cardiac output. If cardiac output is diminished, tissue hypoxia may result. Oxygen consumption in the normal adult man at rest is about 250 cc/min. With a cardiac output of 5 l/min, each liter of blood will have to provide 250/5 = 50 cc of oxygen to the tissues. Since the arterial blood O_2 content is 20 volumes percent or 200 cc/liter, then the venous blood returning from the tissues will have 200 − 50 = 150 cc O_2 per liter or 15 volumes percent. Therefore, with the same arterial O_2 content, venous O_2 content and P_{O_2} will fall if cardiac output falls and will increase if cardiac output rises, provided oxygen consumption remains constant. Thus in assessing tissue

oxygenation, measurement of oxygen content and P_{O_2} in the mixed venous blood can be quite helpful in evaluating the adequacy of therapy in patients with cardiopulmonary disorders.

Hypoxemia and Its Causes

Hypoxemia is present when arterial P_{O_2} ($P_{a_{O_2}}$) is less than the expected normal. Under ideal circumstances of gas exchange the arterial P_{O_2} should equal the alveolar P_{O_2} ($P_{A_{O_2}}$). However, because of the normally occurring venous admixture and some ventilation/perfusion imbalance, the $P_{a_{O_2}}$ is 10–15 mm Hg less than $P_{A_{O_2}}$. The normal $P_{a_{O_2}}$ falls with age. In the young healthy man $P_{a_{O_2}}$ should be about 95 mm Hg or higher. The regression of $P_{a_{O_2}}$ with age is such that at age 80 a $P_{a_{O_2}}$ of 80 mm Hg is normal in the sitting position. This value may be 5 or 6 mm Hg lower in the supine position.

Hypoxemia occurs because of disease of the cardiorespiratory system or when there is reduction in the inspired P_{O_2}. Inspired P_{O_2} is diminished when oxygen content of inspired air is less than 20.9 percent (normal room air) or when there is a fall in atmospheric pressure as at altitude—both rather special circumstances. If the arterial P_{O_2} is less than the expected normal, with the subject breathing room air at 1 atm pressure, then hypoxemia is present because of one or more of the *three* primary causes of hypoxemia (Fig. 4). They are (1) alveolar hypoventilation, (2) increased venous admixture (right-to-left shunts), and (3) ventilation/perfusion imbalance. Diffusion impairment could also be included in this list, but it is best to consider it as a subgroup of ventilation/perfusion imbalance.

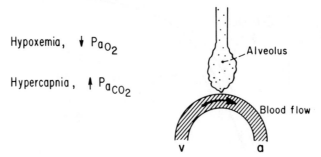

(1) ALVEOLAR HYPOVENTILATION

Hypoxemia, ↓ Pa_{O_2}

Hypercapnia, ↑ Pa_{CO_2}

Alveolus

Blood flow

v   a

(2) VENOUS ADMIXTURE
(Right-to-left shunt)

Hypoxemia, ↓ Pa_{O_2}

Alveolus

Pulmonary capillary blood flow

Shunt flow

v   a

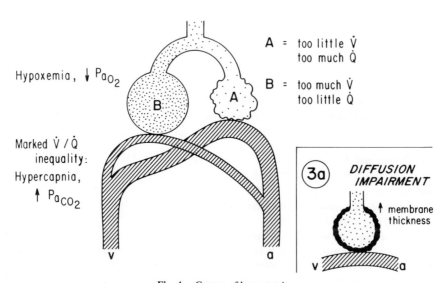

(3) VENTILATION/PERFUSION IMBALANCE
($\dot{V}/\dot{Q}$ inequality)

Hypoxemia, ↓ Pa_{O_2}

Marked $\dot{V}/\dot{Q}$ inequality:
Hypercapnia,
↑ Pa_{CO_2}

A = too little $\dot{V}$
too much $\dot{Q}$

B = too much $\dot{V}$
too little $\dot{Q}$

v   a

(3a) DIFFUSION IMPAIRMENT

↑ membrane thickness

v   a

Fig. 4. Causes of hypoxemia.

Alveolar hypoventilation. Alveolar ventilation is inversely proportional to $P_{a_{CO_2}}$ (see section on CO_2 transport). Alveolar hypoventilation is present when $P_{a_{CO_2}}$ is elevated and alveolar hyperventilation is present when $P_{a_{CO_2}}$ is diminished. Therefore, for hypoxemia to be caused by alveolar hypoventilation there must be elevation of arterial P_{CO_2}. If $P_{a_{CO_2}}$ is normal (38–42 mm Hg) then alveolar ventilation is normal and hypoxemia cannot be attributed to it.

Alveolar hypoventilation can occur because of primary disease of the lungs and because of muscle, neuromuscular, or central nervous system disorders, as well as with administration of depressant drugs and anesthetics.

Venous admixture. About 3–5 percent of the cardiac output in normal man bypasses ventilating alveoli, and thus a portion of venous blood returns to the arterial blood without participating in gas exchange in the lungs. This is the venous admixture or right-to-left shunt. Addition of venous blood to blood from the pulmonary capillary bed reduces the arterial P_{O_2} but leaves the arterial P_{CO_2} unaltered. The arterial P_{O_2} is reduced because the venous blood has a P_{O_2} of 40 mm Hg and the blood leaving the pulmonary capillary bed a P_{O_2} of better than 100 mm Hg; with this large a difference in P_{O_2} mixture of the two bloods results in a lowered arterial P_{O_2}. The final $P_{a_{O_2}}$ depends on the relative size of the venous admixture; the larger the venous fraction the lower the $P_{a_{O_2}}$. In addition, because of the shape of the oxyhemoglobin dissociation curve, the low P_{O_2} of the venous blood is more influential in determining the final $P_{a_{O_2}}$ than the higher P_{O_2} in the pulmonary capillary blood. This phenomenon is discussed further in the next section on $\dot{V}/\dot{Q}$ inequality.

Arterial P_{CO_2} is not significantly altered by venous admixture, first because the P_{CO_2} difference between mixed venous blood and pulmonary capillary blood that is in equilibrium with alveolar P_{CO_2} is small at 6 mm Hg, $P_{\bar{v}_{CO_2}} = 46$ mm Hg and $P_{A_{CO_2}} = 40$ mm Hg. Second, any elevation in arterial P_{CO_2} because of addition of venous blood to pulmonary capillary blood is sensed immediately by the respiratory centers and ventilation is increased and $P_{a_{CO_2}}$ brought back to normal.* This increase in ventilation will increase alveolar P_{O_2} by a few millimeters Hg also, but the elevation of $P_{A_{O_2}}$ is not sufficient to counteract the lowering effect of the venous P_{O_2} on the final arterial P_{O_2}.

*This is due to the extreme sensitivity of the respiratory control mechanisms to the level of $P_{a_{CO_2}}$, so that ventilation is increased or decreased to maintain $P_{a_{CO_2}}$ within a narrow limit (see chapter on the control of ventilation).

The normally occurring venous admixture takes place through the thebesian venous system of the left ventricle, through bronchial vein–pulmonary vein anastomoses, and through direct channels between the pulmonary arteries and veins. Venous admixture is increased in cyanotic congenital heart disease or in lung disease when alveoli become atelectatic or obliterated but continue to have some blood flow. Increase in venous admixture leads to elevation of the alveolar–arterial O_2 gradient (A–aD_{O_2}) on room air. Presence of venous admixture is best demonstrated by measuring the A–aD_{O_2} on 100 percent O_2; it is discussed in greater detail in the section on assessment of hypoxemia. The absolute magnitude of the shunt (venous admixture) can be calculated by using the shunt equation that relates the shunt flow $\dot{Q}_s$ to total cardiac output $\dot{Q}_t$ as a function of the difference in oxygen content of pulmonary capillary blood ($C_{c_{O_2}}$) and arterial blood ($C_{a_{O_2}}$) and the oxygen-content difference between pulmonary capillary blood and mixed venous blood ($C_{\bar{v}_{O_2}}$):

$$\dot{Q}_s/\dot{Q}_t = \frac{C_{c_{O_2}} - C_{a_{O_2}}}{C_{c_{O_2}} - C_{\bar{v}_{O_2}}} \times 100$$

With a relatively normal cardiac and O_2 consumption, using this equation it can be calculated that 1 percent shunt reduces the arterial P_{O_2} by 1 mm Hg.

In primary lung disease, increased venous admixture is a contributing factor to development of hypoxemia, but it is rarely the sole cause of hypoxemia and in most instances does not exceed 20 percent of the cardiac output.

Ventilation/perfusion imbalance ($\dot{V}/\dot{Q}$ inequality). $\dot{V}/\dot{Q}$ inequality is the most common cause of hypoxemia in cardiorespiratory disorders and is the major factor in development of hypoxemia in almost all forms of lung disease. There are at least 300 million gas-exchanging units in the lung, each unit consisting of the alveolus and its capillary meshwork. Each unit is capable of gas exchange, since it has both ventilation and blood flow. The task of the lung is to coordinate blood flow and ventilation to all these units, so that ideally each unit will receive a proportionate fraction of blood flow and ventilation. For the system as a whole the $\dot{V}/\dot{Q}$ ratio is 0.8, i.e., 4/5 = 0.8, where alveolar ventilation is 4 l/min and pulmonary capillary blood flow is 5 l/min. This is the $\dot{V}/\dot{Q}$ ratio for the entire system, and each subunit will have its own $\dot{V}/\dot{Q}$ ratio. It is the sum of $\dot{V}/\dot{Q}$ ratios of all these gas-exchanging units that determines the final composition of gases in the arterial blood.

In normal man in the erect position, distribution of ventilation and perfusion is not evenly matched to all parts of the lungs. There is more ventilation to the base of the lung than to the apex, with a ratio of approximately 1.5:1. Distribution of perfusion is also uneven, the base receiving more blood flow than the apex, the

DISTRIBUTION OF VENTILATION AND PERFUSION AT A–C MEMBRANE

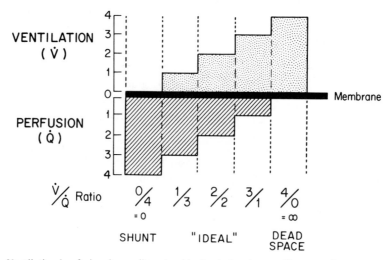

Fig. 5. Ventilation/perfusion inequality. An idealized alveolar–capillary membrane separates ventilation $\dot{V}$ from perfusion $\dot{Q}$. Numbers on the vertical axis represent arbitrary units of flow. Ventilation increases from left to right and perfusion from right to left. At the extreme right there is dead space (ventilation but no perfusion) and at the extreme left there is shunt (perfusion but no ventilation). Shunt and dead space bracket the spectrum of $\dot{V}/\dot{Q}$ inequality with an "ideal" $\dot{V}/\dot{Q}$ ratio in the center of the diagram.

ratio being about 3:1. Thus gradients of $\dot{V}/\dot{Q}$ ratios exist from apex to base, the apex having a high $\dot{V}/\dot{Q}$ ratio of 3.3 and the base a low $\dot{V}/\dot{Q}$ ratio of 0.63. These inequalities in distribution of blood flow and ventilation are due to the effect of gravity on the lung and are discussed in greater detail in the chapter Physical Factors in Lung Function.

In view of the large number of gas-exchanging units in the system and various factors affecting the distribution of both ventilation and blood flow, a spectrum of $\dot{V}/\dot{Q}$ ratios can exist in the lung. A simplified approach to $\dot{V}/\dot{Q}$ ratios is depicted in Fig. 5. An idealized alveolar–capillary membrane separates ventilation from perfusion. Ventilation increases from left to right and perfusion from right to left. On the extreme right there are areas of ventilation with no blood flow. This by definition is dead space. On the extreme left there are areas of perfusion with no ventilation. This by definition is shunt. In between are areas of varying $\dot{V}/\dot{Q}$ ratios. Thus the spectrum of $\dot{V}/\dot{Q}$ ratios is bracketed on one side by dead space and the other by shunt. The ideal $\dot{V}/\dot{Q}$ ratio is in the middle where ventilation and perfusion are evenly matched. Areas of high $\dot{V}/\dot{Q}$ lie between the $\dot{V}/\dot{Q}$ ratio of unity and dead space and those with low $\dot{V}/\dot{Q}$ between that of unity and shunt.

The effect of $\dot{V}/\dot{Q}$ inequality on gas exchange can best be assessed by first considering high $\dot{V}/\dot{Q}$ and then low $\dot{V}/\dot{Q}$. Assuming that the capillary blood leaving an alveolus is in equilibrium with gas tensions in that alveolus, in areas of high $\dot{V}/\dot{Q}$ there is an excess of ventilation in relation to perfusion; so the alveolar gas composi-

tion will be closer to that of the inspired air than that of the mixed venous blood. This results in a relatively high P_{O_2} and relatively low P_{CO_2} and P_{N_2}. The total pressure of the three gases will have to obey the law of partial pressures and add up to the atmospheric pressure minus the pressure for water vapor at 37°C, i.e., 760 − 47 = 713 mm Hg at sea level. Therefore, blood leaving areas of high $\dot{V}/\dot{Q}$ will have high P_{O_2} and low P_{CO_2} and P_{N_2}.

In areas of low $\dot{V}/\dot{Q}$ there is an excess of perfusion in relation to ventilation, and therefore the composition of alveolar air in these areas will move in the direction of mixed venous blood. The net result is that pulmonary capillary blood leaving areas of low $\dot{V}/\dot{Q}$ will have relatively low P_{O_2}, but high P_{CO_2} and P_{N_2}. Theoretical and experimental data confirm these assumptions, and in the normal lung in the erect position (Table 1) it has been shown that the apex with relatively high $\dot{V}/\dot{Q}$ of 3.3 has a P_{O_2} of 132, P_{CO_2} of 28, and P_{N_2} of 553 mm Hg. The base, with a relatively low $\dot{V}/\dot{Q}$ of 0.63, has a P_{O_2} of 89, P_{CO_2} of 42, and P_{N_2} of 582 mm Hg; intermediate areas have gas tensions between the two extremes of apex and base.

The final composition of arterial blood gases depends on the relative preponderance of areas of high and low $\dot{V}/\dot{Q}$. In any given setting, the areas of low $\dot{V}/\dot{Q}$ will predominate in determining the final $P_{a_{O_2}}$. Areas of low $\dot{V}/\dot{Q}$ will have lower P_{O_2}'s, which because of the shape of the oxyhemoglobin dissociation curve fall on

Table 1
$\dot{V}/\dot{Q}$ Ratios and Gas Tensions in Three
Lung Zones of Erect Man

	$\dot{V}/\dot{Q}$ Ratio	P_{O_2}*	P_{CO_2}*	P_{N_2}*
Apex	3.3	132	28	553
Mid-lung zone	0.90	102	40	571
Base	0.63	89	42	582

*In millimeters Hg.
Modified from West JB: J Appl Physiol 17:893, 1962.

the steep portion of the curve and pull down the higher P_{O_2}'s from areas of high $\dot{V}/\dot{Q}$. The net result is development of hypoxemia. This can be demonstrated best by the following example. Let us assume that one-half of the pulmonary capillary blood comes from areas of low $\dot{V}/\dot{Q}$ and its P_{O_2} is 50 mm Hg. Its oxygen saturation will be 83 percent (Fig. 2). The other half of the pulmonary capillary blood comes from areas of high $\dot{V}/\dot{Q}$ and has a P_{O_2} of 110 mm Hg, and it is 100 percent saturated with oxygen (Fig. 2). When these two samples of blood are mixed the final arterial oxygen saturation will be 91.5 percent, which is the arithmetic mean of the two saturations. With an O_2 saturation of 91.5 percent the arterial P_{O_2} will be 63 mm Hg (Fig. 2), which is closer to the P_{O_2} of the blood from areas of low $\dot{V}/\dot{Q}$. It should be apparent that in any given setting the $P_{a_{O_2}}$ will be determined by the relative fractions of blood coming from areas of low and high $\dot{V}/\dot{Q}$ and the oxygen saturation of hemoglobin in each area, which in turn is a function of P_{O_2} in that area. However, because of the S shape of the oxyhemoglobin dissociation curve, the low blood P_{O_2} from the area of low $\dot{V}/\dot{Q}$ that falls on the steep part of the dissociation curve will have more influence on the final arterial P_{O_2} than the high P_{O_2} of the high $\dot{V}/\dot{Q}$ area that falls on the flat part of the dissociation curves. Similarly, with venous admixture, hypoxemia develops because the mixed P_{O_2} of 40 mm Hg significantly reduces the high P_{O_2} of the blood leaving the pulmonary capillary bed.

Areas of high $\dot{V}/\dot{Q}$ do not cause hypoxemia, but they do increase the relative dead-space ventilation, and this "wasted" ventilation increases the work of the respiratory system. Recently it has also been shown that in CO_2 transport marked $\dot{V}/\dot{Q}$ inequality can lead to CO_2 retention and elevation of $P_{a_{CO_2}}$ (hypercapnia). Areas of low $\dot{V}/\dot{Q}$ are again predominant in development of hypercapnia, provided alveolar ventilation increase is limited (see section on CO_2 Transport below).

The normally occurring $\dot{V}/\dot{Q}$ inequality in man in the erect position, despite its relatively large magnitude (Table 1), leads to a fall in $P_{a_{O_2}}$ of about 4 mm Hg. Therefore when hypoxemia develops in lung and heart disease, marked derangements in the $\dot{V}/\dot{Q}$ ratios must be present in the gas-exchanging units. The normal lung has potent neural and humoral mechanisms that control

distribution of blood flow and ventilation and match one for the other. Presence of hypoxemia, therefore, implies significant impairment of these controls as well.

Assessment of Hypoxemia

$\dot{V}/\dot{Q}$ inequality leads to accentuation of the alveolar–arterial gradients for O_2, CO_2, and N_2. By measuring these gradients under appropriate conditions one can assess the relative magnitudes of areas of high and low $\dot{V}/\dot{Q}$ ratios as well as venous admixture and their relative contributions to development of hypoxemia. The alveolar–arterial O_2 gradient (A–aD_{O_2}) on room air is increased with both shunt and $\dot{V}/\dot{Q}$ inequality. The arterial–alveolar CO_2 gradient (a–AD_{CO_2}) is increased primarily with high $\dot{V}/\dot{Q}$ ratios, and the arterial–alveolar nitrogen gradient (a–AD_{N_2}) primarily with low $\dot{V}/\dot{Q}$ ratios. The alveolar–arterial O_2 gradient on 100 percent O_2 is increased principally with venous admixture. From a practical standpoint the measurements of a–AD_{CO_2} and a–AD_{N_2} are difficult; therefore the A–aD_{O_2} is measured on room air followed by measurement of the A–aD_{O_2} on 100 percent O_2.

The A–aD_{O_2} on 100 percent O_2 is due to venous admixture (shunt). If a subject breathes 100 percent O_2 from a closed system, nitrogen concentration in the lungs falls progressively and eventually reaches values of less than 2 percent (usually 7–10 min in normal subjects and 15–20 min or more in those with obstructive lung disease). At this point the entire lung is filled with O_2 and the partial pressure of O_2 everywhere is greater than 600 mm Hg regardless of the distribution of ventilation, since the only other gas in the lung is now CO_2 and its maximum partial pressure anywhere is not greater than that in mixed venous blood. Therefore all the blood leaving the pulmonary capillary bed will have a P_{O_2} in excess of 600 mm Hg. In this manner, by breathing 100 percent O_2 the effect of regional ventilation inequality in determining the arterial P_{O_2} is negated. If the entire venous return went to the ventilating alveoli, then the alveolar P_{O_2} and arterial P_{O_2} would be identical. Any difference between $P_{A_{O_2}}$ and $P_{a_{O_2}}$ in these circumstances is then due to venous blood not going to ventilating alveoli, which by definition is shunting. Therefore measurement of A–aD_{O_2} on 100 percent O_2 reflects the shunt, and an estimate of the shunt as a fraction of total cardiac output can be made. Using the shunt equation and assuming a normal cardiac output and O_2 consumption it can be calculated that an A–aD_{O_2} of 16 mm Hg on 100 percent O_2 results from a shunt of 1 percent. With a normally occurring shunt of 3 percent, therefore, an A–aD_{O_2} of 50 mm Hg is normal in man.

The shunt can be estimated from the A–aD_{O_2} on 100 percent O_2, and since each 1 percent shunt will contribute 1 mm Hg to the A–aD_{O_2} on room air, the part of the A–aD_{O_2} on room air that cannot be accounted for by venous admixture is ascribed to $\dot{V}/\dot{Q}$ inequality.

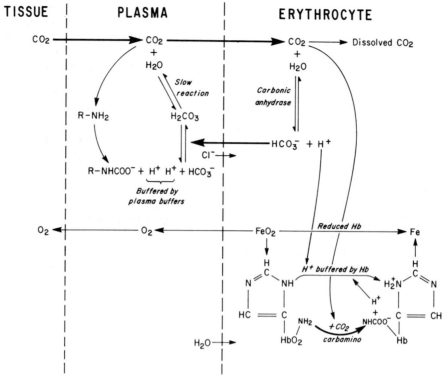

Fig. 6. Schematic presentation of CO_2 transport in blood by plasma and erythrocyte. [Modified by permission from Davenport HW: The ABC of Acid–Base Chemistry (ed 5). Chicago, University of Chicago Press, 1969.]

The other cause of hypoxemia, alveolar hypoventilation, does not increase the $A-aD_{O_2}$, and its presence is determined by measuring the arterial P_{CO_2}.

This approach to hypoxemia looks at a complex problem from a pragmatic point of view, and a number of assumptions are made in so doing. This should be kept in mind in applying this to clinical situations, particularly when cardiac output and/or hemoglobin content are low or when marked alterations in O_2 consumption are believed to exist.

Diffusion Impairment

In any discussion of hypoxemia, one must consider the problem of diffusion impairment for oxygen across the alveolar–capillary membrane. There are numerous disorders that affect the alveolar–capillary membrane and increase its thickness and therefore the diffusion distance for oxygen from the alveolar air to the pulmonary capillary bed. Until recently physiologic thinking held that a physical barrier to passage of oxygen at the alveolar–capillary membrane was a significant factor in development of arterial hypoxemia. Evidence now suggests that increasing the thickness of the alveolar–capillary membrane does not in itself reduce the arterial P_{O_2} significantly at rest. The measured diffusing capacity of the lung for oxygen or carbon monoxide is reduced in these states, but this does not imply that there is a physical barrier to passage of oxygen from air to blood. $\dot{V}/\dot{Q}$ inequality, primarily, and some increase in venous ad-

mixture, are the factors in development of hypoxemia in disorders where there is disease of the alveolar–capillary membrane. Diffusion impairment, therefore, may be classified as a subgroup of $\dot{V}/\dot{Q}$ inequality in causes of hypoxemia.

CO_2 TRANSPORT
Partial Pressure of CO_2 Blood and Air

Carbon dioxide is produced by the tissues and is transported by blood to the lungs, where it diffuses out of blood into the alveolar gas and is exhaled in the gas form. In normal man at rest 200 cc of CO_2 (8.98 mmoles) is exhaled per minute. As with oxygen, CO_2 must diffuse across several membranes to reach the alveolar gas from tissue cells. Transfer of CO_2 across the membranes requires pressure gradients. For CO_2 these pressure gradients are small as compared with those for oxygen. The arterial P_{CO_2} ($P_{a_{CO_2}}$) is about 40 mm Hg, and tissue P_{CO_2} is about 46 mm Hg. Thus a gradient of 6 mm Hg is available for diffusion of CO_2 from cells into blood. Mixed venous P_{CO_2} ($P_{\bar{v}_{CO_2}}$) is in equilibrium with tissue P_{CO_2} at 46 mm Hg. The alveolar P_{CO_2} ($P_{A_{CO_2}}$) is 40 mm Hg, and thus a P_{CO_2} gradient of 6 mm Hg exists for transfer of CO_2 from pulmonary arterial blood into alveolar air. Transfer of CO_2 across the alveolar–capillary membrane is almost instantaneous, and equilibration between blood and air P_{CO_2} is complete in much less than 0.01 sec. In the normal lung in the erect position an arterial-alveolar P_{CO_2} gradient (a–AD_{CO_2}) of 1 mm Hg exists because of the normally present $\dot{V}/\dot{Q}$ inequality. However, for practical purposes one can assume that no a–AD_{CO_2} is present in the normal lung and that $P_{a_{CO_2}}$ and $P_{A_{CO_2}}$ are identical.

CO_2 Transport in Blood

CO_2 is carried in blood in three forms: (1) dissolved CO_2, (2) bicarbonate, and (3) bound to hemoglobin as carbamino-CO_2.

Dissolved CO_2. CO_2 diffuses from cells into plasma and into erythrocytes. The CO_2 in plasma stays primarily as dissolved CO_2, although a minute quantity of it becomes hydrated to form carbonic acid, which then dissociates to form hydrogen ions and bicarbonate ions.

$$CO_2 + H_2O \rightleftharpoons H_2CO_3 \rightleftharpoons H^+ + HCO_3^-$$

The quantity of CO_2 in dissolved form is about 1000 times greater than the quantity of carbonic acid. The H^+ formed by this reaction are buffered by the weak plasma buffers (Fig. 6). A very small quantity of CO_2 is also carried by plasma proteins in direct combination. The amount of carbon dioxide in solution depends on the partial pressure of CO_2 (P_{CO_2}) and its solubility coefficient α, which is 0.0301 mM/l/mm P_{CO_2}. Thus with a venous P_{CO_2} of 46 mm Hg, 46×0.0301 (or 1.38) mM of CO_2 is carried in the dissolved form in 1 l of blood (both plasma and red blood cells).

The major role in CO_2 carriage is played by reactions that take place within the erythrocyte. Some CO_2 is carried in the dissolved form in the erythrocyte, but its quantity is small. There are two primary reversible chemical reactions in the erythrocyte that lead to formation of bicarbonate ions and carbamino-CO_2 compounds.

Bicarbonate formation. CO_2 becomes hydrated in the erythrocyte to form carbonic acid, which then ionizes to form hydrogen ions and bicarbonate ions. These reactions within the erythrocyte are catalyzed by the enzyme carbonic anhydrase, which is present in blood only in the erythrocyte. Because of the presence of carbonic anhydrase these reactions are extremely rapid as compared to CO_2 hydration in plasma, and large quantities of H^+ and HCO_3^- are formed. The hydrogen ions are buffered by hemoglobin, and the bicarbonate ions leave the erythrocyte and go into the plasma. In order to maintain ionic equilibrium a negatively charged ion (Cl^-) moves into the erythrocyte, the so-called chloride shift. The events in this transfer and other aspects of CO_2 transport are summarized schematically in Fig. 6. The erythrocyte, therefore, plays a singularly important role in the transport of CO_2 because of the presence of carbonic anhydrase, which catalyzes the hydration reaction of CO_2, and of hemoglobin, which buffers the hydrogen ions formed.

Carbamino-CO_2. Hemoglobin, in addition, is important in transport of CO_2 in another form. CO_2 reacts directly with the NH_2 groups of the hemoglobin molecule to form carbamino-CO_2, and thus CO_2 is carried directly on the hemoglobin molecule. The hydrogen ions formed by this reaction are again buffered by hemoglobin itself. Formation of carbamino-CO_2 is dependent on the degree of oxygenation of hemoglobin. The more desaturated the hemoglobin, the greater the quantity of carbamino-CO_2 that can be formed. At the same time desaturated (reduced) hemoglobin becomes a better buffer, and the hydrogen ions formed are buffered more effectively.

CO_2 Dissociation Curve

The amount of CO_2 carried in blood is a direct function of the partial pressure of CO_2 (P_{CO_2}) in blood; the higher the P_{CO_2} the greater the total quantity of CO_2 carried. This relationship is defined by the blood CO_2 dissociation curve (Fig. 7), and it is essentially a linear function over the physiologic ranges of P_{CO_2}. This is in contrast with the oxyhemoglobin dissociation curve, which is S-shaped with a flat portion on the top. The linear shape of the CO_2 dissociation curve allows for elimination of CO_2 from blood to the same extent by lowering of P_{CO_2} at a host of points above and below the normal arterial and venous points (Fig. 7).

Shifts in the CO_2 dissociation curve occur as a function of the level of oxygenation. Reduced hemoglobin is a better buffer and carries more CO_2 for a given P_{CO_2} than oxyhemoglobin. The CO_2 dissociation curve shifts to the right when hemoglobin becomes saturated with oxygen and to the left when reduced hemoglobin is formed—the Haldane effect (Fig. 7). These shifts in the CO_2 dissociation curve are of significant physiologic value in CO_2 transport. Reduction of hemoglobin at the tissue level to an oxygen saturation of 75 percent allows for more CO_2 to be carried for any given P_{CO_2}—the venous point v on the CO_2 dissociation curve in Fig. 7. In the pulmonary capillary bed oxygenation of hemoglobin shifts the curve to the right, and CO_2 is driven off the hemoglobin, facilitating elimination of CO_2 from blood; the final arterial point a is established on the dissociation curve (Fig. 7). If no shift in dissociation curve occurred when the partially reduced hemoglobin became oxygenated, the mere reduction in P_{CO_2} from 46 to 40 mm Hg, i.e., going from venous to the arterial point, would significantly reduce the amount of CO_2 eliminated from blood. Reduction in P_{CO_2} from 46 to 40 mm Hg would result in a loss of almost 5 volumes percent CO_2 with the shift in the dissociation curve, but without the shift the CO_2 elimination would be only about 3 volumes percent, as shown in Fig. 7.

CO_2 Elimination

The total amount of CO_2 in arterial and venous blood depends not only on the level of tissue P_{CO_2} and alveolar P_{CO_2} but also on the hemoglobin and its state of oxygenation. Table 2 gives measured values for the three forms of CO_2 present in arterial and venous blood when the hematocrit is 45 percent and $P_{a_{CO_2}}$ and $P_{\bar{v}_{CO_2}}$ are 41 and 47.5 mm Hg, respectively. It is

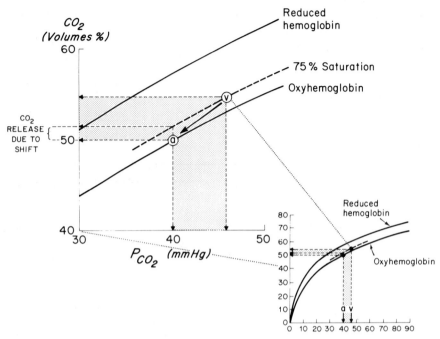

Fig. 7. CO_2 dissociation curves of reduced hemoglobin and oxyhemoglobin, as well as when hemoglobin is 75 percent saturated with O_2, which is normal mixed venous blood, are shown in this diagram. The CO_2 dissociation curves for the usual physiologic ranges of P_{CO_2} are enlarged in the upper diagram. More CO_2 is carried for a given P_{CO_2} when oxyhemoglobin becomes reduced hemoglobin (a shift to the left), and less CO_2 is carried when reduced hemoglobin is oxygenated (a shift to the right). The shift to the right allows for more CO_2 to be eliminated from blood when going from the venous point *v* on the 75 percent O_2 saturation curve at a P_{CO_2} of 46 mm Hg to the arterial point *a* at a P_{CO_2} of 40 mm Hg. If the right shift did not occur, then the mere reduction in P_{CO_2} would result in less CO_2 being eliminated from blood in going from a P_{CO_2} of 46 to 40. Therefore CO_2 release from blood is enhanced when blood becomes oxygenated in the pulmonary capillary bed.

Table 2
CO_2 of Arterial and Venous Blood

	Arterial	Venous
P_{CO_2}	41 mm Hg	47.5 mm Hg
Red cells		
Hematocrit	44.8 %	45.1 %
Dissolved CO_2	0.48 mM*	0.56 mM*
HCO_3^-	5.7 mM	6.11 mM
Carbamino-CO_2	1.09 mM	1.72 mM
Total CO_2	7.34 mM	8.39 mM
Serum		
Dissolved CO_2	0.71 mM	0.81 mM
HCO_3^-	13.83 mM	14.85 mM
Carbamino-CO_2	–	–
Total CO_2	14.54 mM	15.66 mM
Total CO_2 for whole blood	21.88 mM	24.05 mM

*All CO_2 values presented as mM/l whole blood.
Modified from Roughton FJW: in Fenn WO, Rahn H (eds): Handbook of Physiology, Respiration, vol I. Baltimore, Williams & Wilkins, 1964, p 767.

apparent that of the total CO_2 in blood approximately two-thirds is in the serum, and bicarbonate constitutes more than 85 percent of the total CO_2 in blood. Of the total veno-arterial CO_2 difference of 2.17 mM/1 of blood, i.e., the amount of CO_2 given off in the lung, 63 percent is given off from bicarbonate, 29 percent from carbamino-CO_2, and 8 percent from dissolved CO_2 (Fig. 8), thus pointing out the significance of both bicarbonate and carbamino-CO_2 in elimination of CO_2 from the system.

When venous blood reaches the lung, all the chemical reactions described earlier in the process of CO_2 transport are reversed, and CO_2 diffuses from the pulmonary capillary plasma into the alveolar air and is eliminated from the alveolar gas by ventilation.

Alveolar Ventilation and CO_2 Elimination

How much CO_2 is removed is a function of the level of alveolar ventilation. The relationship between alveolar ventilation (in l/min) $\dot{V}_A$, CO_2 production (in cc/min) $\dot{V}_{CO_2}$, and partial pressure of CO_2 in the alveolar air or arterial blood, $P_{A_{CO_2}}$ or $P_{a_{CO_2}}$ (in mm Hg), is given

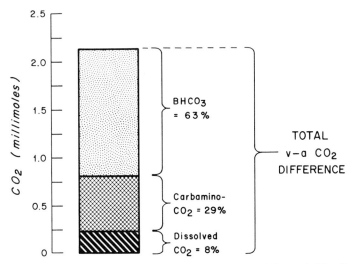

Fig. 8. CO_2 eliminated in the lung from 1 l of blood. The fraction of the total CO_2 eliminated from each of the three forms of CO_2 brought to the lung is given by the relative percentages on the right and the absolute quantities on the left.

by the equation

$$\dot{V}_A = \frac{\dot{V}_{CO_2} \times 0.863^*}{P_{a_{CO_2}} \text{ or } P_{A_{CO_2}}}$$

Since the amount of CO_2 produced by the body is relatively constant and does not vary from minute to minute, the numerator of the equation ($\dot{V}_{CO_2}$) becomes a constant. Therefore alveolar ventilation becomes inversely related to arterial P_{CO_2}. There is increased alveolar ventilation (alveolar hyperventilation) when $P_{a_{CO_2}}$ is reduced; there is decreased alveolar ventilation (alveolar hypoventilation) when $P_{a_{CO_2}}$ is elevated. Since the level of $P_{a_{CO_2}}$ is maintained normally within a narrow range by the respiratory control mechanisms, any deviation from the normal range of 38–42 mm Hg signifies alveolar hyperventilation or hypoventilation. Therefore measurement of $P_{a_{CO_2}}$ is the best means of assessing the adequacy of alveolar ventilation.

Marked derangements of $\dot{V}/\dot{Q}$ ratios may also lead to CO_2 retention and elevation of $P_{a_{CO_2}}$. The main reason for $P_{a_{CO_2}}$ elevation in $\dot{V}/\dot{Q}$ inequality is that disease of the respiratory system does not allow an adequate increase in the level of ventilation to compensate for the elevated $P_{a_{CO_2}}$. In other words, the $\dot{V}/\dot{Q}$ inequality causes an increase in $P_{a_{CO_2}}$, and the normal response of

*The correction factor 0.863 is introduced in this equation because $\dot{V}_A$ is measured at body temperature and pressure, saturated with water vapor (BTPS), and $\dot{V}_{CO_2}$ at standard temperature and pressure, dry (STPD).

increasing alveolar ventilation when $P_{a_{CO_2}}$ is increased is inadequate because of disease of the respiratory system, so CO_2 retention ensues.

In the large majority of patients with lung disease, elevation of $P_{a_{CO_2}}$ is due to alveolar hypoventilation, and even when $P_{a_{CO_2}}$ is increased because of $\dot{V}/\dot{Q}$ inequality there is inadequate alveolar ventilation. Therefore, in management of patients with CO_2 retention, improvement in alveolar ventilation is the critical factor.

Blood pH

The acidity of blood, i.e., its pH, is determined by the Henderson-Hasselbalch equation, which relates plasma pH to its dissociation constant pK, and the ratio of plasma bicarbonate to dissolved CO_2:

$$pH = pK + \log \frac{HCO_3^-}{\alpha \times P_{CO_2}}$$

In acid–base homeostasis the level of alveolar ventilation determines the partial pressure of CO_2 (P_{CO_2}), which will in turn influence the pH. Therefore changes in the level of alveolar ventilation whether due to primary lung disease or to processes elsewhere are of prime importance in hydrogen-ion homeostasis. These and other aspects of acid–base balance are discussed in detail in the chapter on physiology and disorders of hydrogen-ion metabolism.

REFERENCES

Comroe JH, Forster RE, Dubois AB, et al: The Lung. Chicago, Year Book Medical Publishers, 1962

Davenport HW: The ABC of Acid-Base Chemistry (ed 5). Chicago, University of Chicago Press, 1969

Farhi LE: Ventilation-perfusion relationship and its role in alveolar gas exchange, in Caro CG (ed): Advances in Respiratory Physiology. Baltimore, Williams & Wilkins, 1966, p 148

Kazemi H: Pulmonary function tests. JAMA 206:2302, 1968

Lenfant C, Ways P, Aucutt C, Cruz J: Effect of chronic hypoxic hypoxia on the O_2–Hb dissociation curve and respiratory gas transport in man. Respir Physiol 7:7, 1969

Rahn H, Fenn WO: Graphical Analysis of the Respiratory Gas Exchange: The O_2–CO_2 Diagram. Washington, American Physiological Society, 1955

Riley RL, Cournand A: "Ideal" alveolar air and the analysis of ventilation–perfusion relationships in the lung. J Appl Physiol 1:825, 1949

Roughton FJW: Transport of oxygen and carbon dioxide, in Fenn WO, Rahn H (eds): Handbook of Physiology, Respiration, vol I. Baltimore, Williams & Wilkins, 1964, p 767

West JB: Regional differences in gas exchange in the lung of erect man. J Appl Physiol 17:893, 1962

West JB: Effect of slope and shape of dissociation curve on pulmonary gas exchange. Respir Physiol 8:66, 1969/70

CONTROL OF VENTILATION

Homayoun Kazemi

It is a fact that the level of alveolar ventilation is precisely controlled. To establish this control a complex host of impulses and feedback mechanisms arising from different sources are coordinated by the respiratory centers in the medulla and higher centers, and the level of ventilation appropriate for the demand is set by the respiratory muscles (the intercostals and the diaphragm). Broadly speaking these impulses fall into two main groups: (1) chemical and (2) neural. The chemical stimuli arise from changes in the arterial P_{O_2}, P_{CO_2}, and pH. The neural stimuli arise from the lungs, pleura, muscles of respiration, joints, and other structures as well. Although these controlling mechanisms are necessarily involuntary, there is voluntary control of the level of ventilation, and one can increase or decrease the level of ventilation to a point at will.

The known mechanisms that enter into control of ventilation are depicted graphically in Fig. 1, without any attempt to give the relative magnitude of each stimulus.

CHEMICAL FACTORS

The chemical factors in control of respiration are the more critical of the two, since the level of ventilation is adjusted to maintain metabolic homeostasis, i.e., normoxia and acid–base balance. There are two groups of chemoreceptors active in the chemical control of ventilation. The peripheral chemoreceptors are located in the carotid and aortic bodies, distinct anatomic structures at the bifurcation of the carotid artery and at the arch of the aorta, respectively. They are highly vascular structures with a very high rate of blood flow. Afferent nerve fibers from the carotid body join the glossopharyngeal nerve (IXN), and those from the aortic body join the vagus (XN). The peripheral chemoreceptors are sensitive to changes in arterial pH, P_{O_2}, and P_{CO_2}.

In terms of chemical control of respiration, the peripheral chemoreceptors may be thought of as the secondary line of control, since relatively large changes in arterial pH, P_{O_2}, and P_{CO_2} are necessary before changes in the level of ventilation are brought about.

Arterial pH

Fall in arterial pH stimulates ventilation, and a rise in arterial pH depresses ventilation. For significant changes in ventilation to occur the pH must vary from the normal value of 7.40 by about 0.15–0.20. That is, increases in ventilation take place when arterial pH reaches 7.25 or less, and ventilation decreases when arterial pH exceeds 7.55.

Arterial P_{O_2}

The ventilatory response to hypoxemia (fall in $P_{a_{O_2}}$) is variable. In most normal individuals ventilation increases when $P_{a_{O_2}}$ falls below 65 mm Hg in the adult and less than 55 mm Hg in the newborn. But there is a wide scatter of this threshold. Since no change in ventilation can be consistently demonstrated when $P_{a_{O_2}}$ lies between 65 and 95 mm Hg, it has been postulated that in normal man with a normal $P_{a_{O_2}}$ above 85 mm Hg there is no oxygen drive in control of ventilation. This is a controversial point, but the current knowledge would indicate that some oxygen drive is present even with a normal $P_{a_{O_2}}$, particularly since raising $P_{a_{O_2}}$ above 100 mm Hg by only one or two breaths of pure oxygen will depress ventilation transiently by as much as 20 percent.

The oxygen drive of ventilation may be important in disease states. In respiratory failure with CO_2 retention, where the CO_2 drive is significantly blunted, the hypoxic drive becomes dominant, and administration of oxygen can cause further ventilatory depression. The hypoxic drive is absent or markedly depressed in individuals who are hypoxic at birth and remain so at least for the first 5 years of life. Two groups fall in this category, those born at high altitude who continue to reside there and those with cyanotic congenital heart disease. Reasons for this paradoxic lack of hypoxic drive are unknown.

Ventilatory depression may be seen with marked hypoxemia because of general depression of all CNS function in face of significant oxygen lack.

Arterial P_{CO_2}

The peripheral chemoreceptors respond to increases in arterial P_{CO_2} by increasing ventilation and to decreases in arterial P_{CO_2} by decreasing ventilation. Again, as with changes in arterial pH and P_{O_2}, relatively large changes of about 5 mm Hg or more in P_{CO_2} are necessary for ventilation to increase and decrease as the result of peripheral chemoreceptor response to $P_{a_{CO_2}}$. The effect of CO_2 on the peripheral receptors probably is due to changes in hydrogen-ion (H^+) concentration at these sites because of changes in P_{CO_2}. About 10 percent of the overall CO_2 ventilatory response can be ascribed

CONTROL OF VENTILATION

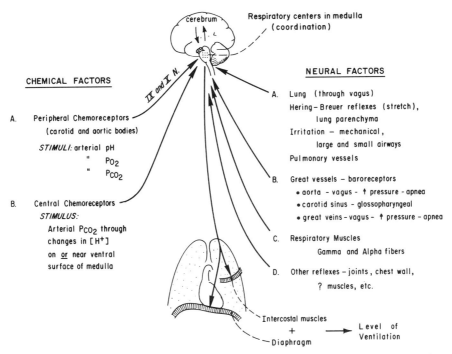

Fig. 1. Schematic presentation of both chemical and neural mechanisms in control of ventilation.

to the action of CO_2 on the peripheral chemoreceptors. The primary site of action of CO_2 is on the central chemoreceptors. The central chemoreceptors are located on or near the ventral surface of the medulla at the point of exit of the IX and X cranial nerves. These chemosensitive areas are not distinct histologic entities, and some controversy exists about their exact nature and location. Nonetheless, in this region of the medulla small changes in hydrogen-ion concentration of fluids bathing them have profound effects on the level of ventilation.

CO_2 can be considered the primary agent in chemical control of ventilation. Because of the rapid diffusibility of CO_2 any change in arterial P_{CO_2} is immediately reflected in all tissues including the brain and cerebrospinal fluid (CSF), where it will alter (H^+) and thus affect the level of ventilation. The level of arterial P_{CO_2} is extremely well controlled within a very narrow limit in any individual, and changes of only 1 mm Hg in $P_{a_{CO_2}}$ are appreciated by the respiratory system, with ventilation being appropriately increased or decreased. The ventilatory response to increase in $P_{a_{CO_2}}$ is rather brisk, and as a rule ventilation increases by 2.5 l/min for each 1 mm Hg increase in $P_{a_{CO_2}}$. The ventilatory response to alterations in arterial P_{CO_2}, P_{O_2}, and pH in normal man is given in Fig. 2. The CO_2 ventilatory response curve is not uniform for all individuals, and a reasonable scatter of responses exists.

Considerable experimental and clinical evidence exists to indicate that the H^+ of the fluids bathing the chemosensitive areas on the medulla can be the single

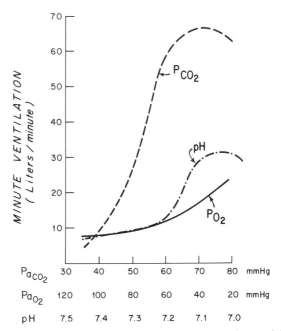

Fig. 2. Ventilatory response in man to changes in arterial P_{CO_2}, P_{O_2}, and pH when each variable is changed singly with the other two kept constant. (Adapted from data of Comroe JH Jr: in: Physiology of Respiration. Chicago, Year Book Medical Publishers, 1965, and Guyton AC: in: Textbook of Medical Physiology. Philadelphia, WB Saunders, 1956.)

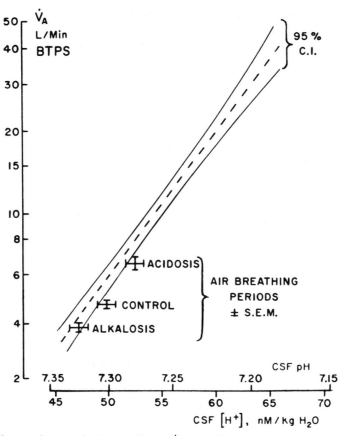

Fig. 3. Resting steady-state alveolar ventilation $\dot{V}_A$ in relation to CSF H⁺ in alkalosis, acidosis, and normal conditions. Changes in alveolar ventilation during CO_2 breathing are given by the dashed line with the 95 percent confidence interval (C.I.). Data from unanesthetized goats. (Reproduced by permission from Fencl V, Miller TB, Pappenheimer JR: Am J Physiol 210:459, 1966.)

most significant determinant of ventilation in the steady state. The pH of the CSF in the steady state may be accepted as closely approximating the H⁺ of fluids in the chemosensitive areas, and ventilation can be expressed as a function of CSF pH in the steady state different states of acid–base imbalance (Fig. 3). Small changes in CSF pH will alter the level of ventilation profoundly. This is to be contrasted with rather large changes in arterial pH (0.15–0.20 pH units or more) necessary to have any effect on ventilation.

Brain and CSF are unique in their ability to maintain a relatively normal pH in various states of acid–base imbalance by changing their bicarbonate concentrations by greater quantities than plasma to bring their pH back to normal values. All the mechanisms responsible for this difference between the brain–CSF system and blood are not known but probably include an active bicarbonate regulation in the brain–CSF system and impermeability of cell walls to charged ions, as well as specific metabolic changes in the brain. The net result, as far as control of ventilation is concerned, is that the CSF pH will be the significant factor in setting the level of ventilation. The CO_2 ventilatory response curve in chronic respiratory acidosis and alkalosis may be examined to illustrate this point. The CO_2 ventilatory

response curve is depressed in subjects with chronic CO_2 retention, i.e., for a given increase in $P_{a_{CO_2}}$ they do not increase their ventilation as much as subjects with normal $P_{a_{CO_2}}$. The opposite holds true for subjects with chronic hyperventilation (respiratory alkalosis at altitude, for example). These subjects have an enhanced CO_2 ventilatory response curve. CSF bicarbonate concentration is markedly increased in those in chronic respiratory acidosis and is greater than that in blood, with the result that the CSF pH is better compensated. CSF bicarbonate concentration is lower than that in blood in respiratory alkalosis, and again the CSF pH compensation is better. Now, if the $P_{a_{CO_2}}$ is increased by the same amount in normal subjects, those in chronic respiratory acidosis, and those in chronic respiratory alkalosis the relative increase in CSF H⁺ will be greater in those with the least amount of bicarbonate, which are the subjects in chronic respiratory alkalosis, and these are the ones that increase their ventilation the most. Those in chronic respiratory acidosis will increase their ventilation least, since the relative increase in CSF H⁺ in these subjects will be least because of their high initial CSF bicarbonate. The normal subjects will occupy an intermediate position.

The CSF bicarbonate changes are relatively slow to evolve in states of acid–base imbalance, and usually several days (2 or more) are needed to reach a new steady state; by the same token they are slow to disappear when the systemic acid–base imbalance has been corrected. This disparity between CSF and blood has to be borne in mind in management of patients with chronic acid–base imbalance.

Since the H^+ of the CSF is important in control of ventilation, any event in the CNS that leads to changes in CSF H^+ can alter the level of ventilation. CSF acidosis and thus hyperventilation is a common accompanying event of reduced cerebral blood flow (e.g., strokes), cerebral hemorrhage, and possibly meningitis and encephalitis.

Despite the paramount role of the chemosensitive areas in control of ventilation, man can function without them at the cost of depressed alveolar ventilation with the accompanying hypoxemia and hypercapnia. Total lack of central response to CO_2 exists in a condition known as central alveolar hypoventilation (Ondine's curse), where no specific anatomic lesion has been described in the medulla but no ventilatory response to CO_2 can be demonstrated. These subjects have hypoxemia and hypercapnia, and ventilation is probably maintained through the interaction of peripheral chemoreceptors and neural factors. Relative insensitivity of the central chemoreceptors to CO_2 exists in the Pickwickian syndrome, where obesity and alveolar hypoventilation are prominent features.

NEURAL FACTORS

Neural factors, although of significance in control of ventilation, are most likely of secondary importance to chemical factors in control of ventilation. They may become predominant in certain disease states or under special circumstances. The role of the vagus nerve is of singular importance in transmission of afferent impulses (Fig. 1). The vagus is also important in modulating the ventilatory response to CO_2.

An increase in the transmural pressure of the aorta and carotid sinus may lead to apnea, whereas congestion and distention of the pulmonary vessels will cause hyperventilation. Hyperventilation may also occur when the great veins are distended. The exact role of these reflexes in control of ventilation is under investigation. Two categories of reflexes arising from the lungs and the respiratory muscles will be discussed in greater detail.

Hering-Breuer (Stretch) Reflexes

These reflexes arise primarily from the lung parenchyma, and the two significant ones are the inhibito-inspiratory (inflation) reflex and the excito-inspiratory (deflation) reflex. The afferent stimuli travel in the vagus nerve. When the lung is inflated to a given volume, the inhibito-inspiratory reflex is stimulated and electrical activity in the inspiratory muscle ceases and inspiration is inhibited. The excito-inspiratory reflex is stimulated when lung volume is reduced and force and frequency of inspiration are increased. These reflexes are important in modulating the respiratory cycle. The receptors for them are within the lung parenchyma. They are stimulated not only by changes in lung volume but also by congestion of the pulmonary parenchyma, and by other pathologic processes in the lung interstitium. Bronchoconstricting drugs such as acetylcholine, pilocarpine, and histamine can increase stretch receptor discharge. These reflexes are stimulated in lung disease and are of importance in the newborn and in many animals. They may not have a significance in maintaining minute ventilation in normal adult man.

Irritant and Mechanical Reflexes

The receptors for these reflexes are located near the mucosal surface of the tracheobronchial tree, and their stimulation leads to sudden expiratory effort for the mechanical reflex and inspiration followed by expiration for the irritant reflex.

Respiratory Muscles

There is evidence that the respiratory muscles (diaphragm and intercostals) have a stretch reflex similar to that in other striated muscle. This reflex through the gamma system interacts with impulses to the alpha fibers coming from the anterior motor neurons in the spinal cord to maintain appropriate tone and muscle contraction. Thus a local reflex arising from the respiratory muscles interacts with impulses arriving from higher centers to set the level of muscular contraction and thus ventilation.

Other Reflexes

Proprioceptive impulses arising from joints and other muscle groups, as well as impulses from other visceral organs, can and do influence the level of ventilation, but their roles have not been completely understood.

Control of ventilation at exercise still remains a mystery, since none of the control mechanisms described in this section can adequately explain the prompt and marked increase in ventilation seen with exercise.

REFERENCES

Burwell CS, Robin ED, Whaley RD, Bickelmann AG: Extreme obesity associated with alveolar hypoventilation—A Pickwickian syndrome. Am J Med 21:811, 1956

Comroe JH Jr: Regulation of respiration, in Comroe JH (ed): Physiology of Respiration. Chicago, Year Book Medical Publishers, 1965, p 28

Fencl V, Miller TB, Pappenheimer JR: Studies on the respiratory response to disturbances of acid–base balance, with deductions concerning the ionic composition of cerebral interstitial fluid. Am J Physiol 210:459, 1966

Guyton AC: Regulation of Respiration, in Guyton AC (ed): Textbook of Medical Physiology. Philadelphia, WB Saunders, 1956, p 590

Kazemi H, Shannon DC, Carvallo-Gil E: Brain CO_2 buffering capacity in respiratory acidosis and alkalosis. J Appl Physiol 22:241, 1967

Leusen I: Regulation of cerebrospinal fluid composition with reference to breathing. Physiol Rev 52:1, 1972

Mitchell RA, Carman CT, Severinghaus JW, et al: Stability on cerebrospinal fluid pH in chronic acid–base disturbances in blood. J Appl Physiol 20:443, 1965

Mitchell RA: Cerebrospinal fluid and the regulation of respiration, in Caro CG (ed): Advances in Respiratory Physiology. Baltimore, Williams & Wilkins, 1966, p 1

Strieder DJ, Baker WG, Baringer JR, Kazemi H: Chronic hypoventilation of central origin. Am Rev Respir Dis 96: 501, 1967

Wichser J, Kazemi H: CSF bicarbonate regulation in respiratory acidosis and alkalosis. J Appl Physiol 38:504, 1975

EXAMINATION OF PATIENT WITH RESPIRATORY DISEASE

Neil S. Shore

and

Homayoun Kazemi

The clinical assessment of the patient with respiratory disease begins with eliciting his symptoms. The cardinal symptoms of respiratory disease are excessive nasal secretions, cough, expectoration of sputum or blood, dyspnea, wheezing, and chest pain. The patient's background, living habits, and environment may have bearing on his illness. There is a higher incidence of chronic bronchitis in urban areas. Certain areas are notorious for endemic disease, especially those that are fungal in origin. Histoplasmosis is endemic in the valleys of the great rivers, and coccidioidomycosis is found in arid deserts. A detailed and complete occupational history may point to the pattern of disease that is present. Occupational lung disease may present years after the first exposure, as in silicosis or asbestosis, long after the patient may think it irrelevant to his present problem. Since the patient may be exposed without realizing it, one should record the occupations of others with whom the patient lived and such facts as manufacturing plants in the area. Cigarette smoking is important in the pathogenesis of chronic bronchitis and bronchogenic carcinoma. A history of the patient's smoking habits is essential and should include the age at which smoking began, the current daily usage of cigarettes, cigars, or pipe, and the total number of cigarettes smoked during his lifetime. If the patient has stopped smoking, his reasons should be noted, since it may have been because of cough, dyspnea, or wheezing. Close contact with pets or flowering plants may be important. Attacks of bronchial asthma may be precipitated by exposure to dander or pollen.

Certain respiratory diseases have familial incidence, such as asthma, cystic fibrosis, or familial emphysema; it is important to ascertain the familial occurrence of respiratory and allergic disease.

Past illnesses and injuries may be important. For example, childhood measles or pertussis may have led to bronchiectasis; a previous injury may be important as a cause of a fibrothorax. Recurrent pulmonary infections may indicate an underlying immunologic or anatomic cause. An inquiry into nonrespiratory symptoms is necessary since there are respiratory symptoms that result from illnesses primarily of other organs. Respiratory diseases, on the other hand, may have extrathoracic manifestations that help point to the proper diagnosis.

SYMPTOMS AND DIFFERENTIAL DIAGNOSIS

Excessive Nasal Secretions

Nasal secretions are normally swept backward to the pharynx by ciliary action, and one is usually unaware of this. Infection of the upper respiratory tract, irritants, or allergens that induce an allergic response characteristically produce obstruction of the nasal passages, congestion of the nasal mucosa, and outpouring of mucus and frequent sneezing. In allergic states the mucosa appears pale and boggy and the discharge is thin and watery. In infection, the nasal mucosa is hyperemic and the discharge is usually purulent. If the paranasal sinuses are involved, pain may be felt over the corresponding areas of the face and scalp. Excessive nasal secretions may occur premenstrually, during pregnancy, and in males treated with estrogen.

If excessive secretions accumulate, they may be felt in the back of the throat as a "postnasal drip." They may induce coughing or frequent throat clearing. Persons exposed to dry air in heated environs commonly have excessive postnasal secretions. A postnasal discharge is also a complaint of patients with nasal obstruction due to a deviated nasal septum or obstruction and in patients exposed to the chronic irritation of smoke, dust, or fumes.

Cough

A cough may be either a voluntary act or a reflex response to irritation of the respiratory system mediated through the medullary cough center. It consists of a forceful expiratory effort with the glottis closed followed by the sudden explosive release of the pent-up air along with sputum or other matter. Cough may be stimulated by impulses that arise in nerve endings located in the mucous membrane of the pharynx, the esophagus, the pleural surfaces, and the external auditory canal. The smaller bronchi are relatively insensitive, and irritation leads to cough only from stimulation in the larger bronchi.

One must differentiate the cough due to respiratory disease states from the habitual cough of a neurotic patient. Further, while the cough may be initiated in the tracheobronchial tree, the primary cause of the cough may be nonpulmonary; for example, pulmonary congestion due to cardiac failure is often associated with a cough. Since cough occurs in a wide variety of respiratory diseases, it has relatively little differential diagnostic value beyond pointing to the presence of respiratory disease.

Certain characteristics of the cough may be helpful, however. Any tendency of the cough to occur at certain times and the time course of the cough should be noted. Cough and expectoration of sputum are often most troublesome on arising in the morning and going to bed at night, especially with chronic bronchitis and bronchiectasis. A cough awakening the patient at night while lying in bed, although quite common in chronic bronchitis, always suggests the possibility of left ventricular failure. Secretions running down from the posterior nares is another cause of nocturnal cough. A cough occurring on exposure to certain irritants such as smoke or dusts or allergens such as pollen suggests that it is due to that external cause. A cough of recent onset suggests an acute infectious process. Recurrent episodes of cough are a feature of chronic bronchitis. Paroxysms of cough are common in obstructive lung disease. A severe paroxysm of prolonged coughing may result in dizziness, faintness, or even syncope due to the decreased blood return to the heart during the paroxysm. Cough is the most common symptom of pulmonary neoplasm. Involvement of the lung parenchyma is usually accompanied by cough. Cough in interstitial lung disease is usually nonproductive and quite dry and has a tendency to be spasmodic. Pleural disease and pulmonary emboli may also cause a nonproductive cough.

Expectoration of Sputum

Expectoration is the act of producing material by coughing that has originated within the trachea or chest. Postnasal drainages cleared from the pharynx in the morning may be difficult to differentiate from true expectoration. Children and women often swallow any sputum brought up into the pharynx, making it difficult to ascertain that they are expectorating. Healthy people do not expectorate sputum except on exposure to irritants; hence its diagnostic value in pointing to pulmonary disease.

Whenever a patient produces sputum, it is important to determine its color, volume, consistency, and odor. Thick, yellow sputum indicates a bacterial infection. Green sputum from verdoperoxidase from the polymorphonuclear cells indicates stagnant pus in sputum. Viral bronchitis usually causes a white, thin, mucoid sputum. In chronic bronchitis the sputum is usually white or grey, mucoid, and sticky. A change from mucoid to purulent sputum may be the only clinical evidence that an acute infection has occurred in a chronic bronchitic patient. In lung abscess and bronchiectasis, several ounces of purulent, usually foul-smelling sputum are produced daily. Bronchorrhea (the daily expectoration of large quantities of watery sputum) is suggestive of alveolar cell carcinoma. A history of expectoration of multiple, small or large, hard, gritty, calcific masses is almost pathognomonic of broncholithiasis. In acute pulmonary edema the sputum is frothy and pink. Patients with asthma usually cough during attacks and produce small amounts of tenacious, clear sputum.

Expectoration of Blood (Hemoptysis)

Hemoptysis is a relatively common respiratory symptom that is of great importance. First, it is often a manifestation of serious pulmonary disease. Second, it usually causes great apprehension in the patient and causes him to seek medical care. It is important to ascertain that the blood is actually expectorated. Bleeding from the nose or gums or from vomitus may be aspirated and then coughed up, simulating true hemoptysis. At times a patient may not be able to differentiate between coughing and vomiting up of blood. The continued staining of the sputum for some time after the initial event is helpful in distinguishing expectoration of blood from vomiting of blood. Once it is definitely established that the blood is coughed up, one should rule out local sites of bleeding in the nose or mouth before being certain that it is true expectoration of blood.

Hemoptysis is seen in bronchitis, bronchiectasis, pulmonary tuberculosis, and a number of bacterial infections. Hemoptysis is also seen in neoplasms of the respiratory tract. Hemoptysis is unusual in most forms of interstitial pulmonary fibrosis and in emphysema and asthma. Hemoptysis can be present in pulmonary emboli and in any form of heart disease where pulmonary venous pressure is elevated, such as mitral stenosis. Hemoptysis is present in pulmonary hemosiderosis, Goodpasture's syndrome, and any of the disorders involving the pulmonary vascular bed. In any hematologic disorder with a bleeding diathesis, hemoptysis can be the major presenting symptom.

Dyspnea

Dyspnea may be defined as an undue awareness of respiratory effort. A person is not usually aware of his breathing except under circumstances in which ventilation is increased considerably, such as in exercise. When assessing the significance of dyspnea it is essential to determine its mode of onset and severity. The severity is determined by the minimal level of activity that is associated with breathlessness on mild exertion, such as (1) climbing a flight of stairs; (2) breathlessness while walking short distances on the level at an ordinary pace; (3) breathlessness while talking, shaving, washing, etc.; (4) breathlessness at rest.

The symptom of dyspnea, or breathlessness, is one of the more difficult symptoms to ascribe to a specific pathophysiologic abnormality. Most patients with lung disease complain of dyspnea at some point during their illness. Dyspnea can occur in lung disease, in heart disease, and in a host of other disorders where weakness is a prominent symptom. Usually dyspnea begins on exertion, with progression to dyspnea at rest. In terms of lung disease, dyspnea can be present in obstructive disease where there is air-flow obstruction, and the dyspnea is thought to be related to the increased work of breathing. Dyspnea can also be a frequent complaint in patients with interstitial lung disease of any etiology. In this group of disorders, lung compliance is diminished, lungs are stiffer, and more work is required for ventilation; therefore whenever increased ventilation is required, as during exercise or effort, the symptom of dyspnea appears.

In addition to its association with diseases of the lung parenchyma or the airways, dyspnea can also be seen in diseases involving the chest cage, such as kyphoscoliosis, or in neuromuscular disorders. Dyspnea is a common finding in cardiac disease, and it may be difficult in many patients to be certain as to whether dyspnea is of cardiac or respiratory origin. Patients with lung disease usually do not complain of nocturnal dyspnea or orthopnea, whereas those with cardiac disease do. Dyspnea can also be seen in anemia because of inadequate delivery of oxygen to the tissue secondary to low hemoglobin level. Although undoubtedly tissue hypoxemia has a role in development of dyspnea, it is difficult to ascribe dyspnea to any given level of arterial blood oxygenation. Finally, in assessing dyspnea it is well to keep in mind that lack of physical conditioning can be the reason for dyspnea.

Chest Pain

Chest pain can be a common complaint in patients with lung disease. Chest pain can also arise from involvement of the intercostal muscles, the costochondral junction, the sternum, and the ribs. Frequently disease elsewhere, particularly in the cervical vertebrae, can be perceived as chest pain. In terms of thoracic structure, the character of chest pain is quite important in distinguishing cardiac from pulmonary disease. The crushing, radiating anterior chest pain of angina and myocardial infarction can usually be distinguished without difficulty from pain secondary to lung disease. The lung parenchyma itself is free of sensory pain fibers. Therefore for chest pain to arise from the lungs either the pleura or the pulmonary vascular bed must be involved. Pleurisy is usually accompanied by chest pain. The pain is usually localized and made worse by inspiration. Any infection (viral, bacterial, fungal, mycobacterial, or parasitic) that has the component of pleurisy can cause chest pain. The pain of pulmonary embolization is usually pleuritic in nature and is made worse by a deep inspiration; it may be present at all times during the respiratory cycle. Pneumothorax can cause chest pain. On the other hand, diseases of the lung parenchyma or airways, such as interstitial fibrosis, asthma, emphysema, and bronchitis, are not usually associated with chest pain. Pulmonary hypertension can cause some substernal chest discomfort, and this should be kept in mind whenever a patient with pulmonary disease complains of chest pain or substernal discomfort. Other structures within the thorax, especially the esophagus, can cause chest pain, and they should be considered in differential diagnosis of pain in the chest. There may be referred chest pain from disease involving structures below the diaphragm.

PHYSICAL EXAMINATION

A complete physical examination is essential in every patient with respiratory disease. It is obvious from the previous discussion that respiratory disease may produce signs that are referable to other systems. In addition, abnormal physical findings in organs outside the thorax frequently yield valuable clues as to the nature of the respiratory illness. This discussion will concern itself only with the examination of the respiratory system

and those other findings that may be helpful in assessing findings in the respiratory system. As with examination of any other system, one must use inspection, palpation, percussion, and auscultation.

The physical examination should answer the following questions:

1. Is there an abnormality in the upper respiratory system?
2. Is there an abnormality in the thorax or diaphragm?
3. If an abnormality is found in the lungs, is it the pattern of airway obstruction, consolidation, atelectasis, interstitial pulmonary disease, pulmonary edema, pleural effusion, and/or pneumothorax?
4. If abnormalities are present in the lungs, what anatomic part is involved?
5. Is pulmonary hypertension present?
6. Is there evidence of pulmonary heart disease?

Further, the physical examination can point out the presence of respiratory distress, respiratory failure, altered central ventilatory drive, and constitutional or systemic derangements.

Signs

Nose. The patency of each nasal passage should be tested by having the patient sniff through one while the other is obstructed. The inside of the nose should be inspected for a deviated nasal septum that could be a cause of nasal obstruction and chronic infection. Healthy nasal mucosa is smooth, pink, and glistening, but an inflamed mucosa is dull and very red. Allergic nasal mucosa is swollen and pale. A thin, watery discharge is present in allergic rhinitis. The nasal discharge is thick and yellow or green in inflammation. Fresh blood in one of the nasal passages may indicate the source of a recent episode of hemoptysis. One should note the presence of a postnasal discharge and whether it is mucoid or purulent.

Mouth. An odorous breath may result from poor oral hygiene and pyorrhea or from chronic infection of the tonsils, adenoids, or nasal mucosa, or from disease of the lungs such as bronchiectasis or lung abscess. The condition of the gums and teeth should be checked for poor dental care, as pyorrhea may be a factor in a lung abscess. The buccal mucosa may show eruptions, petechial pigmentation, cyanosis, or the reddish purple color associated with polycythemia.

Larynx. Involvement of the larynx may be indicated by the presence of hoarseness or stridor, which is a high-pitched harsh inspiratory noise. Aphonia with a type of cough that seems to lose its explosive character suggests vocal cord paralysis.

Trachea. The trachea is normally in the midline position. A shift is indicative of intrathoracic disease. One determines tracheal position at the lowest portion, just before it enters the thoracic inlet. The tip of the examining finger is inserted into the suprasternal notch and gently pressed back, first on one side and then the other. If the trachea is deviated from its normal position the finger will encounter the cartilaginous ring of the trachea on the side to which the mediastinum has shifted.

Chest. When a pathologic process involves either the lung or the chest wall, the properties of the thorax are altered as to size, shape, movement, and sound transmission.

There are wide variations in the general contours of normal thoracic cage, but the bony structure is normally generally symmetric. This symmetry is related to a straight thoracic spine, so that deformities of the spine such as scoliosis or kyphoscoliosis will produce alterations in the chest cage. Kyphosis will produce alterations also, but not right or left asymmetry. Movement of the chest cage may be reduced by the straight spine or ankylosing spondylitis. Such deformities should be sought by both inspection and palpation of the spinous processes. Abnormalities of the chest wall may be of no functional significance, as in pigeon breast in which there is a marked bulging of the sternum, or funnel chest, an exaggeration of the normal depression seen at the lower end of the sternum, although severe grades of funnel chest may so distort and compress the mediastinum that cardiac and respiratory embarrassment may develop.

Localized bulging or recession of the chest wall may result from aneurysm, empyema, enlarged heart, local disease of the ribs or sternum, or fibrotic changes in the lungs and pleura. Evidence of obstructive lung disease is seen in the barrel-shaped chest caused by hyperinflation of the lungs. There is an increased anterior-posterior diameter, a more horizontal position of the ribs, and an obtuse sternal angle. The chest tends to move up and down en bloc. The diaphragms are percussed low and move little. Movement of the diaphragms may be detected by percussion. Lack of movement or paradoxic rise with inspiration may indicate phrenic nerve paralysis.

Engorged superficial veins over the chest wall, neck, and upper extremities are indicative of an elevated venous pressure resulting from superior vena caval obstruction.

Tender areas should be searched for when the patient complains of chest pain.

It is important to note the movement of the chest cage. Diminished movement of a part of the chest is one of the earliest evidences of localized pulmonary disease. This is best detected by palpation of the thorax during deep breathing.

Lungs. Abnormalities in the lungs may produce no abnormality on physical examination of the chest, as in a solitary neoplastic mass or a viral pneumonia. However, certain pathologic processes can be detected on physical examination and can provide important information not obtainable from the chest x-ray. The abnormal findings so elicited indicate only certain categories of disease and their approximate location. These findings do not yield any information as to the exact etiology or nature of the disease. However, certain morphologic changes usually result in fairly character-

istic abnormal physical signs. The effect on chest size, shape, and movement has already been discussed. The effect on sound transmission provides the remaining information.

Fremitus. Vibrations that are produced over the thoracic wall as a result of the conduction of vocal sounds through the tracheobronchial tree and lung parenchyma are known as vocal fremitus. The traditional method of detection is palpation. The intensity of the fremitus is normally uniform over healthy lungs, except for the apex of the right lung, where intensity is increased because the bronchi are closer to the chest wall. Women, children, and obese patients have less intense fremitus, but this reduction is uniform. Fremitus increases in intensity wherever the density of the underlying lung is increased, as in consolidation or extensive pulmonary fibrosis, so long as the underlying bronchi are patent. Fremitus is decreased or absent when there is fluid or air in the pleural space or when bronchial obstruction leads to atelectasis.

Auscultation. Auscultation with a stethoscope may point to a lung lesion and point to the morphologic type. In addition, it can give important information as to the presence of airway obstruction and the relative ventilation of different parts of the lung.

Breath sounds. Normally one hears the soft rustling quality of vesicular breath sounds with an expiratory phase heard only about one-third as long as the inspiratory phase over the entire chest, except in the right supraclavicular area that overlies the apex of the right lung, where the bronchi, being closer, give a bronchovesicular quality to the breath sounds. In bronchial breathing, such as is normally heard over the trachea, inspiratory and expiratory notes are equal in pitch, intensity, and duration and are separated by a silent interval. Bronchial breath sounds occurring abnormally imply loss of air-containing alveoli surrounding a patent bronchus. Pneumonic consolidation is the classic cause of bronchial breathing. Various forms of bronchial breathing occur in an open pneumothorax (amphoric) and cavities (cavernous). The pitch or tone of the bronchial breathing is like blowing over a narrow bottleneck in amphoric breathing and like breathing in a tumbler in cavernous breathing, but otherwise it has the characteristics of bronchial breathing.

Diminished breath sounds occur with increased distance between the lung and stethoscope, as in obesity. They also occur with emphysema and markedly decreased ventilation. Localized areas of diminished or absent breath sounds point to localized atelectasis.

Whispered pectoriloquy. Normal lung parenchyma does not transport high-frequency vibrations set up by whispering "one, two, three." However, when lung tissue is consolidated it loses this quality, and the whispered sound is transmitted to the chest wall with great clarity. This is helpful in detecting small consolidated lesions.

Egophany. A peculiar form of voice transmission is sometimes heard over solid lung or more frequently at the upper limit of a pleural effusion. It has a high-pitched nasal quality likened to the bleating of a goat and is called egophany. In particular, a spoken E is heard as A.

Adventitious sounds. Abnormal vibrations produced by pathologic processes in the tracheobronchial tree or lung parenchyma are called adventitious sounds. Their presence always indicates pathology.

Rhonchi. Rhonchi are prolonged musical or whistling notes produced in the lumen of the tracheobronchial tree. They are indicative of increased turbulence, presumably due to narrowed lumens. Therefore one expects them to be more pronounced during expiration. The pitch of the rhonchus depends on the diameter of the bronchus in which it is produced—the smaller the tube, the higher the pitch. A persistent rhonchus localized to one portion of the chest wall signifies localized partial obstruction. Equal distribution of rhonchi indicates diffuse bronchial obstruction, as in asthma. Wheezes are rhonchi of higher pitch.

Wheezing. Wheezing is present most often in bronchial asthma, but it is well to keep in mind that other forms of obstructive lung disease, such as bronchitis, may also be associated with wheezing. The wheezing of asthma and bronchitis is usually generalized. A localized wheeze usually signifies focal and limited obstruction of a large airway in that part of the lung. This is most often seen with neoplasms, but also may be present with bronchial inflammation. Wheezing can also be seen in cardiac disease with congestion of the pulmonary vascular bed and parenchyma, so-called cardiac asthma. Wheezing may be present in frank pulmonary edema. In addition to the diseases affecting the airways and the lung parenchyma, certain disorders of the pulmonary vascular bed may also be associated with wheezing. In particular, pulmonary embolism may have an associated wheeze. The reasons for this are not entirely clear, but are probably related to bronchoconstriction in the area of the lung supplied by the obstructed vessel secondary to the diminished P_{CO_2} in airways because of absence of blood flow in that part of the lung. In addition, there may be release of certain substances from the thrombus that act on the smooth muscle of the bronchi and bring about bronchospasm. Wheezing may also result from alveolar hyperventilation secondary to exercise or anxiety in some subjects.

Stridor. Stridor may be thought of as a special kind of wheeze brought about by narrowing of the tracheal lumen or larynx, so that air flow through the upper airways makes a noise that is audible to the patient or his physician. It can be best heard by placing the stethoscope over the trachea. In adults stridor usually implies an obstructing lesion of the upper airway that can be a primary neoplasm of the trachea or carcinoma of the thyroid with invasion of the trachea, or other malignant processes in the mediastinum may result in compression of the trachea. Stridor can also be heard in tracheal stenosis, which may occur 6 or more weeks following tracheostomy or endotracheal intubation of several days' duration usually for assisted ventilation.

Râles. Râles are short, disconnected bubbling sounds that are heard most readily during inspiration, in contrast to the musical sounds of rhonchi, which are heard best during expiration. The pitch of the râle depends on the size of the chamber involved, as well as on the type of lesion producing it. Râles may be classified according to pitch and position during inspiration, which in turn may yield information about their site of production. Low-pitched râles heard in the initial third of the inspiratory phase suggest that secretions are present in the large and medium-sized bronchi. Medium-pitched râles heard during the middle third of the inspiratory phase suggest that smaller bronchi are involved. High-pitched or fine râles heard during the terminal third of inspiration suggest that the lung parenchyma (that is, alveoli) are involved. If the disease in the alveoli is very slight, râles may not be elicited by an ordinary deep inspiration. They can often be brought out, however, by having the patient inspire and expire deeply, and then cough. A shower of fine râles may then be heard during the initial phase of the ensuing inspiration. These are called post-tussive râles.

Conversely, râles that are heard during ordinary breathing may disappear following a cough, indicating that the secretions producing the râles have been moved up higher in the tree by active coughing. Dry-end inspiratory râles that are very close to the ear and sound like the crackling of cellophane are usually due to interstitial lung disease, most often interstitial fibrosis of any etiology. Moist râles heard through most of the respiratory cycle usually imply the presence of some fluid and exudate and can be heard in inflammatory disease of the lung, such as pneumonia, as well as in congestive heart failure with pulmonary congestion. Sticky and sibilant râles can usually be heard with inspissation of material in the alveoli or small airways. Such râles can best be heard in infections of the lung parenchyma, such as pneumonitis, as well as in chronic bronchitis. Sticky râles may be heard over areas of atelectasis.

Pleural rub. Pleural rub is a creaking, leathery sound that seems to be close to the examining ear and is heard at the end of inspiration and the beginning of expiration. This friction rub is diagnostic of pleural irritation and is most likely produced by the rubbing of inflamed surfaces of the pleural layers against each other in respiration. Since the excursion of the pleural surface is greatest over the lower lobes, friction rubs are most frequently detected in the lower parts of the chest; only very occasionally are they heard over the upper areas. A creaky, interrupted, dry sound characteristically extends uniformly throughout the whole of inspiration and expiration and may be heard when there is gross fibrosis affecting the lung parenchyma including the peribronchial tissues.

PULMONARY HEART DISEASE

There are no abnormal signs in the lung that are indicative of increased pulmonary vascular resistance. This can only be elicited by examination of the heart. Respiratory disease may lead to an increase in pulmonary vascular resistance, or there may be important changes in pulmonary vascular resistance and consequent development of pulmonary hypertension. It is important that these signs be elicited. The position and character of the cardiac impulse, if visible, should be noted during inspection of the chest. A heave over the hypertrophied right ventricle just to the left of the lower half of the sternum can be felt in cases of right ventricular hypertrophy of pulmonary hypertension. There is often an associated zone and conspicuous retraction over the left ventricle lateral to the heave that gives the pericardium a characteristic rocking motion. In addition, systolic expansion of a dilated pulmonary artery can produce a visible pulsation in the left upper parasternal area.

Palpation, particularly over the pulmonic area, may reveal vibrations associated with an accentuated pulmonic sound, indicating that pulmonary hypertension is present. On auscultation the intensity of a second pulmonic heart sound should be noted because it is increased when pulmonary hypertension is present. The pulmonic second sound is normally split, and this is accentuated during inspiration because of the prolongation of right ventricular systole as a result of its increased filling during inspiration. If this split does not widen during inspiration, this further suggests the presence of pulmonary hypertension. On the other hand, a prolonged split of the second pulmonic sound during inspiration is probably caused by delay in closure of the pulmonic valve that is usually the result of bundle branch block or mild pulmonary stenosis. A high-pitched systolic ejection click in the pulmonic area is also indicative of pulmonary hypertension. This occurs during systole just after the opening of the pulmonic valve at the end of the period of isometric contraction. It is almost invariably found in patients with large left-to-right shunts, mild pulmonic stenosis, or dilation of the pulmonary artery.

EXTRATHORACIC MANIFESTATIONS

Respiratory disease may also be manifested by signs in distant sites, and the most important of these are clubbing of the digits, pulmonary osteoarthropathy, and some systemic manifestations that occur in patients suffering from pulmonary malignancy.

Clubbing of the Digits

Clubbing consists of a painless, nontender enlargement of the terminal phalanges of the fingers and toes and is usually a bilateral condition. Initially there is hypertrophy of the soft tissues covering the root of the nail, so that the angle formed by the root of the nail and the nail bed (normally about 160 deg) becomes 180 deg or more. As clubbing progresses, the skin becomes stretched and glistening. The nail gradually thickens and becomes curved, developing longitudinal ridges; the pulp of the terminal phalanges enlarges and develops a bulbous appearance. Clubbing usually progresses slowly, taking months or years to develop. Occasionally it may develop acutely in a week or so if the underlying intrathoracic lesion is an acute septic process. Regression and even disappearance of digital clubbing may take place if the underlying lesion is eradicated by either medical or surgical treatment.

The exact mechanism leading to clubbing in apparently unrelated diseases is as yet unexplained but is open to conjecture. At present an attractive hypothesis is the liberation of some peptides, which results in the changes seen as clubbing.

Clubbing of the fingers and the toes can be of great diagnostic significance. It is most commonly associated with intrathoracic malignancy, such as bronchogenic carcinoma or pleural mesothelioma. It may also occur with suppurative disease of the lungs such as lung abscess, empyema, and bronchiectasis. It occurs in certain congenital lesions of the heart (pulmonary vascular disease associated with right-to-left shunting), and it occurs in some cases of bacterial endocarditis. Clubbing is seen in patients suffering from disease of the liver or the gastrointestinal tract, such as ulcerative colitis and steatorrhea. It also may occur as a familial form indicating no underlying disease.

Hypertrophic Pulmonary Osteoarthropathy

Hypertrophic pulmonary osteoarthropathy is a condition in which there is clubbing with painful, tender thickening of the wrists, the ankles, and the long bones of the forearms and the legs. The basic pathologic process is proliferating subperiostitis with subperiosteal new bone formation, which involves symmetrically the distal segments of the long bones of the arms and legs and thickening of the connective tissue. The joints of the knees, the ankles, and the wrists often develop an effusion that is clear and viscous and may be associated with a synovitis. It is often associated with pulmonary neoplasms.

Cyanosis

Cyanosis is a common accompaniment of diseases of the lung and the heart and is best perceived by looking at the mucous membranes and the nail beds. Cyanosis is usually appreciated when about 5 g of unsaturated hemoglobin are present. Presence of cyanosis usually means hypoxemia. Cyanosis is usually perceived by most examiners when the arterial oxygen saturation is less than 85 percent. However, significant degrees of hypoxemia can exist with cyanosis not being appreciated by the observer. Cyanosis can also be present with stasis that might occur with a very low cardiac output. With cyanosis present, heart or lung disease should be suspected. However, in the presence of significant heart and lung disease, cyanosis may not be observed, and its absence does not imply the absence of hypoxemia. This is particularly true if anemia is present. Methemoglobi-

Table 1
Patterns of Lung Dysfunction

| TEST | TYPE OF PHYSIOLOGIC IMPAIRMENT | | |
	Obstructive	Restrictive	Interstitial
Ventilatory tests			
Vital capacity (VC)	Normal or decreased	Decreased	Normal
Forced expiratory volume in 1 sec (FEV_1)	Decreased	Normal	Normal
Peak flow rate (PFR)	Decreased	Normal	Normal
Maximum breathing capacity (MBC)	Decreased	Normal	Normal
Lung volumes			
Total lung capacity (TLC)	Normal or slightly increased	Decreased	Normal
Functional residual capacity (FRC)	Increased	Normal or decreased	Normal
Residual volume (RV)	Increased	Normal or slightly decreased	Normal
RV/TLC ratio	Increased	Normal or slightly increased	Normal
Ventilation and air mixing			
Minute ventilation ($\dot{V}_E$)	Increased	Increased	Increased
Alveolar ventilation ($\dot{V}_A$)	Normal or decreased	Normal or increased	Normal or increased
Dead space/tidal volume (V_D/V_T ratio)	Increased	Normal or increased	Normal or increased
N_2 washout or helium equilibration time	Increased	Normal	Normal
Lung mechanics			
Airway resistance	Increased	Normal	Normal
Compliance	Increased	Decreased	Decreased
Gas Exchange			
Arterial P_{O_2} ($P_{a_{O_2}}$) at rest	Decreased	Decreased	Decreased (occ. normal)
$P_{a_{O_2}}$ on exercise	Usually same as at rest or increased	Further decreased	Decreased
Alveolar–arterial O_2 gradient (A-aD_{O_2})			
on room air	Increased	Increased	Increased
on 100% O_2	Slightly increased	Normal; increased late in disease	Normal
Arterial P_{CO_2} (P_{aCO_2})	Normal or increased	Normal or decreased	Normal or decreased
Diffusing capacity (D_L)	Decreased	Decreased	Decreased

nemia of toxic or congenital origin can also cause cyanosis, as well as sulfhemoglobinemia.

FUNCTIONAL EVALUATION
OF THE PULMONARY SYSTEM

The clinical assessment of a patient with respiratory disease needs to include functional evaluation of the lungs just as much as a history and physical examination. This is done using various tests of pulmonary function. No one test alone is able to give an overall assessment of function, for it is the pattern that defines the physiologic abnormalities present. These tests also provide for quantitation of the degree of malfunction, thereby allowing for objective follow-up and for determination of the effect of therapeutic measures suggested by the disturbed pulmonary function. In the case of planned surgery such tests help to assess the patient's ability to tolerate anesthetic and narcotics or the removal of lung tissue, and they serve as a guide in the preparation of postoperative care for the patient. Since groups of diseases many times produce a specific pattern of physiologic impairment, these studies may assist in establishing the correct diagnosis of the respiratory condition. However, different disease processes can produce the same physiologic impairment, and functional evaluation sometimes cannot establish a specific etiologic diagnosis.

Tests of lung function vary from simple measurements of vital capacity to the use of gaseous radioisotopes to determine regional ventilation and blood flow. The tests fall into two general groups: tests relating to the ventilatory function of the lungs and chest wall mechanics and tests relating to gas exchange.

Three principal patterns of lung dysfunction have been identified by physiologic testing: (1) obstructive, as in chronic bronchitis, emphysema, and asthma; (2) restrictive, which includes all those processes causing a reduction in lung volume; (3) interstitial, where there is an abnormal pattern of gas exchange without obstruction to air flow or reduction in lung volume. The interstitial pattern often becomes restrictive as the disease progresses. The major patterns of abnormalities are summarized in Table 1.

Lung function tests can be divided into major groups.

Ventilatory Tests

Ventilatory tests are relatively easy to perform. They provide significant information as screening tests or for evaluation of patients with lung disease. They

LUNG VOLUMES

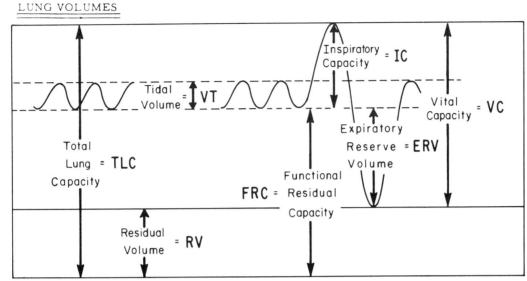

Fig. 1. Schematic presentation of total lung capacity (TLC) and its subdivisions. Vital capacity (VC) and its subdivisions are measured directly by spirometry. The residual volume (RV) is measured indirectly by dilution of an inert gas, such as helium, or by plethysmography.

require the cooperation of the patient and must be interpreted in that light.

Vital capacity is the volume of air exhaled after a full inspiration. Normal values have been established by measurements of large groups of healthy subjects. The normal value is a function of the person's height, age, and sex. The measured value is compared with the predicted normal, and values within 20 percent of the predicted are accepted as normal. Vital capacity can be diminished by congestive heart failure, pulmonary fibrosis, and obstructive emphysema, as well as a host of other disorders; it is thus nonspecific as far as particular disease entities are concerned, but is helpful in quantitating the degree of impairment. It rarely is increased beyond the upper limits of predicted.

Information about airway resistance may be obtained from tests based on determining the rate at which air flows out of the lungs during expiration. A simple test is the analysis of the forced expiratory vital capacity maneuver (FVC). The analysis of the forced vital capacity is commonly done by calculating the volume of air expelled during a particular period of time. The first-second volume is most commonly used (FEV$_1$). In normal individuals this may vary from 70 percent to 85 percent of vital capacity, the value normally falling with age. Reduction in FEV$_1$ means airway obstruction and is abnormal in persons with obstructive lung disease, but usually normal in those with restrictive lung disease. In adults, an FEV$_1$ of less than 1 l signifies severe ventilatory impairment.

Other common measures are those of expiratory air flow rates that can be measured at various points in the respiratory cycle, one of the easiest being the peak expiratory flow rate (PFR) measured by the peak flow meter. The maximum mid-expiratory flow rate (MMFR,

the velocity in liters per second of expiration over the middle third of the total volume expired) is another measure and is perhaps more sensitive.

Not all of these analyses are equally informative, however. It appears that the MMFR is more sensitive than the PFR, which is more sensitive yet than the FEV$_1$ in detecting obstructive disease.

In obstructive airway diseases these indices of air flow resistance are all sharply reduced. On the other hand, in patients with a reduced compliance but no associated airway obstruction, as in diffuse pulmonary fibrosis, flow rates are usually normal.

Measurements of air flow rates at large lung volumes reflect mainly the resistance in the large airways. Flows at low lung volumes, such as 25 percent of vital capacity, are sensitive to changes in the small airways. This information can be obtained most readily by recording the flow-volume loop.

The maximum breathing capacity (MBC) is another test of lung function that depends to a great extent on adequate air flow rates. The test is performed by asking the patient to breathe as hard and as fast as possible for a given period of time, usually 15 sec. Then the volume of expired air is collected and measured and the final value expressed as liters per minute. Since maximum ventilation can be obtained only by voluntary effort, the subject must be encouraged constantly during the performance of the test, and the examiner must be convinced that the patient has made a maximal effort before interpreting a low value as being abnormal. The relationship between MBC and FEV$_1$ is moderately close. A reduced MBC points to obstructive lung disease. In fact, in restrictive lung disease the MBC is usually normal, and even a reduction of vital capacity to 50 percent of predicted may not reduce the MBC. The MBC may be reduced in neuromuscular disorders such as myasthenia gravis, in which muscle fatigue is the causative factor.

If the ventilatory tests give abnormal results, the patient should be given a bronchodilator such as isoproternol by inhalation and the tests repeated to check the presence of a reversible component in the obstructive phenomena.

Static Lung Volumes

Static lung volumes can be measured by means of the body plethysmograph or, except for the residual volume, by means of simple spirometry. The residual volume (RV, volume of gas left in the lungs after full expiration) can be measured by dilution techniques using either helium or nitrogen as a reference gas. In practice one usually measures the functional residual capacity (FRC), that is, the volume of gas in the lungs at the end of tidal expiration. Residual volume is then calculated by subtraction of the expiratory reserve volume (ERV) from the FRC (Fig. 1). The total lung capacity (TLC), that is, the total volume of gas in the lung, is calculated either by addition of the vital capacity to the residual volume or by addition of the FRC and the inspiratory capacity (IC). Lung volumes vary with age, height, and sex. Tables of normal predicted values are available, and measured values differing by more than ±20 percent of predicted are considered abnormal.

A reduction in lung volume would suggest the presence of restrictive lung disease, which may be due to either reduced distensibility of the lung, as in pulmonary fibrosis, or reduced distensibility of the chest wall, as in kyphoscoliosis. An increase in lung volume indicates that the lungs are hyperinflated because of obstruction of the airways, as in asthma, or because of a loss of elasticity in addition to airway obstruction, as in obstructive emphysema. The residual volume normally increases with age from approximately 20 percent of total lung capacity in a young person to as high as 40 percent of total lung capacity in an elderly healthy person. An increase in the residual volume or in the ratio of residual volume to total lung capacity (RV/TLC ratio) beyond that predicted for one's age reflects hyperinflation of the lung. Hyperinflation is present in emphysema, but not all patients exhibiting hyperinflated lungs have emphysema.

Pulmonary Mechanics

Resistance and compliance. Airway resistance (the pressure required to move a given volume of air through the airways per unit time) is increased in patients with obstructive lung disease and is normal or slightly diminished in patients with restrictive lung disease. Compliance of the lung (the amount of air introduced into the lung for a given pressure) is a reflection of the distensibility of the lung. The lung becomes stiffer and compliance is therefore decreased in restrictive lung disease, such as interstitial fibrosis or pulmonary edema. Static compliance is increased in obstructive emphysema, i.e., the lungs are more distensible because of destruction of tissue and loss of elastic recoil.

Resistance of airways and to a lesser extent compliance of the lung and the thorax are reflected in the ventilatory tests, particularly the timed vital capacity and maximal breathing capacity. Direct measurement of these parameters has value in specific instances. Obstruction of small airways will alter the distribution of mechanical time constants in the lung and will influence the distribution of inspired gas, particularly when the respiratory frequency is increased. Thus changes in dynamic lung compliance with increasing respiratory frequency are indicative of uneven distribution of the time constant throughout the lung; therefore, in the absence of large-airway disease, it is a reflection of small-airway disease. Small-airway disease also leads to premature airway closure, i.e., airways collapse at a higher transpulmonary pressure than normal. Therefore a greater than expected closing volume is measured in subjects with obstructive disease affecting the small airways (see the chapter Physical Factors in Lung Function).

Ventilation. Minute ventilation (volume of air exhaled or inhaled per minute) is increased when metabolic demands increase and when there are pulmonary pathologic findings. The amount of ventilation in relation to oxygen uptake (ventilatory equivalent) is an index of the efficiency of the respiratory system, and its increase suggests abnormalities in the lungs.

The volume of air inhaled per breath is the tidal volume, V_T. The fraction of V_T that does not participate in gas exchange because it goes to areas of the respiratory tract where there is no pulmonary blood flow is known as dead-space volume, V_D. Trachea and bronchi, as well as alveoli devoid of blood flow, constitute the dead space. Minute ventilation minus dead-space ventilation equals alveolar ventilation, $\dot{V}_A$, which is the fraction of ventilation utilized in gas exchange.

Elevation of the ratio of dead space to tidal volume (V_D/V_T ratio) means increased wasted ventilation and work of breathing. Normally the V_D/V_T ratio is less than 35 percent. It is significantly increased in pulmonary embolization and may be increased in other diseases of the pulmonary vasculature, as well as obstructive lung disease and late in restrictive lung disease.

Distribution of inspired air. Minute ventilation is a measurement of volume of air entering and leaving the lungs per unit time. How well this volume of air mixes in the lungs is of critical importance in pulmonary gas exchange. Poor mixing of inspired air leads to maldistribution of ventilation and to ventilation/perfusion inequality and thus ultimately to gas-exchange impairment. Adequacy of mixing of inspired air can be evaluated by several techniques. The two most commonly used are the nitrogen washout time and the helium equilibration time. In the former, the patient breathes pure oxygen in a closed system, and nitrogen concentration of expired air is monitored at the expiratory port. The concentration of end-tidal nitrogen falls to less than 2.5 percent in normal subjects after 7 min of oxygen breathing.

The helium equilibration time is determined by

having the subject rebreathe in a spirometer that has the inert gas (helium) in it. At the beginning the helium is present in the spirometer only, but as rebreathing continues the concentration of helium in the spirometer falls, since a larger volume, the volume of air in the lungs, is added to the system. Eventually helium becomes completely equilibrated in the lung–spirometer system, and a helium analyzer in line with the spirometer records no further fall in the helium concentration. The time taken to reach the equilibration point is a function of mixing of the inspired air in the lungs, and in normal subjects less than 2.5 to 3 min are required for this to occur. Both the nitrogen washout time and the helium equilibration time are prolonged in obstructive lung disease but normal in restrictive and interstitial disorders.

Gas exchange. Abnormalities in gas exchange are reflected in abnormal values of arterial P_{O_2} and P_{CO_2} or both. In many patients abnormality in gas exchange may be slight while at rest and become apparent only during exercise. Assessment of gas exchange should therefore be carried out both at rest and during exercise. Partial pressures of oxygen and carbon dioxide and the pH in the arterial blood are measured directly by appropriate electrodes. The bicarbonate concentration of plasma is calculated using the Henderson-Hasselbalch equation.

Normally $P_{a_{CO_2}}$ is kept at 36 to 44 mm Hg throughout adult life, with arterial pH at 7.36 to 7.44 and plasma bicarbonate at 24–26 meq/l. The normal value for $P_{a_{O_2}}$ varies with age. The normal value for a 20-year-old is approximately 95 mm Hg, with a rate of decline with advancing age of approximately 0.4 mm Hg per year in the supine position after age 20.

A decrease in the partial pressure of oxygen in arterial blood is a common feature in patients with cardiorespiratory disease. Although its specific causes are many, a lowered arterial oxygen tension is due to three pathophysiologic mechanisms: alveolar hypoventilation, right-to-left shunting (venous admixture), and ventilation/perfusion inequality. The first is accompanied by elevation of arterial carbon dioxide tension. The other causes of hypoxemia require careful evaluation, which can be done by measuring the alveolar–arterial oxygen tension difference ($A-aD_{O_2}$). The $A-aD_{O_2}$ is increased with both right-to-left shunting and ventilation/perfusion inequality. When breathing room air the normal $A-aD_{O_2}$ is up to 15 mm Hg in a young individual and increases with age up to 25 mm Hg at 70. The $A-aD_{O_2}$ on breathing 100 percent O_2 reflects right-to-left shunting, and its value can be used to calculate the fraction of cardiac output being shunted (see the chapter Oxygen and Carbon Dioxide Transport).

Another possible pathophysiologic mechanism of hypoxemia is reduction in diffusing capacity of the lung or the transfer factor (see the chapter Physical Factors in Lung Function, section on diffusion). Transfer factor of the lung can be measured by using oxygen or carbon monoxide as the reference gas. The carbon monoxide diffusing capacity ($D_{L_{co}}$) is commonly used, and there are several available techniques. The $D_{L_{co}}$ decreases with age, partly because of increasing ventilation perfusion inequality. It also decreases with anemia, because hemoglobin is necessary for removal of carbon monoxide. Diffusing capacity may be diminished in obstructive lung disease and is invariably diminished in interstitial and restrictive disorders.

The level of arterial P_{CO_2} is governed by the alveolar ventilation. Elevated P_{CO_2} indicates alveolar hypoventilation, and reduced P_{CO_2} indicates alveolar hyperventilation.

Hypoxemia may be present in all forms of lung disease, whereas hypercapnia is more often associated with obstructive lung disease.

Regional function. Assessment of regional blood flow, volume, and ventilation in lungs can be made by use of radioactive isotopes and appropriate external detection devices. These measurements are of value in localizing disease process in the lungs or in evaluating the effects of generalized disease on regional function. Abnormalities of regional function can be present in both obstructive and restrictive lung disease and when the pulmonary vascular bed is involved. These are discussed in detail in the chapter Radioisotopes in Lung Diseases.

REFERENCES

Bates DV, Macklem PT, Christie RV: Respiratory Function in Disease. Philadelphia, WB Saunders, 1971, chapters 2 and 3, p 10

Boren HG, Kory RC, Snyder JC: The Veterans Administration-army cooperative study of pulmonary function: II. The lung volume and its subdivisions in normal men. Am J Med 41:96, 1968

Chamberlain EN, Ogilvie C: Symptoms and Signs in Clinical Medicine. Baltimore, Williams & Wilkins, 1967

Cherniak RM, Cherniak L, Naimark A: Respiration in Health and Disease. Philadelphia, WB Saunders, 1972

Comroe JH Jr, Nadel JA: Screening tests of pulmonary function. N Engl J Med 282:1249, 1970

Kazemi H: Pulmonary-function tests. JAMA 206:2302, 1968

Kory RC, Callahan R, Boren HG, Snyder JC: The Veterans Administration-army cooperative study of pulmonary function. I. Clinical spirometry in normal men. Am J Med 30:243, 1961

RADIOLOGY OF CHEST DISEASES

Reginald Greene

RADIOLOGIC TECHNIQUES

The marked differences in the radiation absorption characteristics of air and soft tissue make the lungs ideally suited to examination by radiologic techniques. Plain chest radiographs obtained using 6- to 10-ft tube-film distances keep distortion and magnification to a minimum. Maximal sharpness and minimal magnification (about 10 percent) are obtained for those chest parts closest to the film.

A normal examination consists of two radiographs obtained at right angles to each other which give three-dimensional information. A lateral view complements the frontal radiograph by clearly showing the large volume of the lower lobes which extend deeply below the domes of the diaphragm. Various other views have particular uses. The lordotic view minimizes the obscuring effects of the ribs and clavicles at the lung apices by passing the horizontal x-ray beam from front to back with the patient standing in a hyperlordotic posture. It is useful for detecting apical tuberculosis or demonstrating abnormalities in the right middle lobe and lingula. Lateral decubitus examinations with a horizontal beam can detect small pleural effusions by layering them out in the deep sulcus along the lateral chest wall. When pleural fluid is suspected both left and right decubitus views ought to be obtained to establish the fluid nature of the abnormality and to provide a clear view of the lung, which is obscured by the pleural fluid (Fig. 1).

The appearance of the chest radiograph depends critically on the lung volume at which it is obtained, and consistency of interpretation requires that a standard degree of inspiration is used. A most convenient lung volume is maximum inspiration, since this is the most easily reproducible maneuver for patients to make and provides the maximum contrast between air and soft tissue. Extreme caution should be taken in the interpretation of radiographs obtained after shallow inspirations, because what appear to be consolidations frequently turn out to be normal crowded pulmonary vessels (Fig. 2). Maximum-expiration radiographs, which indicate the configuration of the chest at residual volume, are useful in detecting trapped gas (Fig. 3) and diaphragmatic paralysis. Radiographic measurements of

thoracic gas volume have been found to correlate well with body plethysmographic measurements and can be used to calculate the residual volume when the vital capacity is known. When maximum inspiration is used for chest radiography, reduced lung volume indicates a fall in total lung capacity. This can be a reflection of restriction of chest wall movement as in pleural diseases, reduced lung compliance as in interstitial lung diseases, or reduced muscle power as in neuromuscular disorders.

A great deal of anatomic and physiologic information can be obtained from the careful use of plain chest radiography, but other kinds of radiologic studies such as fluoroscopy yield dynamic information by providing continuous imaging during respiration. For example, inspiration and expiration radiographs may show a totally paralyzed hemidiaphragm, but fluoroscopy can also show varying degrees of diaphragmatic paresis and dyskinesia that would otherwise be missed. Areas with air trapping are easily shown by inspiration–expiration radiographs, but areas of increased airway resistance without air trapping can be detected only by fluoroscopy. The regional deflation (or inflation) of the lung as seen on radiographs after a slow expiration (or inspiration) primarily reflects regional compliance. During these slow maneuvers there is enough time for regions with increased airflow resistance short of air trapping to empty. Radiographs obtained after 1 sec of a full maximum expiration would reflect regional variations in air-flow resistance and be the radiographic analogue of the FEV_1 (first-second vital capacity). Fluoroscopic studies during rapid inspiration (sniffing) or rapid expiration indicate regional variations in resistance. If, for instance, there is a nonobstructing mass in the right mainstem bronchus that increases air-flow resistance short of air trapping, radiographs may detect no abnormality but a fluoroscopic examination during a rapid in-

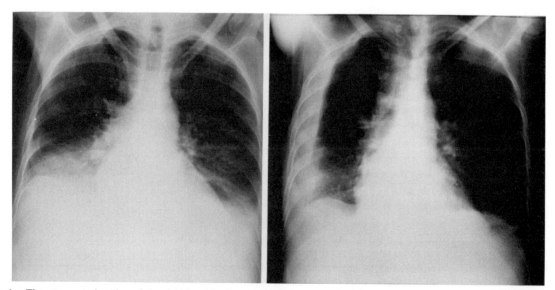

Fig. 1. The apparent elevation of the right hemidiaphragm on the x-ray on the left is actually pleural fluid on which the lung is floating and is clearly shown by the lateral decubitus on the right. Notice the layer of pleural fluid separating the lung from the rib cage. There is also a small left pleural effusion.

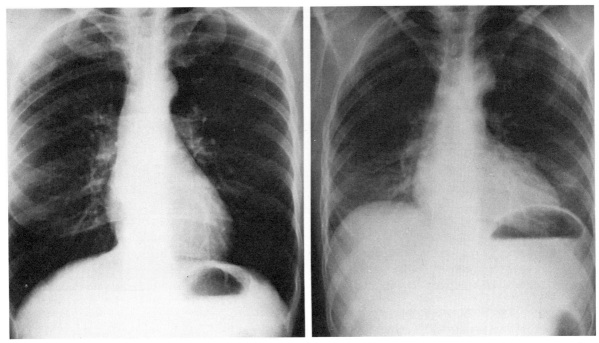

Fig. 2. On the left is a radiograph taken after maximum inspiration, and on the right is one taken of the same normal individual after maximum expiration. Notice the illusionary cardiac enlargement and basal consolidations in the expiration film.

spiration may show a sudden temporary shift of the midline structures to the right, reflecting better air movement into the left lung.

Tomography allows clear visualization of poorly defined densities that are obscured by overlying structures. The combined movement of the x-ray tube and film

is arranged so that the tube–object and object–film distances are kept constant only for a certain plane through the chest. Structures outside the plane of interest are blurred, and those within the plane are sharply defined. Cavities, blood vessels, airways, and fine calcifications can be well shown in this way (Fig. 4). The

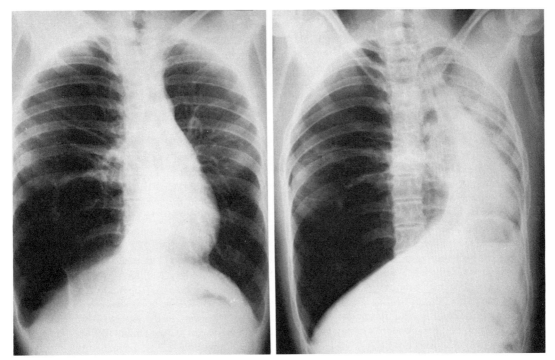

Fig. 3. The maximum inspiratory film on the left shows noticeable bullae at the right base, but the extent of air trapping is surprising in the expiratory film on the right. Notice the marked mediastinal shift to the left after emptying of the normal left lung.

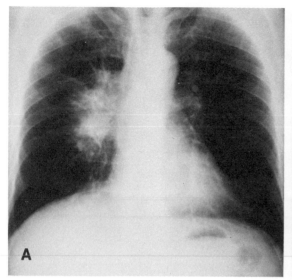 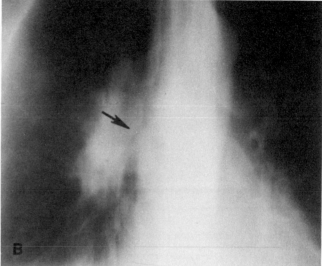

Fig. 4. *A.* A frontal view of the chest demonstrates a right hilar mass. The detailed configuration of the right bronchial tree is not evident from this study. *B.* A tomographic section through the bronchial tree shows marked irregular narrowing of the intermediate bronchus (arrow) by a bronchogenic carcinoma.

careful use of tomography can reduce the number of more complicated and hazardous studies of the lungs.

All of the radiographic procedures described thus far are noninvasive. For detailed visualization of structures with very poor intrinsic contrast, artificial contrast may be required. During bronchography contrast material is used to outline the normally thin-walled air-filled bronchi. For this purpose agents generally composed of liquid iodine are introduced via the nose, mouth, or cricothyroid membrane into the bronchi. The technique is useful for demonstrating the bronchial distortions of bronchitis, bronchiectasis, tumors, and foreign bodies. Liquid contrast agents temporarily interfere with gas exchange in the filled lung segments, and as a result care must be taken in examining patients with impaired lung function.

Anomalous pulmonary vessels can frequently be very well defined by tomography, but various dynamic data such as the patency of vessels to blood flow can only be shown by arteriography. Serial radiographs obtained after the rapid injection of an iodinated contrast medium into the pulmonary artery reflect grossly the regional distribution of pulmonary blood flow. The detailed opacification of pulmonary vessels is particularly useful in detecting intravascular clots and blood-vessel invasion by tumors.

Bronchial brushing and aspiration needle biopsy can provide material for culture and cytology. Both procedures require high resolution fluoroscopic imaging and are best done with a biplane fluoroscope. Brushing procedures are carried out with bronchographic catheters through which fine nylon or steel brushes are inserted to obtain samples. With fluoroscopic imaging directable catheters and brushes can be introduced directly into the precise bronchus or area in question (Fig. 5). It is particularly useful for obtaining cytologic material from central or peripheral endobronchial lesions that are beyond the

view of the bronchoscope. Aspiration biopsy through a fine-gauge needle is a direct, relatively safe, and expeditious way of obtaining material from pulmonary parenchymal lesions. It is a particularly suitable biopsy method in patients in whom surgical or other treatment would be expedited by a precise cytologic or bacteriologic diagnosis. Aspiration needle biopsy has been used primarily in patients for whom diagnostic thoracotomy carries a substantial risk and those in whom incurable cancer is the likely but not established diagnosis.

AIRSPACE DISEASE

The airspaces include the conducting airways and the peripheral gas-exchanging spaces with their covering epithelia. Conducting airways extend from the larynx and cartilaginous trachea to the small (0.5 mm) terminal bronchioles that are devoid of cartilage. The peripheral airspaces include all lung units distal to the terminal bronchioles (acini).

Abnormalities of the conducting airways include bronchial masses, foreign bodies, thickening, irregularity, ectasia, and unusual flaccidity. Intraluminal masses may be seen as opacities in the central airways on well-penetrated radiographs. The thickening of bronchial walls in bronchitis and bronchiectasis is difficult to detect on plain radiographs, but bronchography is diagnostic. In bronchitis the necks of enlarged mucous glands may fill with contrast material, and in bronchiectasis localized widening of the airways can be seen. The two lower lobes and right middle lobe and lingula are most frequently involved in bronchiectasis. Tuberculosis and cystic fibrosis often cause upper lobe bronchiectasis. Bronchography is necessary to estimate the extent of bronchiectasis prior to surgery. The bronchographic findings in bronchiectasis include diminution in the normal number of bronchial generations, lack of normal tapering, and abrupt or enlarged terminations of bronchi.

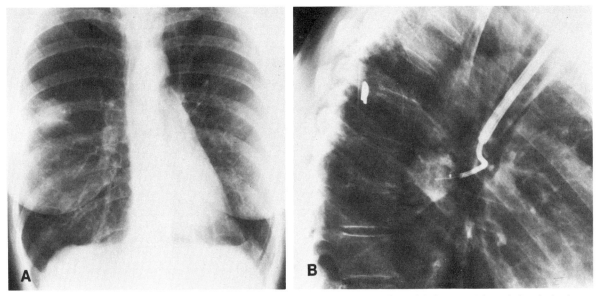

Fig. 5. *A.* Frontal view demonstrates a slightly lobulated mass in the mid portion of the right lung. *B.* A lateral view during bronchial brushing shows a brush extended into the lesion which proved to be an undifferentiated carcinoma of the lung.

Abnormalities of the peripheral airspaces consist primarily of consolidations or alterations in inflation. Underinflation can vary from total airlessness (atelectasis) to slightly diminished inflation. Atelectasis results from total airway obstruction, partial airway obstruction, or increased lung stiffness with patent airways. When gas

absorption by blood exceeds fresh gas delivery, atelectasis is the net result. If airway obstruction occurs in a small conducting airway or if a small area of the lung has increased stiffness, a small portion of the lung may become airless, resulting in platelike atelectasis (Fig. 6). When segments, lobes, or whole lungs become atel-

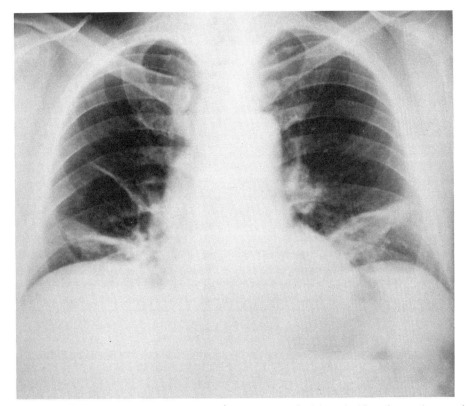

Fig. 6. Several linear areas of platelike atelectasis are present at both bases in this patient on the second postoperative day after cholecystectomy. Notice the high diaphragmatic level as a result of shallow inspiration.

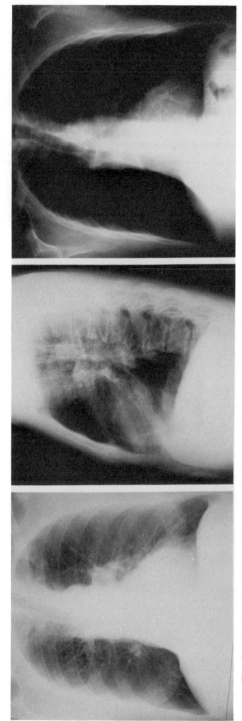

Fig. 7. Atelectasis of the right lower lobe has caused overexpansion of the remaining inflated right lung and a slight shift of the mediastinum to the right. The airless lobe can be seen as a triangular density obscuring the right heart border and the posterior portion of the elevated right hemidiaphragm. The atelectasis is the result of carcinoma of the right intermediate bronchus. There is a pneumonia of the right upper lobe.

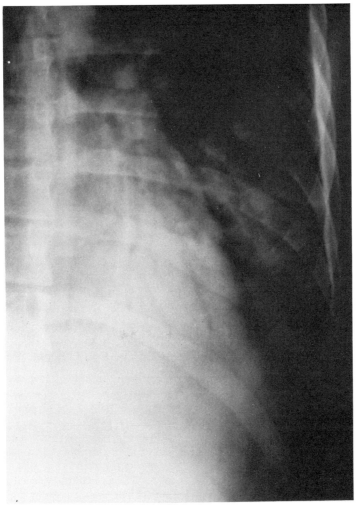

Fig. 8. An air bronchogram can be seen as branching lucent shadows through the cardiac silhouette as a result of pneumonia of the left lower lobe.

ectatic, large uniformly radiopaque areas of airless lung are seen. The shapes of atelectatic lobes are quite predictable because of the limited way in which the remaining lung can expand to fill the thorax (Fig. 7). Normal lung surrounding atelectatic areas hyperexpands because the restriction on inflation provided by the previously expanded lung is lost. Similarly, the diaphragm may elevate and the ribs may come together on the side of atelectasis. If large enough, atelectasis may result in enough overexpansion of the normal lung to shift the mediastinal structures toward the abnormal lung. If the underinflation is slight it may be manifested only as slight crowding of bronchovascular structures, and no compensatory overinflation of the remaining lung may be recognized.

A mass completely obstructing a large conducting airway will generally result in atelectasis, but a mass partly filling the lumen may become completely occlusive only on expiration when the intrathoracic airways diminish in caliber. This ball-valve mechanism may result in hyperexpansion of the lung by allowing air to enter

faster than it can be resorbed. The radiographic signs of localized overinflation consist of spread-out, elongated, sparse-appearing bronchovascular structures, and occasionally compression of adjacent lung. At times the air trapping which does not result in overinflated lung is only recognized by fluoroscopy or expiration radiography as a failure of normal regional deflation (Fig. 3). Although total obstruction of a lobar bronchus will lead to airlessness, obstruction one or two generations more distally may not cause atelectasis because collateral ventilation between the segments of a lobe is adequate to prevent it.

Consolidation of the lung periphery indicates an abnormal solidity of the lung parenchyma and implies replacement of air by liquid or semiliquid material. Pneumococcal pneumonia is a classic example. The radiopacity of consolidation results from the confluence of many fluid-filled acini. When the conducting airways remain gas-filled, they are seen in sharp contrast with the opacified lung. This phenomenon has been called the air bronchogram (Fig. 8). When the lung is not totally consolidated individual fluid-filled acini may be recognized as

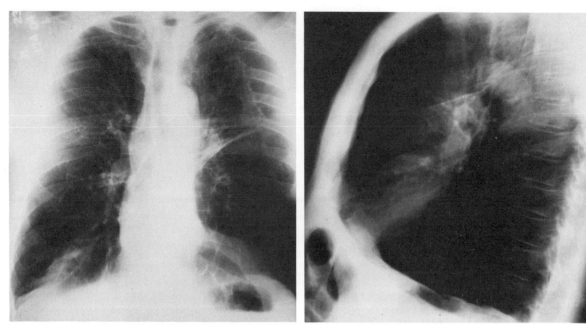

Fig. 9. There is generalized overinflation of the lungs and a large bulla in the left lower lobe. The top of the bulla is indicated by the curvilinear density lateral to the left hilus.

distinct but slightly irregular 5–8-mm-diameter densities. This is best seen in bronchogenic tuberculosis when mycobacteria are aspirated from one portion of the lung to another. The loss of normally sharp interfaces between solid structures such as the heart and diaphragm and aerated lung as a result of consolidation is called the silhouette sign.

OBSTRUCTIVE AIRWAY DISEASE

Advanced forms of emphysema can be diagnosed radiographically, but milder forms are recognized less often. The primary radiographic signs in emphysema are the result of overinflation and destruction of lung parenchyma. The overinflation may be diffuse or regional. In regional disease such as bullous emphysema large areas of overexpansion may be seen and expiration radiographs often demonstrate regional air trapping (Fig. 9). A special unilateral form of overexpansion occurs in the MacLeod (Swyer-James) syndrome, which represents the final result of a bronchiolitis obliterans. Congenital lobar emphysema is a similar condition of childhood in which air trapping generally occurs in the upper or right middle lobes.

Generalized overinflation in emphysema can be recognized by diffusely spread-out, elongated bronchovascular structures, widened intercostal spaces, bulging sternum, and depressed diaphragm. Downward convexity of the diaphragm is generally a reliable sign of overinflation, whereas "blackening" of the lungs is a notoriously unreliable sign.

In the group of emphysema patients classified as "pink puffers" overinflation is often diffuse or most extensive in the anterior and basal portions of the lung (Fig. 10). Lung destruction and overinflation in this type of emphysema is manifested by thin, sparse, spidery pulmonary vessels. The heart generally is small, and there is little evidence of pulmonary hypertension until significant hypoxemia occurs. Familial α_1-antitrypsin deficiency, which is associated with panlobular emphysema, causes severe overinflation of the lower lobes in young patients similar to that found in the older "pink puffers." Less marked evidence of overinflation is the rule in the "blue bloater" type of emphysematous patient who exhibits prominent irregular peripheral vessels, bulging central pulmonary arteries, and evidence of right heart failure (Fig. 11). Overinflation occurs primarily in the upper lobes, and bronchitis is frequently present. The "tram lines" of thickened bronchial walls may be detected in chronic bronchitis, but the primary abnormalities seen are generally the result of coexisting emphysema.

Episodic overinflation is generally the only radiographic finding in asthma unless it is complicated by infection, emphysema, or mucoid impaction. The latter occurs in hypersensitivity aspergillosis, asthma, and cystic fibrosis and tends to occur in subsegmental bronchi which become dilated with semisolid mucoid material. Mucoid impactions are recognized as elongated branching densities, and because collateral ventilation is generally well developed distal to the impaction atelectasis is not commonly seen. Cystic fibrosis is frequently associated with marked overinflation, irregular scarlike strands, tram lines, bronchiectasis, and upper-lobe atelectasis. Central-airway obstruction may result from tracheobronchopathia osteochondroplastica, in which submucosal nodules of cartilage may be seen to project into the airways. Tracheobronchomalacia and tracheobronchomegaly cause expiratory collapse of central airways.

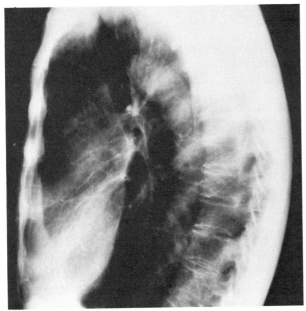 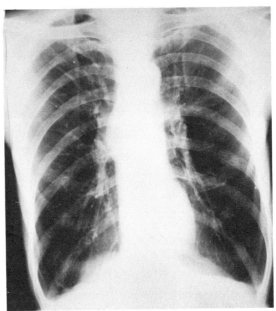

Fig. 10. General overinflation in this "pink puffer" is indicated by the elongated spidery pulmonary vessels, the increased sagittal chest diameter, and the flattened downward convex diaphragm.

SPECIFIC AIRSPACE DISEASE

Pneumonia is generally considered to be an airspace process, but it is always accompanied to a greater or lesser extent by an interstitial component. Some acute pneumonias such as those caused by *Diplococcus pneumoniae, Klebsiella* species, and *Mycobacterium tuberculosis* are characterized primarily as airspace diseases. These pneumonias tend to originate at the lung periphery and spread away from their point of origin via collateral pores. In this way the exudate bypasses bronchial routes so that consolidation does not conform to bronchopulmonary segmental anatomy. Because of their peripheral origin the conducting airways tend to remain patent, air bronchograms are frequent, and atelectasis is uncommon. In contrast to the latter group of pneumonias, those caused by viruses, *Mycoplasma pneumoniae, Staphylococcus aureaus,* and *Streptococcus pyogenes* have a significant interstitial component. They

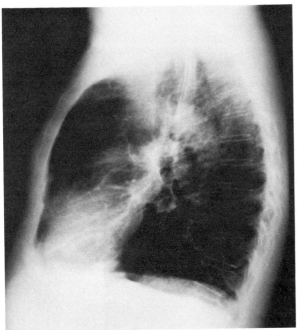 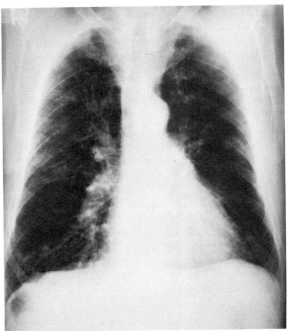

Fig. 11. There is general overinflation of the lungs of this "blue bloater" who also has marked enlargement of the pulmonary arteries and many irregular densities in the lungs. Notice the large cardiac silhouette and bulging vessels compared to their thin counterparts in the "pink puffer."

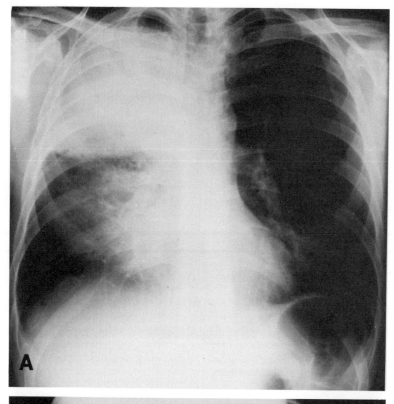

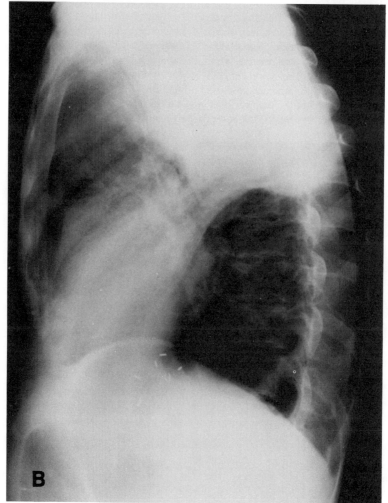

74

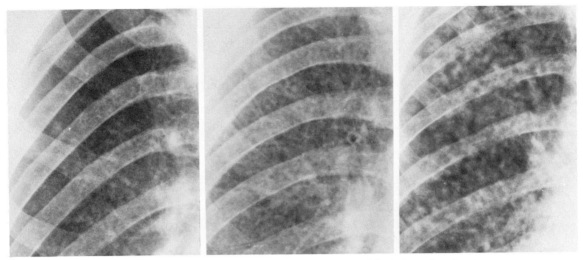

Fig. 13.   Three cases of anthracosilicosis with interstitial nodular lesions of varying size.

generally have their origins in the central peribronchial airspaces and spread peripherally along the bronchovascular bundles. As a result of early bronchial involvement airways are frequently blocked, causing atelectasis. The consolidations correspond to bronchopulmonary segments, and air bronchograms are infrequent.

The specific bacteriologic identity of a pneumonia is not generally possible from the radiographic appearance alone, but clues are frequently provided by the constellation of radiographic findings. Pleural effusion and empyema frequently accompany pneumonias caused by *Klebsiella* and *Aerobacter* species, *Staphylococcus aureus, Streptococcus pyogenes, Bacteroides* species, *Actinomyces* and *Nocardia* species, *Entamoeba histolytica,* and *Mycobacterium tuberculosis.* These same organisms are also frequent causes of cavities. Hilar lymph node enlargement occurs commonly in association with measles, varicella, primary tuberculosis, coccidioidomycosis, histoplasmosis, and anthrax pneumonias. Pneumothorax is a particularly common complication of *Staphylococcus aureus* pneumonia. The "bulging fissure" is a special sign associated with the swollen lung involved in *Klebsiella* pneumonia (Fig. 12). Upper-lobe involvement and involvement of the superior segment of the lower lobe is the rule in *Klebsiella* and reinfection tuberculous pneumonia, while the basal portions of the lower lobes are most commonly involved in *Streptococcus pyogenes* and *Hemophilus influenzae* pneumonia.

Other causes of airspace disease include fat emboli, noxious fumes, aspiration pneumonia, alveolar proteinosis, and Löffler's syndrome. Infant respiratory distress syndrome (IRDS), bronchoalveolar carcinoma, and pulmonary hemorrhage and cardiogenic pulmonary edema can also cause prominent airspace densities, but there is generally some evidence of coexisting interstitial lung abnormality.

INTERSTITIAL DISEASE

The interstitium lies between the airspace epithelium and the vascular structures. This potential space can be enlarged, distorted, or infiltrated by inflammatory or neoplastic cells, fluid, scars, or granulomas. The resulting radiographic appearances vary greatly and differentiation from airspace disease is not always possible. The radiographic appearance of interstitial lung disease can be nodular, linear, or both. Nodules may vary in size from the limits of discernment to several centimeters. Linear densities vary from distinct lines to a honeycomb appearance (Fig. 13 and 14). Honeycombing is the most dependable sign of interstitial disease but none of these appearances is specific for any of the numerous causes of interstitial lung disease. Nor is any interstitial lung disease limited to a single type of appearance during its course. Fluid accumulation, scar, or hemosiderin deposition in the interlobular lymphatic septae (septal lines) may result in linear shadows of about 1 cm in length that extend perpendicularly to the lung surface (Fig. 15). These lines are sure signs of interstitial lung disease. Interstitial pulmonary edema from heart failure can closely mimic interstitial fibrosis (Fig. 16). The interstitial edema fluid accumulates around the central pulmonary vessels and distends the limiting membrane around the perihilar arteries, veins and bronchi. As a result there is obliteration of the normally sharp outline of vessels, causing a perihilar haze.

Generally all of the available clinical data are needed before a specific or etiologic diagnosis of interstitial lung disease can be made. The diagnosis frequently awaits lung or lymph node biopsy. Some radiographic appearances are fairly characteristic, however. Histiocytosis, for instance, frequently has a 0.5–1.0-cm-diameter coarse cystic or honeycomb appearance, while other idiopathic pulmonary fibroses generally have a microcystic appearance (0.2–0.3 cm in diameter). The changes of

Fig. 12.   The opacification of the right upper lobe that bulges the major fissure on the lateral film is the result of *Klebsiella pneumoniae.*

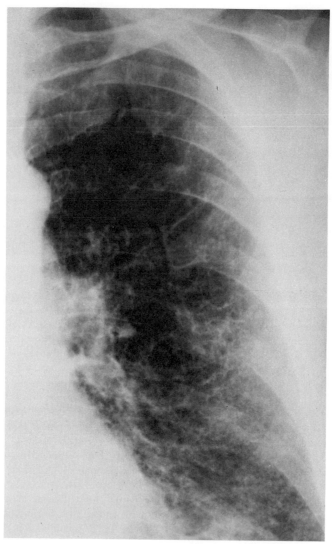

Fig. 14. Linear densities in this case of interstitial lung disease causes a honeycomb appearance. The honeycomb size tends to be larger at the apex where the distending pressure of the lung is greatest.

scleroderma are predominantly basal, while those of early silicosis are evenly distributed (Fig. 17). Sarcoidosis is suggested by the combined finding of interstitial lung change and bilateral hilar and right paratracheal adenopathy (Fig. 18). "Eggshell" calcification of hilar lymph nodes suggests silicosis, and calcified diaphragmatic pleura in the presence of basal interstitial changes suggests asbestosis. Associated pleural changes are not uncommon in silicosis, rheumatoid disease, and alveolar cell carcinoma, and asbestosis.

It is often possible to conclude that a honeycomb or micronodular disease of the lung is primarily interstitial in location. It is somewhat more difficult to decide that 7-mm diameter densities are opacified acini or interstitial nodules. Combinations of interstitial and airspace disease are also difficult to recognize. A number of interstitial diseases are known to desquamate material into the peripheral airspaces, and a number of airspace diseases are known to be associated with prominent interstitial abnor-

malities. Conditions that combine interstitial and airspace disease include bronchoalveolar carcinoma and desquamative interstitial pneumonias, idiopathic pulmonary hemorrhage, hemosiderosis, cytomegalovirus and pneumocystis carinii pneumonia, congestive heart failure, and uremia.

PULMONARY VASCULAR ABNORMALITIES

Pulmonary vascular abnormalities consist primarily of alterations in vessel size, distribution, and configuration.

A change in vessel size is the result of a change in either transmural pressure or vessel compliance. There is a generalized increase in vessel size as a result of increased transmural pressure during high-cardiac-output states such as heavy exercise, left-to-right intracardiac shunts, hypermetabolic conditions, and increased pulmonary venous pressure. An increase in pulmonary driving pressure increases transmural pressure and

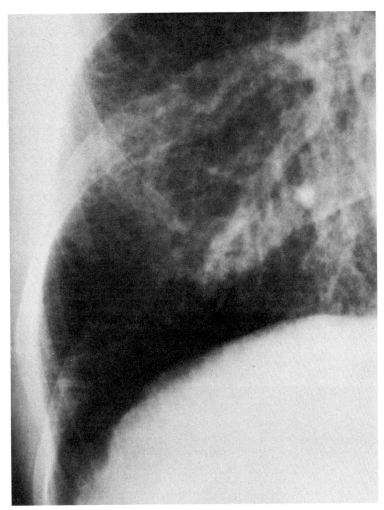

Fig. 15. Multiple thin septal lines are seen extending perpendicularly from the pleural surface in a case of mitral stenosis.

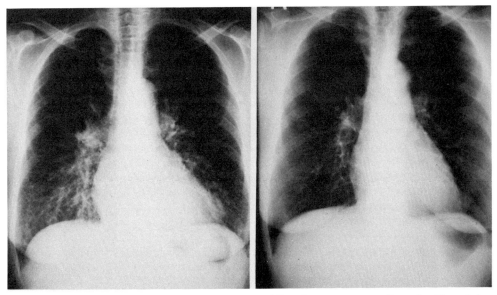

Fig. 16. Interstitial pulmonary edema as a result of congestive heart failure demonstrates many linear densities and shaggy vascular outlines simulating interstitial fibrosis (left). After diuresis the interstitial edema disappeared (right).

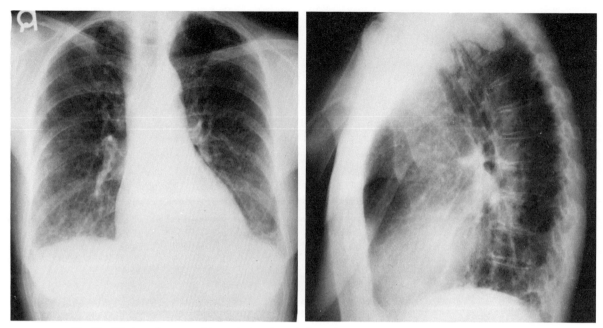

Fig. 17. The hazy linear opacities at the lung bases indicate interstitial lung in a patient with scleroderma.

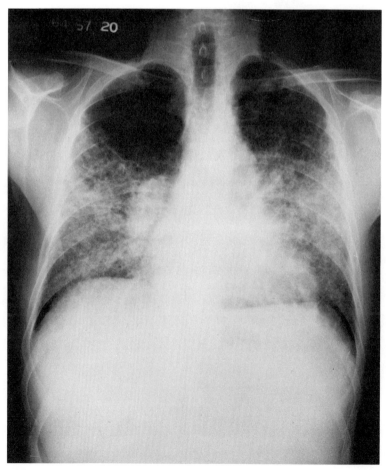

Fig. 18. Linear and nodular lung densities combined with enlarged hilar lymph nodes suggest the diagnosis in this case of sarcoidosis.

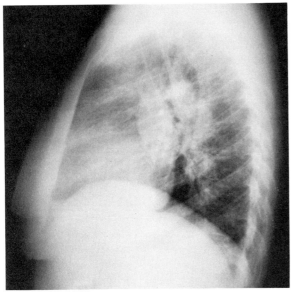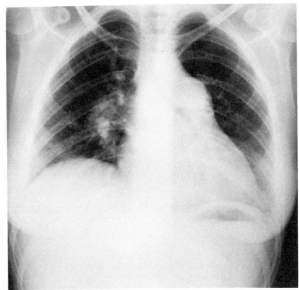

Fig. 19. There is marked enlargement of the central pulmonary arteries and paucity of peripheral arteries in this patent with ventricular septal defect and pulmonary hypertension.

therefore vessel size. The increased vessel size can generally be best appreciated in the larger arteries and veins (Fig. 11). The small vessels of the lungs can also be seen to be enlarged, but their enlargement is less marked. An increase of 10 cm H_2O in the transmural pressure will cause a marked increase in the size of the main pulmonary artery but will hardly affect a 20-μ-diameter pulmonary artery at all. If the pulmonary arterial pressure, which is primarily responsible for the transmural pressure in arteries, remains elevated for long periods then anatomic changes in the small arteries ensue, decreasing their compliance. To maintain the same cardiac output the absolute level of pulmonary arterial pressure must rise. As a result the size of the central pulmonary arteries increases while the stiffer peripheral vessels remain small. Longstanding pulmonary hypertension thus results in large central and small peripheral arteries. (Fig. 19). The anatomic changes in the pulmonary vessels may be regional, such as in mitral stenosis where they occur predominantly at the lung base. The result is that the central- and upper-lobe pulmonary arteries and veins are large, but the lower-lobe vessels are diminutive.

A localized decrease in arterial (and venous) vessel size occurs distal to localized pressure drops, such as in vascular stenosis or intravascular emboli. This is the mechanism of the occasionally observed regional oligemia distal to a pulmonary embolus (Westermark sign). Geometric vascular changes that accompany hyperinflation elongate and compress the vessels.

Unusual vessel configuration may be seen in congenital vascular anomalies. An area of anomalous pulmonary venous drainage may be recognized as an abnormal branching venous structure that extends toward the inferior vena cava instead of the left atrium (Fig. 20). A pulmonary nodule that is connected to a visible artery

and vein is generally an arteriovenous malformation. It can be recognized by its frequent multiplicity, shrinkage on Valsalva maneuver, and configuration on tomography. Occasionally a localized dilation of a pulmonary vein (pulmonary varix) may be recognized, especially in patients with longstanding pulmonary venous hypertension.

Heart failure is a frequent cause of pulmonary vascular abnormality. The early changes of left-sided failure are those of pulmonary venous hypertension which consist of enlargement of the pulmonary arteries and veins, particularly in the upper lobes. Generally the lower-lobe vessels are constricted, probably as a result of microscopic cuffing of lower-lobe vessels with edema fluid, which reduces their compliance. As left-heart failure worsens, the reversal in the normal relationship of upper-to-lower-lobe vessel size may be followed by a perihilar haze and septal visualization indicating an accumulation of edema fluid in the perivascular and peribronchial spaces. In more severe degrees of left-heart failure, frank airspace pulmonary edema fluid may be recognized. Dilatation of the vena cavae or azygos vein reflects systemic venous hypertension which accompanies right-sided heart failure.

Pulmonary emboli frequently show no radiographic signs. In the absence of infarction the primary findings, when present, consist of elevation of the diaphragm, small plates of atelectasis with or without pleural effusion, or a regional decrease in pulmonary vessel size (Fig. 21). Enlargement of pulmonary arteries is rare except when a clot distends the vessel or when there is marked pulmonary hypertension from extensive, recurrent, multiple peripheral pulmonary emboli. Pulmonary infarction, when it occurs, appears as a homogeneous peripheral lung density generally abutting a pleural surface. The constellation of an elevated hemidiaphragm, a

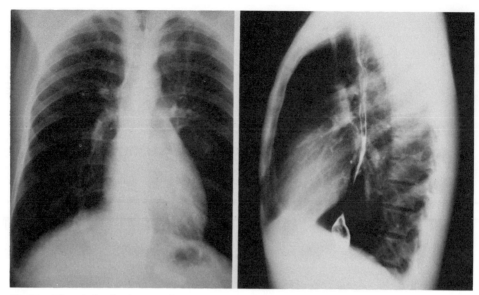

Fig. 20. The tubular density extending toward the right hemidiaphragm, which enlarges as it passes peripherally, is diagnostic of partial anomalous pulmonary venous return to the inferior vena cava.

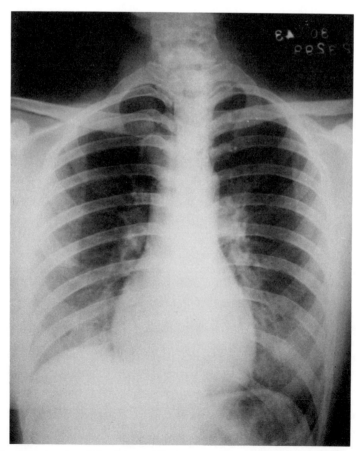

Fig. 21. The slight elevation of the right hemidiaphragm and the hazy density above it are the signs of pulmonary infarct in the right lower lobe.

pleural effusion, and a peripheral lung density should suggest the diagnosis of pulmonary infarct. Macroaggregate isotope perfusion scans are helpful in supporting the clinical diagnosis of embolism when the chest radiograph is normal. When lung densities are present on the plain radiograph, the demonstration of intravascular filling defects with pulmonary arteriography is generally necessary to make a certain radiologic diagnosis. In the presence of chronic obstructive lung disease, regional inhomogeneities in perfusion are common, so that perfusion lung scans are generally unreliable in making the diagnosis of pulmonary embolism. At times ventilation isotope scans with xenon-133 may help to differentiate nonventilated, poorly perfused areas of emphysema from areas of pulmonary emboli which are ventilated but nonperfused.

CHEST CAGE AND PLEURAL DISEASE

Rather large amounts of pleural fluid (300 ml) can be detected in erect plain chest films. Smaller amounts of fluid (<100 ml) can be visualized in the lateral decubitus position when it is layered out in the deep lateral concavity of the chest cage. The fluid density separating the aerated lung from the ribs can then be easily seen. In the erect position fluid tends to accumulate first in the deep posterior costophrenic sulcus, so that it is not always well seen except on lateral films. Fluid frequently accumulates along the diaphragmatic surface causing the lung to float on it. This phenomenon is called subpulmonic effusion and may closely simulate an elevated diaphragm. The careful search for a fluid meniscus extending up the major fissure may help in its detection.

The positive determination that a pleural density is fluid requires either that the density was known not to be present a few days before or that the liquid nature of the fluid is shown by shifting its location with changes in body position. Lateral decubitus studies are convenient not only for demonstrating small pleural effusions but also for clearly visualizing lung formerly obscured by fluid.

The most common cause of bilateral pleural effusions is congestive heart failure. The associated signs of cardiac enlargement and pulmonary venous hypertension or pulmonary edema are generally present. Cardiac enlargement and pleural effusion can also occur in systemic lupus erythematosus.

Bilateral effusions in the absence of cardiac enlargement frequently indicate the presence of metastatic cancer. Isolated pleural effusion can result from tuberculosis and other pneumonias, lymphoma, hepatic cirrhosis, subdiaphragmatic infections, collagen diseases, and ovarian tumors.

The association of airspace disease and pleural effusion occurs in pneumonias, particularly those that tend to form cavities such as tuberculosis, *S. aureus, S. pyogenes, K. pneumoniae,* and *Actinomyces israelii.* Mediastinal adenopathy often coexists with pleural fluid in lymphoma, lung cancer, and matastatic carcinoma. Interstitial pulmonary disease and pleural effusion may coexist in collagen vascular disease. Pulmonary nodular

densities and effusion occur together in metastatic carcinoma.

Some intrapleural fluid densities do not shift with change in body position because of loculation or organization. The latter occurs in empyema and fibrinous bloody collections. Nonfluid pleural densities may coexist with pleural effusion such as mesothelioma and metastatic pleural nodules. Pleural calcification occurs as the late result of intrapleural hemorrhage, tuberculosis, empyema, or asbestos exposure. The latter is particularly associated with bilateral diaphragmatic pleural calcification which is virtually diagnostic of the condition.

Pneumothorax occurs spontaneously in asthenic young males as a result of the spontaneous rupture of apical blebs. It also occurs as a complication of staphylococcal pneumonia, chronic berylliosis, bauxitosis, histiocystosis X, desquamative interstitial pneumonitis and subpleural rheumatoid or metastatic sarcoma nodules. Air entering the potential space between the two pleural surfaces causes the lung to deflate because the negative contact pressure between the two layers of pleura is lost. The space of the pneumothorax is identified by a thin rim of visceral pleura inside the rib cage with a space devoid of lung at the periphery (Fig. 22). Pneumothorax is most easily detected on the expiration radiograph. Spontaneous pneumothorax is frequently associated with small amounts of pleural fluid that form air–fluid levels at the lung base. In uncomplicated pneumothorax the contents of the mediastinum, i.e., heart, great vessels, and trachea, may shift toward the side of the pneumothorax during inspiration because the normal lung expands more readily. Various ball-valve mechanisms can cause air to enter the pleural space with no chance for rapid egress resulting in a "tension" pneumothorax. This condition is recognized by a marked contralateral mediastinal shift and restriction of the opposite lung. An air bronchogram is generally seen in the pneumothorax lung, and its absence should alert the observer to the likelihood of an endobronchial lesion.

Elevation of the diaphragm may occur in phrenic nerve paralysis, subdiaphragmatic inflammation, and basal pulmonary infarcts. A rapid inspiration or sniff will show limited movement of the splinted diaphragm or paradoxical elevation of the paralyzed diaphragmatic leaf.

MEDIASTINAL DISEASE

The mediastinum occupies the space between the parietal pleural surfaces of the two lungs. Displacement of its contents, which include the heart and great vessels, may indicate the presence of air trapping, atelectasis, or a space-occupying lesion. Lack of any shift of the mediastinum in the presence of a large pleural effusion suggests fixation of the mediastinum by involvement with tumor or scar. The differential diagnosis of mass lesions in the mediastinum is based on knowledge of the structures that are normally present in its various parts. The anterior mediastinal compartment, which lies anterior to the pericardium and great vessels, is a frequent site of malignant tumors such as thymoma, teratoma, and lym-

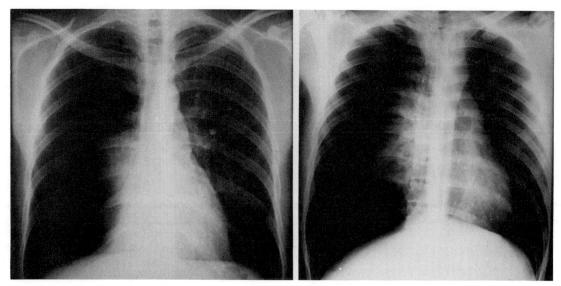

Fig. 22. The absence of peripheral right lung vessels and a perihilar density indicate the presence of a pneumothorax (left). The mediastinum is shifted to the left in another case, indicating a "tension" right pneumothorax (right).

phoma. In addition, thyroid, parathyroid, and aortic aneurysmal masses may be found. The upward movement of an anterior mediastinal mass with swallowing suggests thyroid origin. Calcifications may be found in thyroid tumors, thymomas, and teratomas.

The middle mediastinum extends from the anterior to the posterior extremes of the pericardium and contains many vascular and lymph node structures. The vast majority of the nonvascular masses in this compartment are malignant tumors such as lymphomas, carcinomas, or metastases. Oat-cell carcinomas of the lung often exhibit massive mediastinal adenopathy even when the primary lesion is inconspicuous. Benign middle mediastinal masses include benign lymph node enlargement, bronchogenic and pericardial cysts, aneurysms of the aorta, and distended vena cavae and pulmonary vessels.

Between the pericardium and the thoracic spine lies the posterior mediastinum where neurogenic tumors, neurenteric cysts, and esophageal tumors occur. The most frequently encountered posterior mediastinal mass in clinical practice is the air and fluid-filled hiatus hernia.

MASS LESIONS

Solitary pulmonary nodules are of considerable clinical importance since they may be small lung cancers. The only characteristics of nodules that help in differentiating between benign and malignant nodules are size, stability, and the presence of benign calcification. A determined search for previous chest films is of utmost importance when a nodule is discovered, since its unchanged size over a 2-year period would indicate its certain benign nature. Benign calcification consists of punctate, target or laminated calcification. Common causes of benign solitary nodules that may contain calcium include tuberculoma, histoplasmoma, and hamartoma. Bronchogenic carcinoma, metastatic cancer, and bronchoalveolar cell carcinoma are common malignant causes of solitary nodules. Bronchial carcinoid is an uncommon cause of pulmonary nodules.

Large mass lesions may be caused by bronchogenic carcinoma or metastasis, pulmonary abscess, bronchogenic cysts, and bronchopulmonary sequestration. Any of these lesions may cavitate. Large hydatid cysts tend to have unusual shapes and occur in the right lower lobe. Multiple nodules occur with septic pulmonary emboli, abscesses, various metastases, Wegener's granulomatosis, and amyloidosis.

Bronchogenic carcinoma does not always appear as a pulmonary nodule when first detected. Atelectasis as a result of endobronchial obstruction is a common presentation, as is recurrent pneumonia distal to a partially obstructing endobronchial carcinoma. As a result of collateral ventilation atelectasis may be absent, with total obstruction of segmental bronchi by cancer. In such a case air trapping ought to be detected, but it is frequently missed because it is not looked for with fluoroscopy or expiration radiographs. Hilar adenopathy is often present at the time of diagnosis of lung cancer, and in the case of oat-cell carcinoma may be the only chest abnormality seen. Cavitation of a bronchogenic cancer generally indicates squamous cell histology. Phrenic nerve or recurrent laryngeal nerve involvement by tumor may result in diaphragmatic or vocal cord paralysis. Lesions at the pulmonary apex (Pancoast tumor) frequently involve the rib cage and brachial plexus, causing pain and rib erosion. Pleural effusion generally indicates tumor extension to the pleura.

REFERENCES

Fenessey JJ: Transbronchial biopsy of peripheral lung lesions. Radiology 88:878, 1967

Fleischner FG: Observations on the radiologic changes in pulmonary embolism, in Sasahara AA, Stein M (eds): Pulmonary Embolic Disease. New York, Grune & Stratton, 1965, p 889

Fleischner FG: The visible bronchial tree: A roentgen sign in pneumonic and other pulmonary consolidations. Radiology 50:184, 1948

Fraser RG, Pare JAP: Diagnosis of Diseases of the Chest. Philadelphia, WB Saunders, 1970

Gamsu G, Thurlbeck WM, Macklem PT, Fraser RG: Roentgenographic appearance of the human pulmonary acinus. Invest Radiol 6:171, 1971

Good CA: Roentgenologic appraisal of solitary pulmonary nodules. Minn Med 45:157, 1960

Greene R: Radiographic measurement of thoracic gas volume. Radiol Clin North Am 9:63, 1971

Leigh TF, Weens HS: Roentgen aspects of mediastinal lesions. Semin Roentgenol 4:59, 1969

Nicklaus TM, Stowell DW, Christiansen WR, Renzett AD Jr: The accuracy of the roentgenologic diagnosis of chronic pulmonary emphysema. Am Rev Respir Dis 93:889, 1966

Nordenstrom B: Transthoracic needle biopsy. N Engl J Med 276:1981, 1967

Rabin CG, Blackman NS: Bilateral pleural effusion. Its significance in association with a heart of normal size. J Mount Sinai Hospital 24:45, 1957

Reid L: Reduction in bronchial subdivisions in bronchiectasis. Thorax 5:233, 1950

Robbins LL, Hale CH, Merrill OE: The roentgen appearance of lobar and segmental collapse of the lung. I. Technic of examination. Radiology 44:471, 1945

Robbins LL, Hale CH: The roentgen appearance of lobar and segmental collapse of the lung. II. The normal chest as it pertains to collapse. Radiology 44:543, 1945

Robbins LL, Hale CH: The roentgen appearance of lobar and segmental collapse of the lung. III. Collapse of an entire lung or the major part thereof. Radiology 45:23, 1945

RADIOISOTOPES IN LUNG DISEASES

Reginald Greene

The efficiency of the lung as an organ of gas exchange requires the accurate matching of ventilation and perfusion. In normal man regional inhomogeneities of ventilation and perfusion do not result in significant inefficiencies of gas exchange. In disease, however, there may be gross regional mismatching resulting in the overperfusion of one lung relative to its ventilation and the opposite effect in the other lung.

Prior to the development of radioisotope techniques, regional gas exchange could be studied only by bronchospirometry, which required bronchial cannulation. Radioisotope study provides a safe and accurate method for measuring ventilation and perfusion.

REGIONAL VENTILATION

Xenon 133 is an inert, relatively insoluble radioactive gas that is convenient for making measurements of regional ventilation ($\dot{V}$). The patient sits in front of a stack of scintillation detectors that provide comparative data in each of three zones (top, middle, bottom) in the two lungs.*

After the patient inhales the radioisotope mixed with air, he holds his breath for several seconds while data are

*With appropriate counting devices the lungs may be divided into more zones, or a gamma camera can be used to look at the entire lung.

collected from each of the regional scintillation detectors. The number of counts detected is proportional to regional ventilation. A correction can be made for the large volume of lungs at the bases by having the patient rebreathe xenon 133 for a few minutes until it is equilibrated in all the air spaces according to their volumes. The distribution of activity at the end of equilibration is proportional to the volume of lung "seen" by each of the regional detectors (V). Using this data regional ventilation can be corrected for lung volume and expressed as regional ventilation per unit lung volume ($\dot{V}/V$). Figure 1 illustrates data obtained from normal seated adults.

A significantly greater proportion of a normal slow breath normally goes to the dependent lung. This apex-to-base gradient in regional $\dot{V}/V$ is apparently lost in going from the seated to the supine position, but a similar ventral-to-dorsal $\dot{V}/V$ gradient can be detected. The difference in ventilation of the superior and inferior portions of the lungs appears to be primarily the result of a gravity dependent gradient in pleural surface pressure down the lungs. The reduced distending forces in the dependent portions of the lung cause the lower alveoli to be smaller and more compliant than the superior ones. They can, therefore, accommodate a larger proportion of a slow breath.

A fast breath, in contrast with a slow one will result in considerably less ventilation to the dependent lung. The smaller diameters of the less distended lower lung bronchi result in greater resistance to air flow than in the superior portions of the lung, so that a fast breath encounters more resistance at the base.

If the lung compliance is reduced in the dependent portions of the lung, as with pneumonia or pulmonary edema, then less than the expected amount of a slow breath will reach the lung base. Similarly, reduction in dependent airway caliber by interstitial edema or peribronchial inflammation would reduce ventilation to those areas during rapid, labored breathing. Unless this redistribution of ventilation is matched by like changes in pulmonary blood flow, abnormalities of gas exchange can be expected.

The volume of the lung from which a breath is taken affects the distribution of ventilation. Thus substantially more of a slow tidal breath goes to the lung base when it is taken from residual volume rather than from functional residual capacity. The different distributions of ventilation reflect the steeper gradient of pleural pressure (and therefore smaller volume of the lung base) at residual volume than at functional residual capacity (Fig. 2).

It is paradoxical that while most of a maximum breath from residual volume goes to the dependent lung, the initial part of the breath goes to the lung apex. Studies of the distribution of small (inhaled) boluses (5 ml) of xenon 133 and nitrogen 13 show that 6 to 10 times as much of the bolus goes to the lung apex than base when the breath is taken from residual volume (Fig. 3). Slow inspiration from functional residual capacity shows that the bolus is distributed more like the breath as a whole. The lack of ventilation of the lung base in the initial part of in-

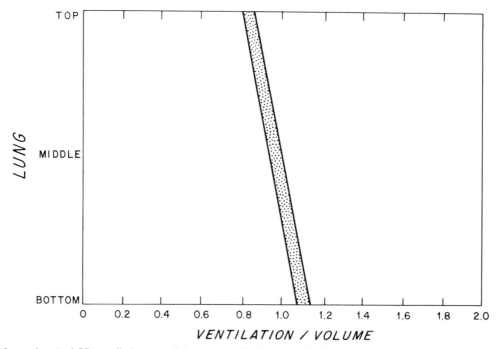

Fig. 1.   Mean values (± 2 SD) ventilation per unit lung volume obtained with tidal breaths of xenon 133 for a group of normal adults. Notice the gradual increase in ventilation from top to bottom of the lung.

spiration from residual volume has led to the important concept of airway closure.

When a patient exhales after having inhaled a small bolus from residual volume, the level of activity in the expirate suddenly increases (Fig. 4), suggesting that the

basal portions of the lungs that have little radioactivity no longer contribute to the expirate. It appears that at residual volume the distending pressure on the basal airways may fall below their critical closing pressures, accounting for the distribution of radioactivity to the lung

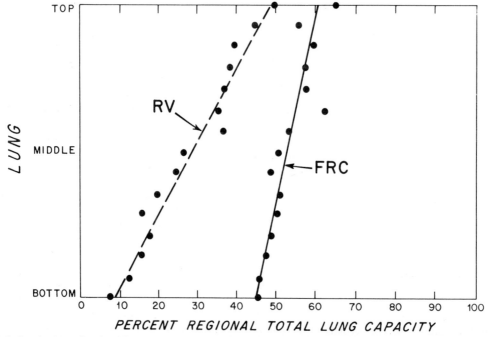

Fig. 2.   Calculated values of regional lung volumes as percentages of their maximal obtained in a normal subject using nitrogen 13. The slightly larger regional volumes at the lung top reflects the pleural pressure gradient down the lung. The difference between the regional lung volume at the top and bottom is more marked at RV and becomes progressively less pronounced at higher lung volumes. The smaller volumes at the lung bases at RV and FRC provide a greater capacity for expansion than at the lung top. Thus there is a basal predominance of slow breaths from RV or FRC.

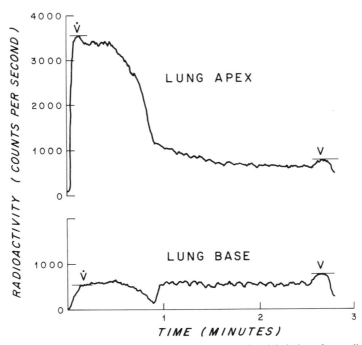

Fig. 3. Comparative data obtained in a normal adult after the slow inhalation of a small bolus of radioactive nitrogen. A scintillation detector at the lung top indicates that substantially more of the gas goes to the lung apex. Compare the activity levels during a breath hold at maximum inspiration ($\dot{V}$). The activity detected after rebreathing the air–^{13}N mixture (V) reflects the volume of the lung "seen" by each scintillation detector. Notice that in spite of the fact that each detector is "seeing" about the same volume of lung, much more of the radioactivity goes to the apex during the first breath.

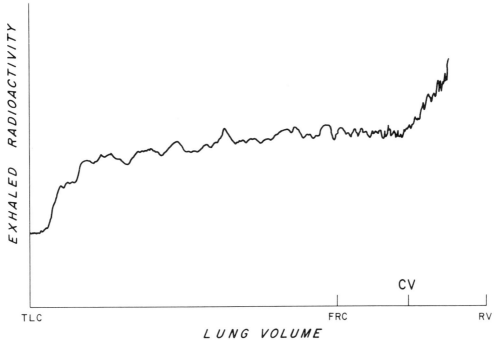

Fig. 4. A plot of exhaled radioactivity in a middle-aged man after slow inhalation of a bolus of radioactive nitrogen from residual volume to total lung capacity. The initial part of the expirate shows a uniform background level of the anatomic dead space. As portions of the lung that contain the inhaled bolus contribute to expirate the activity rises. A plateau of activity with superimposed cardiogenic oscillation is established as a fairly constant proportion of the expirate comes from radioactive and relatively nonradioactive areas. The activity suddenly rises when the radioactively poor areas (lung base) no longer contribute to the expirate near RV. The sudden rise of radioactivity is attributed to airway closure at the lung base, and the lung volume at which this occurs is called the closing volume (CV). With aging and airway disease the CV occurs closer to and ultimately within the normal breathing range (FRC).

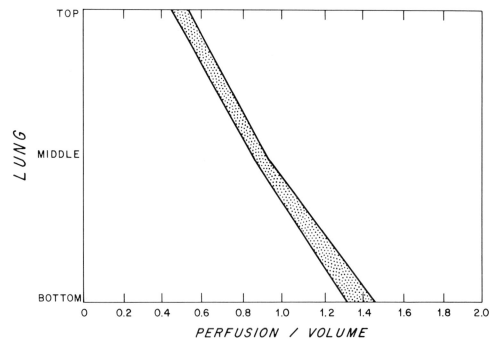

Fig. 5. Mean values ($\pm$ 2 SD) of perfusion per unit lung volume obtained with intravenous injections of xenon 133 in a group of normal adults. Notice the continuous rise in regional perfusion down the lung.

apices. Measurements of the volume of lung at which airways close show that airway closure occurs closer to the normal breathing range with advancing age, cigarette smoking, and bronchitis than in normals. Premature closure of airways has also been described in conditions that favor the formation of basal interstitial edema such as cirrhosis and acute myocardial infarction, suggesting that peribronchial edema may promote airway closure. Abnormalities in gas exchange correlate well with the occurrence of closing volumes above functional residual capacity (FRC). Since there is not generally a corresponding reduction in blood flow in these regions, airway closure results in areas of low $\dot{V}/\dot{Q}$. Abnormalities of airway closure can be detected in the presence of normal air-flow rates, suggesting that the involved areas are the very small airways (less than 2 mm in diameter). It is known that airways less than 2 mm in diameter normally contribute less than 10 percent of total airway resistance.

Changes in body position significantly affect the influence of airway closure on gas exchange. Thus, although the volume at which airways close does not change significantly in going from the seated to the supine position, the volume at which one normally breathes falls rather markedly (about 10 percent of total lung capacity, TLC). Airway closure might be just below FRC in the seated position and therefore not influence gas exchange in the seated position, but may be well above FRC in the supine position and therefore contribute to hypoxemia.

REGIONAL BLOOD FLOW

The regional distribution of xenon 133 that goes into the alveoli after an intravenous injection is proportional to regional pulmonary blood flow and has been shown to increase from the apex to the base of the lung in the seated position (Fig. 5). This gradient in perfusion varies strictly with body position, so that blood flow always increases from the superior to the inferior portions of the lung. The gradient of pulmonary blood flow is the result of a gravity-dependent gradient of pulmonary vascular pressures down the lung equivalent to an increase of 1 cm H_2O pressure for every centimeter of distance down the lung.

One would think that since the arterial and venous pressures increase down the lung that there would be no regional disparity in pulmonary blood flow, because the arterial–venous pressure difference, regardless of the lung region, would remain constant. But pulmonary blood flow does increase down the lungs because (1) the arterial–venous pressure difference is not the gradient responsible for flow in all parts of the lungs and (2) the vascular cross section increases and resistance to flow falls as the absolute levels of pressure rise (arterial and venous).

At the top of the lung there may be no blood flow during part of the cardiac cycle. In this zone the pulmonary artery pressure may fall below atmospheric pressure, so that the vessels collapse and no flow occurs. This is called Zone I, where the alveolar pressure (approximately atmospheric at rest) is greater than both pulmonary arterial and venous pressures. At a more dependent level the arterial pressure will exceed the alveolar pressure but the venous pressure will still be subatmospheric. At this level the arterial–alveolar pressure difference is responsible for flow, and blood flow increases rapidly below this level because both the driving pressure and the transmural arterial pressure are increasing. This is called Zone II.

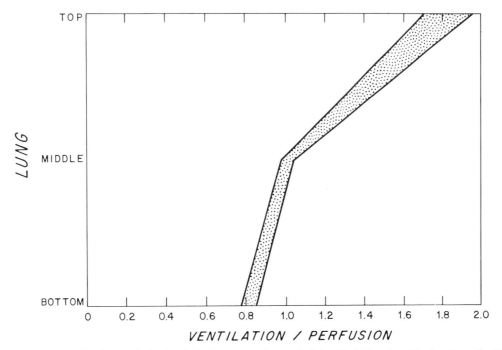

Fig. 6.   Mean values (± 2 SD) for ventilation/perfusion in a group of normal adults. The high ratios at the lung top reflect its relative overventilation (or underperfusion). The lower ratios at the bottom indicate a relative overperfusion (or underventilation).

When venous pressure exceeds alveolar pressure farther down the lung, then the arterial–venous pressure difference is responsible for flow. This is called Zone III. Flow increases down this zone less rapidly than down Zone II because the arterial–venous pressure difference remains constant. Only the transmural pressure (and vascular cross section) increases to reduce resistance to flow.

Pulmonary blood flow normally increases down the lung, as does ventilation, but the former does so at a faster rate. As a result there is less perfusion than ventilation at the lung apex, high $\dot{V}/\dot{Q}$, and more perfusion than ventilation at the lung base, low $\dot{V}/\dot{Q}$ (Fig. 6). This regional inhomogeneity in $\dot{V}$ and $\dot{Q}$ however, has only a slight effect on overall gas exchange in normals.

ABNORMALITIES OF REGIONAL VENTILATION, PERFUSION, AND $\dot{V}/\dot{Q}$ RATIOS

Although the primary cause of abnormal gas exchange in chronic obstructive pulmonary disease is the marked $\dot{V}/\dot{Q}$ inequality within very small gas-exchanging units, accentuated regional inhomogeneities in $\dot{V}$ and $\dot{Q}$ in other disease states can substantially affect gas exchange. Vascular muscular hyperplasia in mitral stenosis, or interstitial edema in congestive heart failure can increase vascular resistance at the lung base enough to cause the blood flow to the apices to exceed that to the bases. The result may be relative underperfusion or overventilation of the lung bases with a dead-space effect. Under special circumstances, e.g., low cardiac output states and low lung volumes, the accumulation of interstitial fluid as in congestive heart failure may reduce the cross section of extraalveolar vessels enough to result in a zone of decreased blood flow below Zone III. This has been called

Zone IV. Unless this local reduction in blood flow is matched by local reduction in ventilation, evidence of $\dot{V}/\dot{Q}$ inequality can be expected.

In obstructive lung disease the amount of lung at the extremes of $\dot{V}/\dot{Q}$ ratios is increased. In areas with bullae, regional ventilation/perfusion ratios approach zero. In other areas ventilation may far exceed local perfusion. In addition to these regional abnormalities, marked $\dot{V}/\dot{Q}$ inhomogeneities occur within very small lung units which cannot be detected by radioisotope studies. Regional ventilation/perfusion ratios approach infinity in areas that are devoid of blood flow but continue to be ventilated. Pulmonary embolism is such an example. It is apparent that unless compensatory mechanisms are complete (and they are not) atelectasis results in a very low regional $\dot{V}/\dot{Q}$ and embolism results in very high regional $\dot{V}/\dot{Q}$.

Abnormally high regional $\dot{V}/\dot{Q}$ ratios at the lung apices have been found in pulmonary hypotension, positive-pressure ventilation, and acceleration. Abnormally low $\dot{V}/\dot{Q}$ ratios particularly at the bases have been found in patients under prolonged anesthesia or with obstructed airways, as in aspiration of liquid material into the airways and in patients with abdominal distension.

The detection of variations of $\dot{V}/\dot{Q}$ within small regions of the lung requires radioisotopic "cameras" or arrays of scintillation detectors that view small areas of the lungs. The detector array systems generally lack resolution, and cameras are not efficient detectors of the widely available xenon-133 emissions. The development of more suitable isotopes for the cameras and the continued development of the positron cameras using ^{13}N gas promise to provide more information about varia-

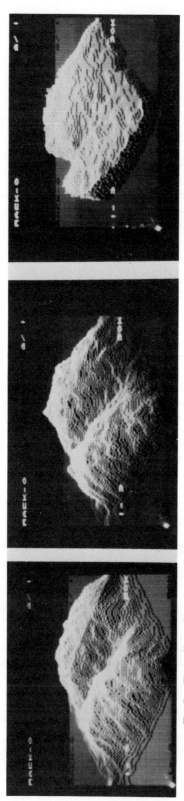

Fig. 7. Three-dimension representations of ventilation data obtained from radioactive nitrogen studies in a normal man using a positron camera. The left figure indicates the levels of activity throughout the lungs at total lung capacity after equilibration with radioactive nitrogen. This is proportional to the distribution of regional lung volume. The left lung is to the left. The deep valley indicates the location of the heart and great vessels. The middle figure indicates the distribution of residual volume obtained after equilibration, maximum expiration, and the inspiration of air to total lung capacity. The figure to the right is a representation of RV as a percentage of total lung capacity. Notice the progressive fall in the regional residual volume from top to bottom of the lungs.

tions in ventilation and perfusion within relatively small lung regions. Figure 7 illustrates the maplike data of regional lung volume that can be obtained from such a camera.

RADIOISOTOPE IMAGING

The widespread availability of radioisotope imaging of the lungs after intravenous injection of radioactive particles is particularly useful in the clinical evaluation of pulmonary thromboembolism. Radioactive particles that are large enough to become temporarily entrapped in the pulmonary microcirculation after intravenous injection are distributed approximately in accordance with pulmonary blood flow. Macroaggregates of human serum albumin and ferric hydroxide particles 10 to 30 μ in diameter have been commonly used labeled with technetium 99m, iodine 131, or indium 113. Macroaggregates of human serum albumin temporarily obstruct a very small proportion of the pulmonary vascular bed, and many clinical studies indicate the safety of such studies. Imaging is obtained with rectilinear scanning devices or gamma-detecting cameras during quiet breathing. Injections are generally made in the supine position to obtain adequate activity in the lung apices.

Although attempts have been made to quantitate the results of these studies, most are evaluated by studying the image and comparing it to a chest radiograph. While their primary use is in the clinical evaluation of pulmonary thromboembolism, they have also been used to grossly evaluate the distribution of blood flow in obstructive lung disease. The latter studies are best done, however, by using radioactive gases.

The role of radioisotope imaging as a screening procedure in pulmonary thromboembolism has become preeminent because of the knowledge that a large number of significant pulmonary emboli are not diagnosed in life, that clinical signs may be few, and that chest radiographs generally show no significant abnormalities. Pulmonary infarction, atelectasis, oligemia, and pleural effusion are seen in a small minority of the chest radiographs of patients with pulmonary embolism. The primary value of imaging lies in evaluating the patient suspected of having a pulmonary embolism who has a normal-appearing chest radiograph and no known cause for uneven pulmonary blood flow such as chronic obstructive lung disease, bullous disease, or pneumonia.

The presence of a normal perfusion radioisotopic image excludes the possibility of a large regional embolus. It cannot exclude, however, the presence of multiple small peripheral emboli. An abnormal scan indicates uneven blood flow, and if other causes for it are excluded it is diagnostic of pulmonary thromboembolism. Radioisotopic imaging is a very sensitive test of regional inhomogeneity of blood flow, but it lacks the specificity inherent in the pulmonary arteriographic demonstration of intravascular filling defect. Arteriography is no more specific than radioisotope imaging, however, when the diagnosis of embolism is based on secondary radiographic findings rather than on actual demonstration of the clot.

In the presence of a pulmonary density on the chest radiograph, the finding of other areas of decreased activity in the radioisotope image, particularly peripheral ones, can be diagnostic of embolization. The ease and safety of radioisotope imaging allow it to be used serially in following the resolution, recurrence, or response to therapy of demonstrated lesions.

Quantitative images that can provide data on perfusion per unit lung volume may become available clinically with the development of new isotopes suitable for use with isotopic cameras. Computer programs can then be used to map out ratios of regional perfusion per volume.

Ventilation images obtained with insoluble gaseous isotopes can be used to view the regional distribution of ventilation, and if carefully obtained they can be used in conjunction with macroaggregate perfusion imaging to exclude air trapping or other ventilation abnormalities as causes of regional reduction in pulmonary blood flow. Care must be taken in the performance of these ventilation studies, however, since the image obtained from a single breath depends on the lung volume and the speed of inspiration as well as on the volume of the radioisotope inhaled. Little attention has been paid thus far to these details in imaging studies. Ventilation images based on rebreathing techniques are often more indicative of the distribution of the volume of the equilibrated gas space than ventilation. There are many pitfalls and much misleading information that can result from so-called ventilation images. "Washout" images are probably the most dependable sources of true ventilation data.

Images obtained from inhaled radioactive particles do not seem to provide real ventilation data, nor do they give unique information about patent airways. Their main use appears to be in research related to the distribution of inhaled particulate matter.

PULMONARY EXTRAVASCULAR WATER VOLUME

Estimations of the extravascular water volume of the lung is of interest in evaluation of interstitial pulmonary edema, but thus far it has found only research applications. Intravascular markers such as dyes or radioisotope microaggregated particles have been used to measure the volume of the pulmonary vascular bed during a single transit through the lungs. Measuring the time–concentration (or activity) data of arterial blood of the vascular indicator and subtracting this data from that obtained from the simultaneous intravenous injection of a diffusible indicator such as tritiated H_2O or oxygen-15-labeled H_2O will give a measure of total pulmonary extravascular interstitial water. This has been found to be increased in interstitial pulmonary edema.

REFERENCES

Chinard F, Enns T, Nolan M: Indicator dilution studies with "diffusible" indicators. Circ Res 10:473, 1962

Greene R, Hoop B, Kazemi H: Use of ^{13}N in studies of airway closure and regional ventilation. J Nucl Med 12:719, 1971

Holland J, Milic-Emili H, Macklem PT, Bates DV: Regional distribution of pulmonary ventilation and perfusion in elderly subjects. J Clin Invest 47:81, 1968

Ruff, F, Hughes JMB, Stanley N, et al: Regional lung function in patients with hepatic cirrhosis. J Clin Invest 50:2003, 1971

Shore N, Greene R, Kazemi H: Lung dysfunction in workers after exposure to enzyme of bacillus subtilis. Environ Res 4:512, 1971

West JB: Ventilation/Blood Flow and Gas Exchange (ed 2). Philadelphia, FA Davis, 1970

SURGICAL DIAGNOSTIC PROCEDURES

Hermes C. Grillo

A number of manipulative or surgical diagnostic procedures are useful in obtaining microscopic morphologic diagnoses, either histologic, cytologic, or bacteriologic. These procedures include endoscopic examination of the bronchial tree and the biopsy of lungs, pleura, or thoracic lymph nodes by open intervention or by the use of special needles. The precision, technologic range, and application of all of these methods have increased in the last decade and show promise of further extension. None of these methods should be applied routinely in a predetermined sequence. Those techniques should be selected that give the needed answers as precisely and promptly as possible in a given clinical situation.

BRONCHOSCOPY

There are several variations of the standard bronchoscope. In essence it consists of a rigid tube that is passed directly through the larynx into the tracheobronchial tree. Visualization is direct, with or without the addition of a magnifying lens. The light source at the tip of the instrument was formerly a small electric bulb, but is now more often a fiberoptic light carrier. The bronchoscope may be introduced under either topical or local anesthesia or, with convenience to the patient and operator when extensive manipulations are to be done, under general or dissociative anesthesia. With a sealing window and a ventilating side arm, ventilation may be safely maintained during an examination under anesthesia. By rotating and angulating the head and neck it is possible under direct forward vision to look for short distances into the upper-lobe orifices on both sides and the middle-lobe orifice on the right and to examine the superior and basal segmental orifices of the lower lobes (Fig. 1). With right-angle or Foroblique telescopes it is further possible to visualize the segmental divisions of the upper-lobe orifices. In addition to visualization of gross abnormalities, aspiration of material present in the bronchial tree and washings of selected lobar or segmental orifices may be done. Bronchial brushes developed for radiologic placement are also useful in bronchoscopy. Fine biopsy forceps are also useful, and flexible biopsy forceps that are directable through lens systems are available for the upper-lobe orifices.

Small-diameter (3-5 mm) flexible fiberoptic bronchoscopes are now available. These may be passed directly under local anesthesia through the nasopharynx and into the bronchial tree as far as the subsegmental subdivisions. These instruments may also be passed through endotracheal tubes fitted with special sealing gaskets and through ventilating tracheoscopes, so that manipulation and examination may be done at leisure in a closed system under anesthesia. These instruments permit washing, brushing under direct vision, and direct biopsy with fine flexible forceps. Such flexible equipment has greatly widened the range of application of bronchoscopy to the more peripheral lesions and made possible the pursuit of such special problems as the patient with positive sputum cytology who has normal chest x-rays and no gross lesions on conventional bronchoscopy. As is not the case with esophagoscopy, there are complications of bronchoscopy other than those related to sensitivity to a topical anesthetic agent or to the complications of general anesthesia, but these are few with the adequate oxygenation provided by modern technique.

Bronchoscopic examination is of specific value in certain types of clinical problems. Central lesions may sometimes be visualized directly by conventional bronchoscopy. Upper-lobe lesions, however, are not often available unless a fiberoptic flexible bronchoscope is used. Varying degrees of distortion of the bronchial system, the presence of extrinsic pressure, and suggestions of fixation or blunting of carina due to lymph nodes or direct extension of tumors will be obtained on examination. In otherwise undefined peripheral infiltrates bronchoscopy may reveal the presence of a proximal obstructive lesion or foreign body, of bronchial wall deformation, of mucosal changes, or of a wholly open bronchial tree that is of negative importance. The aspiration, washing, and biopsy techniques mentioned earlier are applicable to these situations. Occasionally bronchoscopy performed in a patient who has recurring episodes of unilateral or bilateral pneumonia without other explanation will reveal partial obstruction due to a tumor of tracheobronchial origin. Bronchoscopy is of little value diagnostically in the patient with a small solitary nodule or multiple peripheral nodules. However, if diagnosis is not obtained by other means, it is advisable that bronchoscopy be performed concomitantly if surgical excision is elected.

Bronchoscopy is clearly indicated in some patients who develop wheezing or shortness of breath but who have normal x-rays. This is the case where the patient has a history of intubation in the recent past. Obstructing lesions, either those that follow the trauma of intubation with or without ventilation or those of primary neoplastic obstruction, may occasionally be discovered. Examination must be done with careful timing if the patient is severely obstructed. In patients with hemoptysis with either normal lung fields or changes due to aspiration of blood, bronchoscopy is important. It serves on rare occasions to identify the source of bleeding from an area of small bronchial vessel erosion and in other cases to localize the source of bleeding to a given segment, so that treatment may be pointed precisely in the event that conservative measures fail. Where hemoptysis is not profuse, the flexible instrument has particular application in this

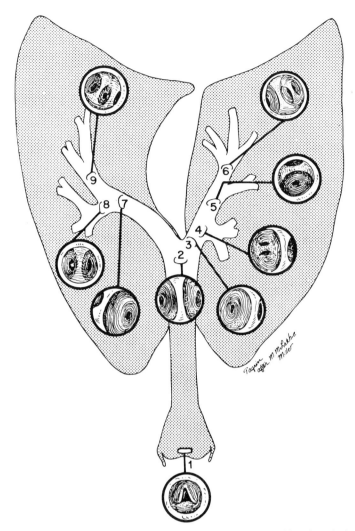

Fig. 1. Bronchoscopic view of the tracheobronchial tree. The tree is positioned as the bronchoscopist views the patient, who is lying supine. The insets show the range of view obtained with a conventional straight bronchoscope and fixed-angle telescopes. (Reproduced by permission from Benedict EB: Endoscopy. Baltimore, Williams & Wilkins, 1951.)

last case. There are multiple therapeutic indications for bronchoscopy also, sometimes in combination with diagnostic manuevers, as in the case of lung abscess or a foreign body. Cultures obtained from bronchoscopic material are often of great diagnostic value.

THORACIC LYMPH NODE BIOPSY

The classic studies of lymphatic drainage by Rouvière demonstrated predominant drainage of the entire right lung and the lower half of the left lung (via the subcarinal lymphatics) to the paratracheal nodes on the right and thence to the right thoracic duct. The upper portion of the left lung was shown to drain from its lobar and hilar nodes to the left paratracheal lymph nodes and thence to the left thoracic duct. Subsequent studies of dye injection into the lower lobes in man and clinical observations of nodal metastases of tumors in various locations have supplemented these findings. Both lower-lobe regions may frequently drain into the left paratracheal

nodes. Upper-lobe lesions may drain down into the subcarinal lymph nodes as well as upward, and crossed metastases from the opposite side have been noted even in the absence of ipsilateral metastases (Fig. 2).

Scalene Node Biopsy

The highest node in the thoracic drainage chain lies at the junction of the subclavian vein and internal jugular vein close to the entry point of the thoracic duct on either side. These nodes frequently show anthracotic pigment, unlike higher nodes in the scalene fat pad area that drain the arm and neck. The deep lymph nodes frequently reflect intrathoracic disease. Patients with carcinoma of the lung who do not have palpable nodes at the base of the neck nonetheless will have positive deep cervical node biopsy in at least 10 percent of cases. The incidence of positive nodes increases further in the hands of skilled operators, where the highest thoracic lymph nodes are truly biopsied, rather than nodes of the scalene fat pad. In

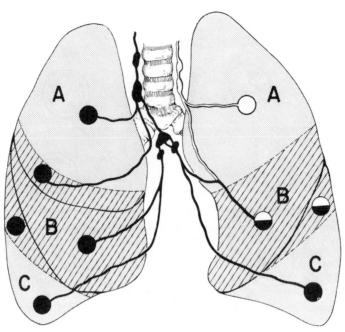

Fig. 2. Lymphatic drainage of the lungs. The principal pathways of drainage as described by Rouvière are indicated by dashed lines. The additional pathways since shown experimentally and clinically are noted by dotted lines. Lymph nodes that are usually examined by mediastinoscopy are solid black. Only the highest of these nodes is accessible by scalene node biopsy.

sarcoidosis or tuberculosis the incidence of positive nodes may run 60 percent or higher. Such biopsies provide diagnoses in systemic diseases or in diseases that involve the lungs and are otherwise difficult diagnostic problems, with little stress to the patient. Involvement of nodes as peripheral as this usually indicates that a malignant lesion is beyond the bounds of cure and may dictate a change in therapeutic plan.

Mediastinoscopy

Since a higher degree of positive diagnosis can be expected by moving more proximally on the lymph node drainage chain toward the lesion, the scalene node biopsy was extended, with a laryngoscope, along the paratracheal chain in the upper mediastinum. This has increased the positive findings in all cases of carcinoma of the lung to above 30 percent, often in situations where the scalene node was still negative. This extension of central nodal biopsy has been widened with the introduction of mediastinoscopy. This procedure is done through a short transverse incision in the suprasternal notch, with dissection along the pretracheal plane to the carina. Through this channel a tubular instrument is passed, and the right and left paratracheal and subcarinal regions are examined. It is possible to pass a short distance out on the right and left main bronchi as well. Biopsies of nodes are taken with forceps in the various locations.

This type of extended biopsy is useful in the cancer suspect where diagnosis alone is desirable because of the patient's medical inoperability, but has been unavailable by bronchoscopy. It is also used as an index of curability and to determine the extent of treatment—whether by surgery, by irradiation, or by a combination of both. In many cases the extent of disease found clearly indicates incurability. In some situations, particularly in the patient with squamous cell carcinoma of the lung, limited metastatic involvement of paratracheal lymph nodes may possibly be an indication for preoperative irradiation and thus still provide a possibility of cure. Patients with bilateral hilar adenopathy will also usually yield a diagnosis on this examination. Sarcoid and lymphoma are leading possibilities in many such cases. The approach has also been extended to mediastinal tumors, making it possible to differentiate mediastinal lymphoma from other lesions that require surgical extirpation.

Approximately 40 percent of patients with carcinoma of the lung demonstrate metastases to the mediastinal lymph nodes (as differentiated from the lobar or strictly hilar nodes). Undifferentiated carcinoma is more likely to be positive, and central lesions are more likely to be so than peripheral lesions. As many as 20 percent of patients with mediastinal node metastases from carcinoma of the lung have been found to have contralateral spread. The careful use of such information has progressively limited the number of the thoracotomies that have ended in exploration only, with their high morbidity and without chance for cure or palliation. As many as 98 percent of patients with sarcoid involving the lung will be positive on mediastinoscopic node biopsy.

In skilled hands the number of complications of scalene node biopsy and of mediastinoscopy are few and usually minor. However, the procedure is not to be underestimated or performed by the unskilled. Another variation of mediastinal exploration is by resection of the second costal cartilage anteriorly with paramediastinal

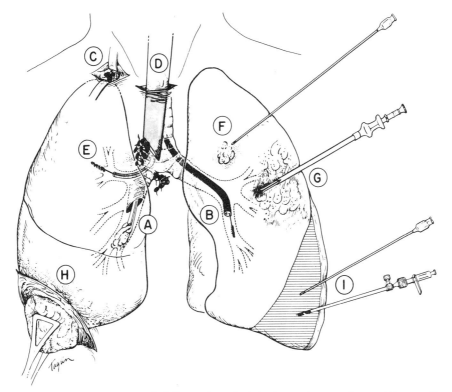

Fig. 3. Summary of principal surgical diagnostic methods in pleuropulmonary disease: (A) conventional bronchoscopy and biopsy, (B) flexible bronchoscopy, (C) scalene node biopsy, (D) mediastinoscopy, (E) bronchial brushing, (F) needle biopsy of pulmonary mass, (G) needle biopsy of diffuse disease, (H) open biopsy of lung, (I) needle biopsy of pleura and thoracentesis.

dissection to the root of the lung. This has the disadvantage of being unilateral and of being in a field of potential resection of neoplasm, but is sometimes applicable where central mediastinal exploration will not permit access to a nonresectable lesion. Such an approach may also be combined with open lung biopsy.

LUNG BIOPSY

Direct biopsy of the lung is frequently necessary for diagnosis, both in cases of mass or nodular lesions and in cases of diffuse pulmonary disease. Increasing diagnostic use has been made of percutaneous needle biopsy in both categories. There are some advantages to open biopsy, usually by very limited thoracotomy for diffuse disease and by more extensive thoracotomy for circumscribed disease where therapeutic as well as diagnostic maneuvers are to be carried out simultaneously.

Needle biopsy of a large intrathoracic mass has long been used in patients who clearly present too great a risk for thoracotomy, who are clearly incurable because of distant metastatic disease, or in whom there is evidence of multiple pulmonary masses of probable metastatic origin. Little hazard has been envisioned or encountered, particularly when such masses are close to the parietal pleura.

Percutaneous needle biopsy of small parenchymal nodules has become increasingly useful. In a large experience, Dahlgren and Nordenström obtained satisfactory material by needle biopsy under fluoroscopic con-

trol in 82 percent of patients. By repetitive biopsy this was increased to over 91 percent. The aspirated material was examined both cytologically and bacteriologically as indicated. Small pneumothorax occurs commonly, but resolves readily. Larger pneumothorax occurs occasionally. Intrapleural hemorrhage is rare, but hemoptysis is not infrequent. There have been few if any instances to substantiate a prior theoretical concern about tumor implantation in needle tracts.

Needle biopsies using such instruments as the Franklin modification of the Vim-Silverman needle, or more recently the high-speed hollow drill, have produced results such as histologically interpretable material in 86 percent of patients and clearly diagnostic material in over 66 percent. Biopsy of diffuse parenchymal disease does not require fluoroscopic control because of its widespread nature. About 20 percent have developed complications, with pneumothorax most common and hemoptysis frequent. Rarely have these been serious complications that required more than a tube for management. Clearly, a patient with extensive cystic disease, a patient with severe and uncontrollable cough, or a patient with pulmonary artery hypertension should not be subjected to such a procedure. In neither diffuse disease nor localized nodular disease is such a biopsy done lightly, since mortality can occur.

Open lung biopsy in diffuse disease is done through a small intercostal thoracotomy, usually in the anterolateral position if the diseased lung is accessible through such an approach. It has the advantages of providing wholly adequate specimens not only for histology and bacteriology but also for metal analysis and other types of study. With meticulous technique it is a safe procedure that is tolerated even by the patient with severe pulmonary dysfunction. Many physicians still prefer that a solitary nodule pulmonary lesion be removed for diagnosis and treatment. Wedge excision or local excision of the nodule is done initially for diagnosis, followed by lobectomy should examination by frozen section prove a primary malignant lesion.

The nature of the lesion and clinical problem must be taken into account in selecting a method of lung biopsy, as well as the availability of diagnosis through the more peripheral means discussed in this section and elsewhere. It is obvious that the needle biopsy, even with diffuse lung disease, is more appealing, since it eliminates the need for limited thoracotomy with its attendant anesthetic risk and postoperative discomfort. It is also possible to perform repeated needle biopsies subsequently to observe the effects of treatment. On the other hand, open biopsy is a sure road to diagnosis. We have frequently combined the two, performing closed biopsy and then proceeding to an early open biopsy if the results of the first are inadequate for diagnosis.

PLEURAL BIOPSY

Pleural biopsy is employed either in the presence of a marked local or diffuse thickening of pleura or very frequently in conjunction with diagnostic aspiration of pleural effusion of unknown etiology. Pleural biopsy should probably be performed more frequently than it is at the time of an initial aspiration of an effusion of puzzling origin. This is an excellent time to perform the biopsy and is especially safe where there is residual fluid. If the problem is obviously purulent infection, pleural biopsy is not indicated. Various instruments are available; the Cope type needle is particularly useful since it invariably provides a specimen. It is well to remove several specimens. The pleural biopsy should be done after the initial aspiration of fluid, since it may cause a little localized bleeding that confuses the cell count in subsequent aspirate. In one series of patients, pleural biopsy in the presence of effusion was diagnostic in 73 percent. If tuberculosis is a possibility, a biopsy specimen should be cultured, since it is more likely in the untreated patient to yield a positive culture than is the pleural fluid. It has proven to be more frequently diagnostic in tuberculosis (60–80 percent) than in malignant disease (40–60 percent). A diagnosis of nonspecific pleuritis, of course, does not rule out either of the other two possibilities mentioned. Thickened pleura alone is less likely to result in a diagnostic biopsy than is the case with concurrent effusion. This is probably due to the fact that the thickened pleura may be residual from a disease that has subsided. Localized deposits along with pleural surface visualized radiologically may be precisely biopsied under fluoroscopic control, and in some cases a Silverman type needle is effectively employed. Multiple diagnostic possi-

bilities exist including metastatic deposits and mesothelioma. Unlike lung biopsy, open biopsy will not often yield more information than pleural biopsy obtained by needle. A summary of surgical procedures in diagnosis of lung disease is presented in Fig. 3.

REFERENCES

Ashbaugh DG: Mediastinoscopy. Arch Surg 100:568, 1970

Benedict EB: Endoscopy. Baltimore, Williams & Wilkins, 1951

Carlens E: Mediastinoscopy: A method for inspection and tissue biopsy in the superior mediastinum. Dis Chest 36:343, 1959

Dahlgren S, Nordenström B: Transthoracic Needle Biopsy. Chicago, Year Book Medical Publishers, 1966

Donohoe RF, Katz S, Matthews M: Pleural biopsy as an aid in the etiologic diagnosis of pleural effusion: Review of the literature and report of 132 biopsies. Ann Intern Med 48:344, 1958

Keltz H, Scerbo J, Stone DJ: A prospective study of closed pleural biopsies. JAMA 218:377, 1971

Krumholtz RA, Manfredi F, Wef VG, Rosenbaum D: Needle biopsy of the lung. Report on its use in 112 patients and review of the literature. Ann Intern Med 65:293, 1966

Skinner DB: Scalene lymph node biopsy: Reappraisal of risks and indications. N Engl J Med 268:1324, 1963

CHRONIC OBSTRUCTIVE LUNG DISEASES (COLD)

Denise J. Strieder

Emphysema, chronic bronchitis, asthma, and bronchiectasis—these four diseases, pathologically different, share the symptoms of shortness of breath, cough, and expectoration, and the signs of hyperinflation of the chest, ronchi, wheezes, and rales, although in varying combinations. Their course is chronic but capricious, with remissions or stabilizations and with exacerbations. They can present each as a single disease and apparently the result of a single cause, but often they appear in some two- or three-way association and as a result of multiple factors. They have a common physiologic defect, airway obstruction, associated with maldistribution and hypoxemia, and a common major complication, respiratory failure. Indeed, the chronic obstructive lung diseases have a great deal in common. Hence the usage of the group name, often by its initials COLD, either as a provisional diagnosis or as a brief notation to indicate that two or more entities are associated in a given instance. But COLD is not a diagnosis, it is a clinical problem that once recognized calls for an appropriate approach to the patient in terms of diagnostic work-up, supportive management and therapy.

In the late 1950s a series of national and international meetings and interdisciplinary studies demonstrated a lack of factual knowledge about these diseases, especially with regard to the boundaries between emphysema, asthma and chronic bronchitis. A consensus was reached on the following terms: (1) emphysema was to be defined by its pathologic changes (dilatation of distal air spaces), (2) asthma by its physiologic abnormalities (variable airway obstruction), and (3) chronic bronchitis by its symptoms of cough and expectoration, with suitable criteria to assess the chronicity of the course. Bronchiectasis was not considered.

These working definitions led to the use of reasonably uniform diagnostic criteria and epidemiologic questionnaires, within and beyond the English-speaking medical community. New correlations were described between the pathology, radiology, physiology and clinical presentation characteristic of patients with chronic obstructive lung disease. Concurrently great progress in immunology and in physiology uncovered some of the basic mechanisms relevant to the pathogenesis and functional defects of emphysema and asthma, and the place of chronic bronchitis in relation to these two entities could begin to be understood.

COMMON ENVIRONMENTAL FACTORS

It became apparent also that environmental factors are particularly important in the case of chronic obstructive lung diseases. Most notable in this respect are socioeconomic circumstances, air pollution and smoking habits.

Poverty brings crowded housing, frequent and prolonged exposures to cold, marginal or deficient nutrition and inadequate health care. Predictably infants and young children show a greater incidence of upper respiratory infections, otitis, bronchitis, infectious asthma, bronchiectasis, and pneumonia. In adults economic factors are partly overshadowed by occupational exposures and personal habits, such as abuse of cigarettes or alcohol.

Air pollution, present in all modern cities, has worsened in recent decades, mostly with increased use of fossil fuels. Differences among cities are due to type and density of industrial plants, number of automobiles, nature of domestic fuel and local climate. A large number of pollutants have been identified. Particulate matter comprises metal, coal, soot, soil, stone and cement dust, and high-molecular-weight hydrocarbons. Gases include the oxidants (NO_2, SO_2, O_3, and a number of less stable molecules), carbon monoxide, and low-molecular-weight hydrocarbons. The oxidants are particularly noxious because of their dual modality of action: mucosal irritation causing cough, hypersecretion and bronchospasm, and cellular toxicity affecting epithelium, macrophages and leukocytes. Decreased bacterial clearance and increased frequency of viral and bacterial lung diseases have been demonstrated in animals when standard infective doses have been coupled with exposure to oxidants. In man increased morbidity for emphysema, chronic bronchitis and asthma occurs as a result of year-round urban air pollution, regardless of age or previous state of health. Increased mortality with peaks of air pollution affects older persons with chronic obstructive lung disease.

Tobacco smoke contains similar toxic agents (CO, hydrocarbons and oxidants) in concentrations well above that of common urban air pollution, as well as variable amounts of tars and nicotine. Emphysema, chronic bronchitis and asthma are among the most common of the many health hazards to which cigarette smokers are exposed.

COMMON PHYSIOLOGIC CHANGES

In chronic airway disease inflammation and mucus hypersecretion are found in airways of all sizes. But mild mucosal edema or a minute amount of mucus, which leaves the resistance of large bronchi nearly unchanged, can close terminal bronchioles. Thus the physiologic changes of airway disease begin with the malfunction of small airways. As an isolated abnormality, small-airway disease is observed at the early stage of chronic bronchitis and during remissions from asthma. It is present, however, in the more severe stages of chronic bronchitis, asthma and bronchiectasis; then it is probably responsible for much of the associated maldistribution of ventilation.

With small-airway disease a reduction of forced expiratory flow rate is demonstrable only at low lung volume: the flow–volume curve becomes convex toward the volume axis, and the maximal mid-expiratory flow rate (MMFR) is slightly reduced. But the forced expiratory volume in the first second (FEV_1) and peak flow rate (PFR) are normal. Because the small airways contribute little to total airway resistance, the latter remains normal. Lung compliance also is normal when measured in static conditions or during tidal breathing at a low frequency. But dynamic compliance, measured during tidal breathing at normal or rapid respiratory rates, falls with increasing frequency, a behavior that reveals a significant inequality in the resistance of individual bronchial pathways. Maldistribution of ventilation/perfusion ratio is appreciable, resulting in increased alveolar–arterial P_{O_2} difference.

Airway obstruction results from advanced airway disease or loss of elastic lung recoil, or both. Suspected on clinical grounds, it can be readily documented and quantitated by tests of forced expiration (Table 1). Direct measurements of airway resistance are used for physiologic investigation rather than for clinical diagnosis or follow-up.

Hyperinflation is reflected in altered lung volumes. Increased total lung capacity correlates with radiologic evidence of hyperinflation and increased functional residual capacity with hyperresonance on physical examination. Increased residual volume is a measurement of air trapping, which in relative value appears as the most striking change (Table 1). When hyperinflation is due to emphysema the elastic recoil of the lung is decreased and a decreased steady-state diffusing capacity is usually observed.

Maldistribution or inequality of ventilation/perfusion ratios, results in increased alveolar–arterial P_{O_2} difference and hypoxemia, of increasing severity with advancing disease. Hypoxemia is associated at first with hypocapnia, then with normocapnia, and finally with CO_2 retention.

PREVALENCE AND MORTALITY

Statistical data regarding the prevalence and death rate of chronic obstructive lung diseases are greatly de-

Table 1
Clinical Tests of Airway Obstruction and Lung Hyperinflation

	Abbreviation	Normal Range	Direction of Change
Forced expiration			
Peak flow rate	PFR	400–600 l/min	Decreased
Forced expiratory volume in 1 sec	FEV_1	3–4 l	Decreased, more than PFR
Maximal mid-expiratory flow rate	MMFR	200–300 l/min	Decreased, more than FEV_1
Timed vital capacity	$(FEV_1/VC)\,100$	70–85%	Decreased
Lung volumes			
Total lung capacity	TLC	5–7 l	Increased
Functional residual capacity	FRC	2.5–4 l	Increased
Residual volume	RV	1–2 l	Most markedly increased
RV/TLC ratio	$(RV/TLC)\,100$	20–30%	Increased
Vital capacity	VC	4–5 l	Decreased
Closing volume	–	less than FRC	Increased for age or above FRC

pendent on the reliability and general acceptance of diagnostic criteria. Asthma and bronchiectasis are diagnosed on the basis of objective findings, easily recognized and generally accepted. Accordingly these diseases are han-

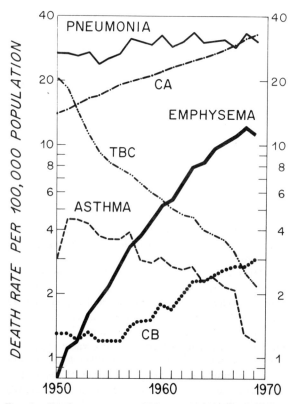

Fig. 1. Death rate among U.S. populations from leading respiratory diseases in the years 1950–1969, showing sustained rise of mortality from neoplasms of the respiratory system (CA) and from emphysema, and the decreasing mortality from tuberculosis of the respiratory system (TBC); there is a slower rise for chronic bronchitis (CB) and a decline for asthma; pneumonia has been stable for the past 10 years. (Data reproduced by permission from: Vital Statistics of the United States, vol 11, Mortality, 1950 through 1969. Washington, U.S. Government Printing Office.)

dled separately in statistical studies whose pertinent results are summarized later in this chapter.

For emphysema and chronic bronchitis, difficulties arise from various sources. First, medical tradition varies from one country to another. For example, patients with similar clinical characteristics are thought to suffer from and eventually to die of emphysema in the U.S. (Fig. 1) but chronic bronchitis in Great Britain. In fact, the diagnosis of emphysema remains tentative in most cases, unless the disease is so far advanced that unequivocal changes are found by x-ray examination and appropriate function tests, or unless postmortem examination is carried out. Defined by a symptom complex, chronic bronchitis is more easily amenable to population surveys in which questionnaires on respiratory symptoms have become a major investigative tool.

Statistical studies in recent years have provided valuable information, although the data are usually divided into prevalence figures for chronic bronchitis and mortality data on emphysema. Thus it has been shown that chronic bronchitis affects nearly 10 percent of non-smoking adult men and over 40 percent of cigarette smokers; intermediate figures are usually observed for pipe smokers and ex-smokers. Regardless of smoking habits and occupation, urban dwellers have a greater incidence of respiratory symptoms than rural residents. Differences also observed from city to city support the concept that air pollution is a major element in the "urban factor" that clearly contributes to the pathogenesis of COLD. Indeed, increasing air pollution probably caused the dramatic rise in mortality due to emphysema in recent years, a trend quite independent of the concomitant aging of population (Fig. 2).

Emphysema, rigorously diagnosed on pathologic evidence, has been found in 48 percent of men over 60 years of age coming to necropsy in a Boston hospital. More importantly, all large pathologic series emphasize the frequent association of emphysema and chronic bronchitis. Such evidence may well dampen the physician's incentive to attempt a differential diagnosis. But the recognition of chronic bronchitis as a distinct entity remains desirable because it promises not only a better understanding of

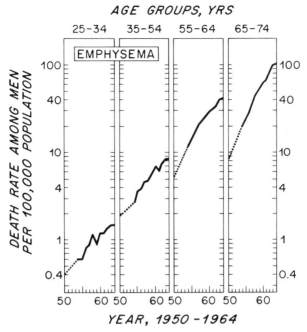

Fig. 2. Age-corrected mortality data for emphysema in men showing a similar trend in all age groups and high mortality rates in the older age groups. (Reproduced by permission from: Mortality from Disease associated with Smoking. Washington, National Center for Health Statistics and U.S. Government Printing Office, 1966.)

COLD but also a greater chance of early diagnosis and active therapeutic approach.

EMPHYSEMA
Definitions

The American Thoracic Society defines pulmonary emphysema as a "condition characterized by the enlargement of air spaces distal to terminal bronchioles, accompanied by destructive changes of the alveolar walls." A similar definition has been adopted by the World Health Organization. However, as judged from the current literature the older usage seems to prevail, whereby emphysema is defined as "enlargement of air spaces beyond the terminal bronchioles, either from dilatation or from destruction of their walls" (Ciba Symposium on Emphysema, London, 1959). The latter definition includes a varied group of disorders, beside the widespread, destructive emphysema that is one of the chronic obstructive lung diseases (Table 2).

The enlargement of distal air spaces in the lung, common to all forms of pulmonary emphysema, arises by three primary mechanisms: (1) Increased transpulmonary pressure causes overdistension of structurally normal lung whenever one lobe stretches out to fill one hemithorax or one lung to fill nearly the whole chest (compensatory emphysema). (2) Loss of lung recoil causes alveolar enlargement even though transpulmonary pressure is low (panacinar emphysema) or normal (Swyer-James syndrome). (3) Air trapping is due to a ball-valve effect whereby air moves more easily into the lung than out of it (obstructive emphysema). In many forms of emphysema more than one mechanism is at work.

The following paragraphs on pathology, pathogenesis and clinical presentation refer to widespread, destructive emphysema, panacinar and centriacinar (Table 2).

Table 2
Classification of Various Forms of Emphysema

Pulmonary emphysema
  Panacinar and centriacinar emphysema
  Focal emphysema
    with the pneumonoconioses
    with healed granulomatous lung disease
  Bullous emphysema
    single bulla (Type I)
    cluster (Type II)
    extreme panacinar (Type III)
  Lobar emphysema
    congenital infantile
    acquired (Swyer-James syndrome)
    obstructive emphysema
  Compensatory emphysema
    with atelectasis
    with S/P lobectomy
    with S/P pneumonectomy
    with agenesis of one lung
Other disorders
  Subcutaneous emphysema
  Mediastinal emphysema (pneumomediastinum)
  Interstitial emphysema

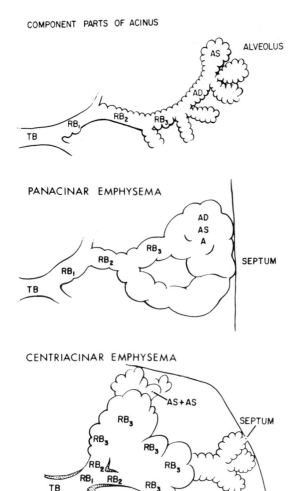

COMPONENT PARTS OF ACINUS

PANACINAR EMPHYSEMA

CENTRIACINAR EMPHYSEMA

Fig. 3. Schematic representation of the normal constituents of the acinus (top), the diffuse dilatation affecting all distal air spaces in panacinar emphysema (middle), and the selective destruction of respiratory bronchioles and alveolar ducts in centriactinar emphysema (bottom). [Reproduced by permission Thurlbeck WM: in Sommers SC (ed): Pathology Annual. New York, Appleton-Century-Crofts, 1968.]

Pathology

Emphysematous lungs fail to deflate in the open chest. They are pale and their weight is normal. For proper evaluation the lungs should be fixed, fully expanded under positive transpulmonary pressure, and prepared in thick (400-μ) sections of a whole lung or lobe (Gough sections). In normal lung so prepared, individual alveoli, less than 0.1 mm in diameter, are barely distinguishable, but the lobules are punctuated with larger air spaces representing cross sections of respiratory bronchioles and alveolar ducts.

In panacinar emphysema all air spaces within the lobule are more or less uniformly enlarged (Fig. 3). Individual alveoli are easily seen on the lung section and the severity of the disease may be evaluated from alveolar diameters, which range from less than 1 mm in mildly

affected areas to 5 mm and over in severely diseased areas.

In centriacinar emphysema the destruction of respiratory bronchioles and of their adjacent alveoli creates a hole in the middle of each acinus (Fig. 3). Such holes, which may reach 5 mm in diameter (the lobule is about 10–12 mm in diameter), have no recognizable wall; they are directly surrounded by normal-looking alveoli. Several holes may be seen in one lobule; if the holes are large, only a rim of preserved alveolar tissue remains around each one. Thin strands of tissue often run across the emphysematous space; they are the acinar arterioles and their branches.

Panacinar and centriacinar emphysema are elementary lesions that may be found in association, each one prevailing in different areas. The lesions may be truly widespread, involving most of the lungs, although often with unequal severity, or they may be localized to one or two lobes. Thus grading emphysema on pathologic specimens must take into account the type, severity, and distribution of lesions, as well as the presence of spared areas.

Evidence of chronic bronchitis is nearly always found in lungs with centriacinar emphysema, less commonly in lungs with panacinar emphysema. The incidence of right ventricular hypertrophy and dilatation of the large pulmonary arteries correlates with that of associated chronic bronchitis rather than with the severity of emphysema itself. In specimens showing severe widespread emphysema without chronic bronchitis (mostly panacinar disease), postmortem pulmonary angiograms show normal arterial size and branching pattern, contrasting with the poor perfusion revealed by angiograms in vivo. Other gross pathologic findings that may be noted in emphysematous lungs are bronchopneumonia and pulmonary embolism.

Microscopic examination of emphysematous areas is comparatively less informative. In centriacinar emphysema the alveoli surrounding the holes are normal or minimally enlarged. Bronchi and bronchioles show chronic bronchitis and arteries show medial and intimal thickening, all of variable severity. In panacinar emphysema alveolar enlargement is striking. Alveolar walls are thin and interrupted in places, as though part of the wall had vanished. Bronchi and arteries may be normal.

Pathogenesis of Emphysema

Epidemiologic studies have left no doubt that a number of environmental factors, particularly cigarette smoking and air pollution, are capable of causing widespread emphysema. Nevertheless it has long been suspected that host defense mechanisms are equally important in determining the occurrence and severity of the disease. Actually emphysema is known to occur without exposure to noxious inhalants, presumably because of failing defense mechanisms whereby the integrity of alveolar structure cannnot be maintained even in a favorable environment. Inherited deficiency of serum antitrypsin is the best known of such host factors.

Alpha$_1$-antitrypsin makes up 90 percent of the α_1

fraction of serum proteins. Decreased levels are therefore recognizable by inspection of the serum electrophoretic pattern (Fig. 4). Synthesized in the liver, the glycoprotein is normally present in serum at a concentration of 210 mg/100 ml and accounts for 90 percent of normal serum trypsin inhibiting capacity (TIC, 1 ml of serum normally inhibits 1 mg of trypsin). α_1-antitrypsin also inhibits plasmin, thrombin, elastase, collagenase and several other enzymes; hence its more general name of proteinase inhibitor (Pi). Further studies of the protein have revealed individual differences in electrophoretic mobility that reflect genetic variations controlled by codominant inheritance. The common type is designated by the letter M (Pi type M). A number of variants are known with normal serum concentration and activity. Others (Pi types S, F, and Z) have a reduced serum concentration with correspondingly low activity. The normal M homozygous phenotype is observed in 80–96 percent of European natives and the MZ heterozygous type in 2 percent or less; the Z genotype, associated with the lowest recorded serum levels (10 percent of normal), is rare. In M homozygotes, antitrypsin levels rise in response to inflammation, corticosteroids and estrogens, up to 200–300 percent of baseline values. In the same conditions MZ heterozygotes show a rise from moderately low to low-normal values and Z homozygotes do not respond.

Patients with Z deficiency develop emphysema. Their disease is remarkable for lack of environmental etiologic factors, for early onset of symptoms (mostly before age 40, sometimes in childhood), for equal involvement of males and females and for absence of associated chronic bronchitis. Available pathologic reports describe widespread panacinar emphysema and confirm the absence of airway disease. Liver biopsies have shown accumulation of the glycoprotein in hepatocytes, from which the aberrant protein fails to be excreted. In a small number of patients the deficiency is associated with juvenile cirrhosis of the liver, and possibly cirrhosis in the adults as well.

MZ heterozygotes do not develop emphysema spontaneously, but they are thought to have increased susceptibility to environmental insults. Because of overlap between normal and heterozygous blood levels, a Pi-type determination is necessary for sure identification of heterozygotes. Known MZ heterozygotes should be strongly encouraged to avoid exposure to noxious inhalants and to select their occupations accordingly.

Experimental evidence thus far suggests that antitrypsin deficiency may be directly responsible for the development of emphysema in affected patients. In animals administration of papain, elastase or other proteolytic enzymes in aerosol causes alveolar destruction, air-space enlargement and loss of lung recoil, i.e., a disorder nearly identical to human emphysema. In man proteolytic enzymes could reach the lung from various sources, particularly from macrophages and polymorphonuclear leukocytes, whose lysosomes and granules release active enzymes after lysis of the cell; destruction of the proteinic framework of alveolar walls would ensue in

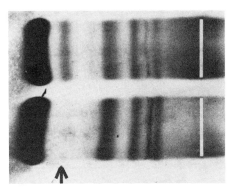

Fig. 4. Protein electrophoresis of a normal serum (upper) and a serum deficient in α_1-antitrypsin (lower); the place of the missing α_1-globulin band in the patient's pattern is indicated by an arrow.

the absence of a proteinase inhibitor. Such a mechanism may well pertain to the occurrence of emphysema in normal hosts, since oxidants are known to injure alveolar macrophages and leukocytes attracted to the lung in increased numbers as a result of chemical inflammation (Fig. 5).

In centriacinar emphysema, however, the destruction of respiratory bronchioles, alveolar ducts and neighboring alveoli, which leaves behind the scattered holes characteristic of the disease, is thought to originate with a lesion of the airway. Inflammation due to chemical injury and superinfection is widespread throughout the bronchial tree, but because of their fragile structure the respiratory bronchioles are a point of least resistance; where the basement membrane has been injured regeneration is impossible and the respiratory bronchiole disappears with or without a scar.

The possibility that tissue stresses contribute to the enlargement of air spaces characteristic of emphysema is suggested by the observation that in autopsy material areas of emphysematous destruction are found preferentially in the regions of the lungs that are normally subjected to greatest traction (Fig. 6). Similarly the excess or the abnormal direction of stress forces could explain the occurrence of focal emphysema in regions where alveolar architecture is distorted by the presence of fibrotic scars and that of destructive emphysema in areas of longstanding compensatory emphysema.

The incidence and severity of emphysema rises with increasing age. Obviously the cumulative dose of noxious inhalants increases with prolongation of exposure. But age alone causes changes in the lungs that resemble panacinar emphysema (enlarged alveoli, air trapping) and whose underlying mechanisms are still poorly understood. Serum antitrypsin level and activity are unaffected by aging.

Clinical Presentation

In early emphysema, as it may be diagnosed in young adults with homozygous antitrypsin deficiency, exertional dyspnea is the only constant clinical finding. It may long go unnoticed unless the patient engages in strenuous work or sport. Physical examination is normal. X-ray films of the chest show large hyperlucent lung fields with scarce

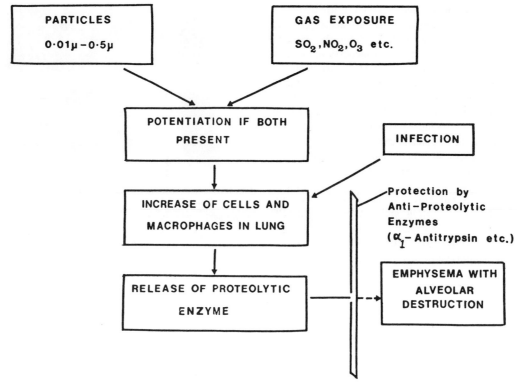

Fig. 5. The roles of environmental insults and host defense mechanisms in the pathogenesis of emphysema. (Reproduced by permission from Bates DV: Am Rev Respir Dis 105:1, 1972.)

bronchovascular markings. On the serum protein electrophoretic strip, the α_1-globulin band is missing (Fig. 3). Pulmonary function tests are characteristic of hyperinflation and airway obstruction, and the arterial blood gases at rest show minimal hypoxemia. Management consists of avoiding exposure to environmental pollutants and preventing or promptly treating respiratory infections in the hope of slowing down progression of the disease.

Most patients with emphysema, however, present

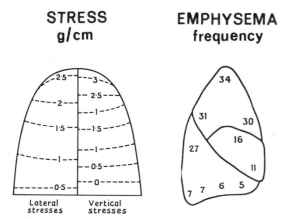

Fig. 6. Distribution of stresses (g/cm²) in the upright lung compared with that of centriacinar emphysema in a random series of 138 patients with the disease. (Reproduced by permission from West JB: Lancet 1:839, 1971.)

past the age of 50 years with a chief complaint of dyspnea on light exertion. Many also complain of fatigue, of loss of appetite and weight, and of orthopnea. Cough and expectoration follow each upper respiratory infection, lasting for weeks rather than days, but unless the patient is currently in the habit of smoking, chronic cough is denied. Pain, felt in the epigastrium and around the base of the thorax, is occasionally mentioned. On physical examination the vital signs are normal. The chest is hyperinflated with elevated shoulders and increased anteroposterior diameter; an association of kyphosis and sternal convexity often produces the well-known barrel shape of the chest. Increased resonance, always present, may be striking in emaciated patients. Breath sounds are decreased throughout the lungs, occasionally with areas of near complete silence. Expiration is prolonged, but there are no adventitious sounds except for wheezing induced by forced expiration. Maximal cardiac impulse is felt against the left sternal border or even in the epigastrium, below and under the xyphoid process; the heart sounds are distant but otherwise normal. While the liver edge is palpable below the right costal margin, the height of hepatic dullness is normal. Cyanosis is absent and clubbing of the fingers is uncommon. During the examination orthopnea is often noted, and in severe cases tachypnea, use of accessory inspiratory muscles, and labored expiration with pursing of the lips become apparent with undressing and dressing or with climbing up and down the examination table. The observation of such

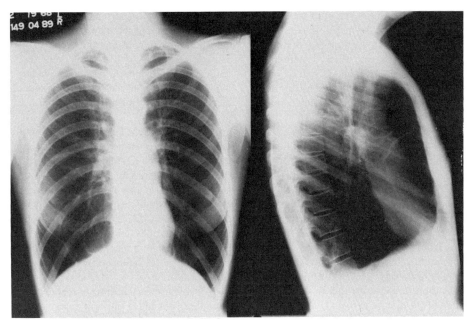

Fig. 7. X-ray films of the chest in a 36-year-old woman with α_1-antitrypsin deficiency and severe airway obstruction attributable to panacinar emphysema (see text).

a "pink puffer" with severe disability immediately suggests that advanced, widespread emphysema is the major component of his chronic obstructive lung disease.

Diagnostic work-up includes a comprehensive evaluation to detect any associated chronic illness that may be overshadowed by the obvious respiratory disease, particularly arteriosclerotic cardiovascular disease. The presence of emphysema is confirmed by radiologic examination of the chest, which is diagnostic in severe cases: the chest is hyperinflated with increased anteroposterior diameter, enlarged retrosternal air space, low straight diaphragms, and narrow mediastinum in which a heart of normal size appears small; the cardiothoracic ratio is decreased. The lung fields are hyperlucent. Vascular markings are decreased beyond the main branches of the pulmonary artery and altogether lost at the periphery of the lungs (Fig. 7).

The electrocardiographic changes associated with emphysema alone include tall and pointed P waves and deviation of QRS axis to the right; signs of right ventricular hypertrophy are inconstant. The hematocrit and blood count are normal; however, the smear may reveal microcytic or macrocytic changes associated with dietary deficiency in erythropoietic factors. In most cases the protein electrophoresis is normal, but some patients have heterozygous MZ or even homozygous Z phenotype.

Pulmonary function tests demonstrate a marked increase of TLC and RV/TLC ratio, and extreme reduction of the forced expiratory flow rates. The association of reduced elastic recoil and low steady-state diffusing capacity is characteristic of emphysema. Arterial blood gases show modest hypoxemia with hypocapnia or normocapnia; in the absence of intercurrent respiratory infection P_{O_2} remains above 60 mm Hg. CO_2 retention is a late finding.

A number of patients present with evidence of chronic bronchitis as well as emphysema. There is a long history of chronic productive cough, and physical examination reveals the additional findings of wheezes, ronchi, and possibly cyanosis and right ventricular failure. The radiologic and physiologic findings are somewhat different. These cases will be discussed in the section on chronic bronchitis.

Clinical Course and Management

The course is one of slow and relentless progression. Therapeutic measures include the discontinuation of smoking habits, yearly immunization against influenza, and prompt treatment of any respiratory infection. Systematic administration of broad-spectrum antibiotics during the winter months has been shown in chronic bronchitis to limit the severity and duration of intercurrent respiratory infections and may also benefit those patients whose dominant problem is emphysema. Prescription of short courses of ampicillin and tetracycline in conventional dosage once a month during the cold season seems preferable to that of small daily doses continually. Bronchodilators are useless, and sedatives are to be avoided. Supportive management is needed in the form of a doctor's availability and understanding, a social worker's intervention for financial and housing problems, and continued treatment programs including physiotherapy, IPPB, and adequate exercise supervised by a nurse or respiratory therapist at home or in the community hospital. O_2 therapy with a portable device often improves exercise tolerance.

The first complications of emphysema are social and

psychological, due to early retirement and to the extreme discomfort that accompanies any physical effort. The patient's chances of adapting to his disability are dependent upon his economic resources, which determine the availability of help and transportation, as well as on his family situation and intellectual resources. All too often the problems of forced inactivity are compounded by old age, isolation, and poverty, and depression is a common occurrence.

Pneumothorax is a fairly frequent complication. Chest pain is accompanied by extreme respiratory distress but little change in physical findings. The diagnosis is made by x-ray examination of the chest, which often shows the degree of lung collapse to be modest. Insertion of a chest tube brings relief, but healing is often delayed and recurrences are common.

Respiratory failure may be precipitated by pneumonia, pulmonary embolism, or any unrelated acute illness. Occasionally, following a respiratory infection or a surgical intervention, respiratory failure occurs as a first manifestation of the disease early in its course, when the baseline impairment of lung function is still moderate; respiratory failure then responds to intensive care as it would any other chronic lung disease. But as a late complication of far-advanced widespread emphysema, respiratory failure has a high mortality regardless of the excellence of care and may lead to chronic tracheotomy and continued need for mechanical ventilation.

Focal Emphysema

The elementary lesion in focal emphysema is a crown of enlarged air spaces surrounding an area of fibrosis, produced by the healing of pyogenic infection, vascular thrombosis, or granulomatous infiltration, or by a reaction to dust deposits. Hence the names of focal or perifocal emphysema and of scar emphysema.

The distribution of focal emphysema reflects that of the initial insult to the lung: apical in tuberculosis, widespread in sarcoidosis and the pneumoconioses. Focal emphysema may involve large areas of the lungs in conditions such as sarcoidosis or beryllium disease, contributing to the obstructive impairment observed in some cases.

Focal emphysema is also found around silicotic nodules. But many patients with micronodular or nodular silicosis have no clinical or physiologic signs suggesting significant emphysema. Obstructive disease, when present in association with silicosis, can generally be related to the presence of chronic bronchitis (whether due to occupational exposure to inert dust besides silica, regional exposure to air pollution, or personal exposure to tobacco smoke); pathologic data in such cases confirm the presence of chronic bronchitis and may reveal centriacinar as well as focal emphysema.

In coalworkers' pneumoconiosis the dust deposits and the emphysema have a predominant centriacinar distribution; the association of chronic bronchitis is nearly constant, and disability correlates best with the presence of obstructive disease. Some authors list emphysema as a complication of coalminers' pneumoconiosis, along with progressive massive fibrosis and cor pulmonale.

Localized Emphysema

Bullous emphysema designates a spectrum of disorders that have in common the presence of bullae, defined as large air spaces (over 1 cm in diameter) limited by distended visceral pleura and interlobular septa. Single bullae (Type I), apparently the remnants of one or a few blown-up lobules and attached to the lung by a narrow neck, are observed occasionally in patients with otherwise normal lungs. These bullae remain asymptomatic unless they grow large enough to fill one hemithorax almost completely. Type II bullae occur in clusters; they are thought to represent alveolar destruction selectively involving part of one lobe, either a superficial layer of alveoli or a whole segment. The remainder of the lung often shows evidence of chronic bronchitis or mild, widespread emphysema, suggesting a relationship between this type of bullae and the chronic obstructive lung disease. Type III bullous disease is characterized by one or several areas of far-advanced panacinar emphysema, each involving a subsegment, segment, or lobe. The remainder of the lungs shows widespread emphysema. Distinction between these three types of bullous emphysema is important because symptomatic patients with large Type I bullae are cured by surgical excision and patients with Type III bullae should not be operated upon. Type II bullous disease is helped by surgery in selected instances.

In infantile lobar emphysema congenital malformation of the bronchi within a lobe produces a ball-valve mechanism and air trapping. Clinically, respiratory distress, bulging and hyperresonance of one hemithorax, and displacement of the heart to the other side suggest lobar emphysema or tension pneumothorax. The chest film is diagnostic, showing the affected lobe, enormously dilated and radiolucent, causing collapse of normal lobes and mediastinal shift. Emergency surgery (lobectomy) is life-saving.

In acquired lobar emphysema (Swyer-James syndrome) the affected lobe has normal or increased volume and diminished breath sounds. The chest film shows hyperlucency, and fluoroscopy reveals localized air trapping with forced expiration. The pathologic findings of widespread bronchiolar obstruction and scarring are consistent with healed obliterative bronchiolitis. The vessels are well developed, but in vivo they are poorly perfused, as shown by angiography or radiospirometry. The alveoli are enlarged in size and often reduced in number. The remainder of the lung is normal. Many patients have a history of severe pneumonia in infancy or childhood, which could account for the bronchiolar lesions and for individual variation in number of alveoli and size of the lobe; the development of new alveoli, which normally continues until 2–5 years of age, would be diversely affected depending upon the severity of the infection and the age at which it occurs. When a whole lung is involved the chest film shows a hyperlucent lung, nonfunctional and often smaller than the normal contralateral lung. Most patients are asymptomatic, and the physical findings are limited to reduced breath sounds over the affected area. Fluoroscopy, radiospirometry, bronchoscopy, or selective pulmonary angiography may be needed to distinguish this benign condition from other causes of hyperlucent lung or lobe that may require prompt treatment such as acquired obstruction of one main-stem bronchus.

Obstructive emphysema, due to incomplete obstruction of a lobar or main-stem bronchus with ball-valve effect, is characterized by locally diminished breath sounds, with or without wheezing. The chest film shows a large hyperlucent lobe (or lung), and fluoroscopy confirms the presence of air trapping. The incomplete obstruction may be due to aspiration of a foreign body (in children) or intraluminal growth of tumor (in adults).

Compensatory emphysema refers to simple overdistension of one lobe or one lung, secondary to loss of volume elsewhere. Thus it occurs with lobar scarring or atelectasis and following a pulmonary resection, lobectomy, or pneumonectomy. The physiologic picture is characterized by mildly reduced TLC and increased RV/TLC ratio, but there is no airway obstruction. After convalescence from surgery, arterial blood gases are normal, unless there is residual disease. The physical findings vary with the etiology. The chest film shows overdistension of the involved lobe or lung, spreading of vascular markings, and hyperlucency due to relative hypoperfusion.

Other Disorders

In subcutaneous emphysema air from the upper airway or the pleural space passes into the surrounding soft tissues, dissecting the anatomic planes defined by aponeuroses and fascias, and infiltrating muscle bundles and subcutaneous fat. The result is a painless swelling, spread over the trunk, neck, and face, that under gentle pressure with the hand gives a characteristic feeling of crepitation. It is an impressive but benign complication, not uncommon after pneumothorax, pneumomediastinum, tracheotomy, tracheal puncture, and thoracic trauma or surgery.

Mediastinal emphysema or pneumomediastinum refers to the infiltration of air into the connective tissue of the mediastinum. Air reaches the hilum either from the upper airway, having traveled down the tracheal sheath, or from ruptured alveoli, having traveled along the interlobular septa and bronchovascular sheaths. The rupture of normal alveoli requires transpulmonary pressure in excess of 60 cm H_2O; this may occur at birth, during asthmatic attacks, with blast injury or blunt trauma to the chest, and with sudden decompression. If the pleura is injured, then a pneumothorax occurs rather than pneumomediastinum, or in association with it. Mild cases of pneumomediastinum are asymptomatic and may be discovered on the chest film, which shows the lungs separated from the mediastinal organs by a clear layer of air. Severe cases present with a superior vena cava syndrome and respiratory distress. Treatment consists of surgical drainage through a suprasternal incision.

Interstitial emphysema is a rare complication of pneumomediastinum in which air infiltrates the bronchovascular sheaths throughout the lungs. Respiratory distress is intense; it is more marked at expiration and therefore resembles an asthmatic attack. Diagnosis depends on the radiologic recognition of the pneumomediastinum, whose treatment slowly brings relief.

CHRONIC BRONCHITIS
Definition

Chronic bronchitis is defined as "a clinical disorder characterized by excessive mucus production in the bronchial tree and manifested by chronic or recurrent productive cough—present on most days for a minimum of three months in the year and for no less than two successive years." Diagnosis is to be made by exclusion of other bronchopulmonary or cardiac disorders that may cause identical symptoms (American Thoracic Society).

Recently it has become apparent that before the patient becomes symptomatic the disease is already manifested by pathologic changes of epithelial metaplasia and physiologic changes of small-airway disease. Simple chronic bronchitis is characterized by chronic cough productive of small or moderate amounts of sputum. Depending upon environment and host factors, the disease progresses slowly to obstructive bronchitis. Disability results from increased susceptibility to acute bronchitis and bronchopneumonia, from progressive impairment of lung function exaggerated by the common association of either emphysema or asthma or both, and from frequent episodes of right ventricular failure and CO_2 retention.

Pathology

Mucous metaplasia is characterized by goblet cell proliferation in the bronchial epithelium. In large bronchi the ratio of goblet cells to ciliated columnar cells rises from the normal one-fourth to one-half and higher. In the bronchioles, where normally goblet cells are absent, they appear in increasing numbers and their secreting activity is apparent from the presence of mucus in the lumen, occasionally backed up into alveolar spaces. Squamous metaplasia, in which normal epithelial cells are replaced by stratified squamous epithelium, is found in patchy distribution, and its prevalence in the bronchial tree correlates with exposure to tobacco smoke and urban air pollution. In advanced cases the metaplastic epithelium becomes hyperplastic. In places the histology is consistent with premalignant proliferation or cancer in situ.

Mucous gland hypertrophy is the best known among the pathologic changes that take place in the bronchial wall. Normal bronchial glands are of the mixed type, with a predominance of mucous over serous cell types; the cells are grouped in acini, and their products are secreted through a fine duct system. In chronic bronchitis the glands are almost exclusively mucus-producing; they seem to undergo both hypertrophy and hyperplasia, and their dilated ducts form wide crypts, large enough at times to be visible on bronchograms. The degree of bronchial gland hypertrophy is usually estimated by measuring the Reid index, or percentage of submucosal thickness occupied by the mucous gland layer (Fig. 8).

Bronchial cartilage atrophy has been recognized in the segmental bronchi and their branches of division. At this level in the bronchial tree cartilage plates are normally discontinuous, but in chronic bronchitis they are fewer, smaller, and thinner than normal. The change is

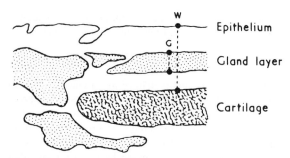

Fig. 8. The Reid index is the ratio of mucous gland thickness (G) to bronchial wall thickness measured from basement membrane to cartilage (W) and gives an estimate of mucous gland hypertrophy. (Reproduced by permission from Reid L: The Pathology of Emphysema. Chicago, Year Book Medical Publishers, 1967.)

rarely reported because its demonstration requires special dissection and staining of the first five or six generations of bronchi, and the adjacent parenchyma is damaged in the process. But it is of considerable significance in that it probably contributes to the occurrence of dynamic compression in the large airways of patients with chronic bronchitis.

Evidence of inflammation is otherwise extremely variable. Often it is limited to intraluminal accumulation of leukocytes, mostly polymorphonuclear, with or without stainable bacteria. Large bronchi may reveal mononuclear infiltrates beneath the basement membrane and around some of the mucous glands. Acute bronchial inflammation is shown by patchy mucosal erosions coated with a fibrinous and purulent exudate and by scattered microabscesses that as a rule do not extend beyond the lamina propria. Patches of scar tissue in the wall of small bronchi are seen as remnants of previous episodes of acute inflammation.

Chronic bronchiolitis has been recognized recently as an important component in the pathology of chronic bronchitis (Fig. 9). Besides the goblet cell proliferation, bronchiolar changes include mononuclear and polymorphonuclear infiltrates within the wall and around it, mucosal erosions, and obstruction by granulation tissue that resembles bronchiolitis obliterans. Insufficient data are available as yet to relate the severity of bronchiolar lesions with the clinical and functional changes of chronic bronchitis.

Pathogenesis

Tobacco smoking is the dominant factor whose role in the pathogenesis of chronic bronchitis is unquestioned. Consequently the preclinical stage of the disease can be studied in asymptomatic smokers, and early discontinuation of the smoking habit is the most useful measure for the prevention of the disabling disease. Urban air pollution causes increased frequency and severity of chronic bronchitis in the general population, children included. The importance of air pollution has been confirmed by the observation of decreasing trends in morbidity and mortality attributable to chronic bronchitis in London since promulgation of the British Clean Air Act.

Air pollutants act in proportion to their concentration and cumulative dose, through bronchial irritation and direct cellular toxicity. Here again individual susceptibility is greatly variable, pointing to the intervention of significant host factors. But hereditary factors, implicated by a number of studies, have remained largely unidentified. Homozygous antitrypsin deficiency may have little bearing on the development of chronic bronchitis, since patients with familial emphysema, as a rule, present without symptoms of airway disease. The incidence of cutaneous hypersensitivity to common antigens

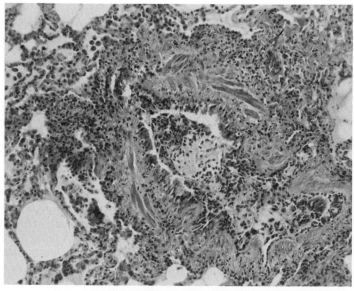

Fig. 9. Terminal bronchiole in a patient with clinical and physiologic evidence of small-airway disease. Histology shows obstruction by mucus, slight goblet cell proliferation and infiltration of the bronchiolar wall by mononuclear cells. (Courtesy of Dr. Gerald Nash, Massachusetts General Hospital.)

is no different in bronchitics than in the general population. Bronchial hyperreactivity manifested by bronchospasm in response to inhalation of histamine or acetylcholine aerosols has been described in bronchitic patients. Normal immunoglobulins have been found in all patients, except for a small number of affected children. Isolated deficiency of IgA, the major immunoglobulin in bronchial secretions, alone does not predispose to chronic bronchitis. The hypothesis that the heterozygous state for cystic fibrosis might contribute to the development of chronic bronchitis in some patients has been disproved.

Whereas the normal bronchial tree is free from bacteria, a variety of organisms are commonly isolated from bronchitic sputum, whether mucoid or muco-purulent, even from clean specimens obtained at bronchoscopy. The bacteria most frequently identified are common elements of the throat flora, pneumococci of a variety of typable strains, α-hemolytic streptococci, *Neisseria catarrhalis, Staphylococcus albus,* and *S. aureus. Hemophilus influenzae* has been reported with widely different frequencies in otherwise comparable groups of patients. The finding of a mixed bacterial flora is common. In most instances there is no evidence of deep infection, and the consensus is that infection remains intraluminal during most of the course of the disease. During clinical exacerbations, however, a dominant organism emerges, usually while systemic evidence of infection becomes apparent. Numerous studies have tried and failed to demonstrate a relationship between the presence of bacteria in sputum, or the frequency of acute exacerbations, and the rate of progression of lung function impairment.

Viral infections are responsible for 50 percent or more of clinical exacerbations, with acute bacterial infection a secondary event. All the known respiratory viruses have been isolated or recognized by rising antibody titers. Persistent high titers are no more frequent in patients with chronic bronchitis than among comparable individuals in the general population; thus persistent viral infection with any of the known agents is unlikely.

The possibility that after repeated environmental insults causing tissue breakdown an autoimmune response might give the disease its self-perpetuating character has been suggested on the basis of animal experiments. At present there is no evidence that such a mechanism intervenes in man.

Clinical Presentation

The early stage of small-airway disease is asymptomatic or accompanied by occasional cough, brief and sometimes productive of small amounts of sputum, such as the well-recognized "smoker's cough," which the patient may deny, even though he coughs in the physician's presence.

Simple chronic bronchitis is manifested by frequent cough and the production of mucoid sputum, mostly upon arising in the morning. Upper respiratory infections are followed by purulent bronchitis, slowly clearing over a period of weeks. The patient, more often a man than a woman and usually a smoker, is often seen for an unrelated ailment and attaches little importance to this aspect of his medical history, which is elicited through persistent interrogation. The examination of the chest is normal except for an occasional wheeze heard during forced inspiration or expiration. The chest x-ray and ECG are normal, but the pulmonary function tests show small-airway disease and mild airway obstruction. Management consists in convincing the patient that he should stop smoking and in promptly treating all bacterial respiratory infections with antibiotics and bronchodilators. At this stage the physiologic manifestations of the disease are largely reversible.

Unfortunately most patients live with simple chronic bronchitis for years without seeking or accepting medical advice. Then exertional dyspnea appears insidiously, but is accentuated during acute respiratory infections. It is often in the aftermath of such an exacerbation that the patient seeks help. He is now over 50 years of age, with a daily cough productive of 1–3 oz of sputum, more often purulent than not. He is short of breath on climbing one or two flights of stairs. He describes wheezing with acute exacerbations, while coughing spells, or on exposure to smoke, fog, or cold air. He has no complaints of chest pain but may have noted blood-streaked sputum on occasion, and even frank hemoptysis. The occupational history may reveal significant exposure to industrial air pollution. A familial history of allergy is not uncommon, but personal history is usually negative for allergy.

On physical examination the patient appears well nourished and often plethoric. The vital signs are normal. The neck veins are full during expiration only. The chest has increased anteroposterior diameter but normal resonance. Diaphragms are in normal position with limited motion. Auscultation reveals scattered ronchi and wheezes without rales. The heart is normal, except possibly for a loud pulmonic second sound. Cyanosis and clubbing of the fingers are commonly noted. The remainder of the examination is normal.

Hematocrit, red-cell count, and hemoglobin are elevated. The white-cell count may show modest leukocytosis but is often normal. On the chest film the cardiothoracic ratio is normal, the lung fields mildly hyperinflated, and the hilar markings increased; in the lung fields the vascular markings can be followed clearly to the periphery. Characteristic physiologic findings include high-normal TLC, increased RV, reduced forced expiratory flow rates by all the usual tests, and moderately severe hypoxemia with low or normal P_{CO_2}.

Mild or moderate centriacinar emphysema, often associated with chronic bronchitis, cannot be ruled out. Its presence would change neither the treatment nor the course of the disease. The association of asthma, when present, is revealed by a personal history of allergy, varying severity of dyspnea, prominent hyperresonance and wheezing, and marked response to bronchodilator therapy. Other disease associations may affect the presentation of chronic bronchitis. With pulmonary venous hypertension, whether due to mitral or left ventricular disease, wheezing, sputum production, and dyspnea are exaggerated. With cirrhosis of the liver the

Table 3
Checklist for the Evaluation and Treatment of Chronic Bronchitis (CB)

Problems	Evaluation	Treatment
Chronic bronchitis		
Etiology	Interrogation: tobacco, heart disease, alcoholism	Stop smoking; treatment of underlying condition
Infection	Gram stain and culture of sputum; WBC; chest x-ray	Chest physiotherapy; antibiotics; influenza immunization
Airway obstruction	Physical examination and pulmonary function tests	Bronchodilators
Hypoxemia	Arterial blood gases on room air and on pure oxygen	Controlled oxygen therapy
Associated diseases		
Asthma	Personal history, physical examination, eosinophilia, response to bronchodilators	Bronchodilators, trial of corticosteroids
Emphysema	α_1-antitrypsin level and Pi type; chest x-ray and pulmonary function tests	—
Complications		
Erythrocytosis	CBC	Treatment of CB
	Red-cell mass	Rarely, phlebotomy and plasma restitution
CO_2 retention	Arterial blood gases	IPPB
	Respiratory infection	Treatment of CB
	Obesity	Weight control
	Use of sedatives	D/C sedatives
Metabolic alkalosis	Serum electrolytes	KCl, acetazolamide
Cor pulmonale	Physical examination	Diuretics
	ECG; chest x-ray	Digitalis
Pulmonary embolism	Physical examination, chest x-ray, lung scan, angiography	Anticoagulants
Respiratory failure	Progressive CO_2 retention in spite of therapy	Tracheal intubation and mechanical ventilation

development of intrapulmonary shunts causes unusually severe hypoxemia. With obesity episodes of severe hypoxemia, CO_2 retention, and right ventricular failure occur with increased frequency, and severity. Alcoholism also contributes to the severity of the disease because of decreased responsiveness of respiratory centers, repeated aspiration, and impairment of lung clearance mechanisms (Table 3).

Clinical Course and Management

Untreated, the disease progresses to dyspnea at rest, severe hypoxemia with erythrocytosis, and cor pulmonale, giving the clinical picture often referred to by the term "blue bloater." Cardiorespiratory failure is precipitated by bronchopneumonia or the use of sedatives, the latter causing depression of respiratory centers. Thus a number of patients first receive medical attention when they present in congestive failure or respiratory distress. Treatment consists of controlled O_2 therapy under surveillance of arterial blood gases, bronchodilators (aminophylline and hydrocortisone i.v., isoproterenol in aerosol), chest physiotherapy, IPPB, and diuretics. KCl is given as needed to correct the hypochloremia and potassium depletion of chronic respiratory acidosis. In the absence of left ventricular disease digitalis may not be needed, since relief of right ventricular failure is best achieved by treating the lung disease. Antibiotics are indicated even when no dominant organism can be identified by sputum smear or culture. Parenteral therapy is preferred at this acute stage and is often given in the form of ampicillin i.v. unless results of culture or known penicillin

sensitivity indicate otherwise. Intubation and mechanical ventilation are needed for those patients who develop progressive CO_2 retention and respiratory acidosis in response to O_2 administration, however careful.

In-hospital treatment of such episodes of cardiopulmonary failure is usually successful. Progress is followed by clinical and radiologic evaluation and frequent determinations of arterial blood gases and serum electrolytes. After recovery the baseline condition of the patient is carefully evaluated with the help of comprehensive pulmonary function tests. The frequent association of emphysema can be recognized only when emphysema is severe enough to cause unequivocal changes in the radiologic appearance of the lungs and a significant decrease of lung recoil and diffusing capacity. The association of asthma is diagnosed from history, from blood and sputum eosinophilia, and by demonstrating marked reversibility or airway obstruction in response to bronchodilators.

A maintenance program appropriate to the severity of the disease is then instituted. In almost every case the first step is the recommendation that the patient should stop smoking. Once this is accomplished, a minimal pulmonary regimen often suffices to bring about considerable symptomatic improvement. This includes bronchodilators p.o. (aminophylline), to be continued for months or years, influenza immunization, and antibiotics (tetracycline or ampicillin p.o.) given for 1 week each month during the cold season. Such administration of antibiotics has been shown to reduce not the number but the severity of clinical exacerbations. Additional courses of appropriate antibiotics are instituted whenever such an exacerbation nevertheless results in fever, leukocytosis, and recrudescence of sputum infection.

More severely affected patients will in addition require long-term diuretic therapy. Most diruetic drugs induce metabolic alkalosis and therefore decreased responsiveness of respiratory centers, an undesirable side effect in patients who are prone to CO_2 retention. The use of acetazolamide and thiazide in a suitable alternate regimen obviates this difficulty while providing sustained, effective diuretic therapy.

Most patients benefit from a continuing program of chest physiotherapy. Postural drainage and voluntary cough once a day upon awakening are often sufficient. More aggressive programs, requiring several daily sessions with a physiotherapist, are occasionally needed but are difficult to institute unless a member of the family can be trained to give the necessary treatment. The value of IPPB in maintenance programs may be due in part to its ability to promote expectoration and substitute for physiotherapy.

Beyond this basic pulmonary regimen, management is adapted to individual needs and community resources. For some patients weight reduction and a change of occupation bring about considerable improvement. Others, whose disease represents an association of chronic bronchitis and asthma, improve only when long-term corticosteroids are added to their treatment, preferably in the form of prednisone on an alternate-day schedule. Yet others see their exercise tolerance greatly increased by continuous O_2 therapy administered from a portable supply of liquid O_2. In some communities rehabilitation programs are offered in which the patients find group support for their efforts to abstain from smoking and are provided facilities for chest physiotherapy, IPPB, and progressive exercise retraining.

Most important of all, chronic bronchitis is a preventable disease. Public information is now widely available, but reinforcement by the smoker's personal physician is bound to be more effective in encouraging better health habits before chronic disability prevails. Early diagnosis of chronic bronchitis depends upon a few pertinent questions and simple lung function tests. Increased awareness and an active therapeutic approach on the part of physicians should bring about a reduction of morbidity due to this disease.

REFERENCES
(EMPHYSEMA AND CHRONIC BRONCHITIS)

Advisory Committee to the Surgeon General of the Public Health Service: Smoking and Health. Washington, U.S. Government Printing Office, Pub 1103, 1964

Bates DV: Chronic bronchitis and emphysema. N Engl J Med 278:546, 600, 1968

Burrows B, Earle RH: Course and prognosis of chronic obstructive lung disease. N Engl J Med 280:399, 1969

Burrows B, Kettel LJ, Niden AH, et al: Patterns of cardiovascular dysfunction in chronic obstructive lung disease. N Engl J Med 286:912, 1972

Deutscher S, Higgins MW: The relationship of parental longevity to ventilatory function and prevalence of chronic nonspecific respiratory disease among sons. Am Rev Respir Dis 102:180, 1970

Epstein RL: Constituents of sputum: A simple method. Ann Intern Med 77:259, 1972

Ferris BG, Whittenberger JL: Environmental hazards: Effects of community air pollution on prevalence of respiratory disease. N Engl J Med 275:1413, 1966

Fletcher CM, Jones NL, Burrows B, Niden AH: American emphysema and British bronchitis. Am Rev Respir Dis 90:1, 1964

Larson RK, Barman ML, Kueppers F, Fudenberg HH: Genetic and environmental determinants of chronic obstructive pulmonary disease. Ann Intern Med 72:627, 1970

Lee DHK: Environmental Factors in Respiratory Diseases. New York, Academic Press, 1972

Lefcoe NM, Paterson NAM: Adjunct therapy in chronic obstructive pulmonary disease. Am J Med 54:343, 1973

Levine G, MacLeod P, Macklem PT: Gas exchange abnormalities in mild bronchitis and asymptomatic asthma. N Engl J Med 282:1278, 1970

Mitchell RS, Filley GF: Chronic obstructive bronchopulmonary disease. Am Rev Respir Dis 89:360, 878, 1964

Reid L, Millard FJC: Correlation between radiological diagnosis and structural lung changes in emphysema. Clin Radiol 15:307, 1964

Talamo RC, Langley CE, Levine BW, Kazemi H: Genetic versus quantitative analysis or serum alpha$_1$ antitrypsin. N Engl J Med 287:1067, 1972

Tandon MK, Campbell AH: Bronchial cartilage in chronic bronchitis. Thorax 24:607, 1969

Thurlbeck WM, Henderson JA, Fraser RG, Bates DV: Chronic obstructive lung disease. Medicine 49:81, 1970

Woolcock AJ, Vincent NJ, Macklem PT: Frequency dependence of compliance as a test for obstruction in small airways. J Clin Invest 48:1097, 1969

ASTHMA

Asthma is a chronic disease characterized by recurrent dyspneic attacks that are reversible, spontaneously or with appropriate treatment. Each attack represents an episode of paroxysmal airway obstruction, produced by contraction of smooth muscle, submucosal edema, and hypersecretion. The disease is the expression of a double hypersensitivity: immunologic hypersensitivity (immediate, Type I), or allergy, and physiologic hypersensitivity of bronchi to normal chemical mediators. The latter distinguishes asthmatics among other allergic patients.

Pathology

The lungs are large and fail to deflate when the chest is open. On the cut section the thick-walled bronchi are filled with mucus and adherent mucus plugs. On microscopic sections mucus, leukocytes, and cellular debris fill the lumen of numerous bronchi in each low-power field, and mucus plugs are seen to undergo organization. Submucosal edema lifts the epithelial lining into deep longitudinal folds that on cross section form a characteristic star pattern. The thickened basement membrane is prominent. Cellular infiltration in and around the bronchi includes numerous eosinophils. Degranulated mast cells, which are not recognizable with usual stains, can be identified with immunofluorescence techniques or electron microscopy.

The parenchyma of the lung is hyperinflated even when no precautions are taken to fix the lungs under controlled transpulmonary pressure. The alveoli show normal structure, but foci of bronchopneumonia and atelectasis are common.

Immunologic Release of Mediators

Innumerable antigens are capable of inducing sensitization of the respiratory tract. Pollen allergy is most easily recognized by the seasonal recurrence of symptoms. Pollens from trees appear in early spring, from grasses and agricultural crops in late spring, and from ragweed in late summer. Also common, hypersensitivity to animal proteins, such as guinea-pig, cat, dog, or horse dander, is revealed by careful interrogation. House dust is a continual source of exposure to antigenic material from molds, mites, and insects as well as wool and feathers. Indoor vacuum cleaning removes large amounts of dust from the environment, but while in use most appliances cause a transient rise in the density of airborne particles. Cotton fibers are not antigenic, but the plant bractae, mixed in the bulk of unprocessed cotton, cause sensitization in susceptible cotton-mill workers. Among other industrial products that also cause sensitization, toluene diisocyanate (TDI) stands out as a particularly potent antigen.

Hypersensitivity to infectious agents, well demonstrated for *Aspergillus* species, remains unproven for the common bacterial invaders of the lower respiratory tract. Hypersensitivity to parasites (*Ascaris lumbricoides, Toxocara canis*) may cause asthmatic attacks and pulmonary infiltrates in infested children.

Food allergy can cause asthma as well as gastrointestinal and cutaneous manifestations. Eggs, milk, and seafood are most commonly implicated. Drug hypersensitivity is an uncommon cause of asthma, except for aspirin.

The immune response to allergens is singular in that its end product is the formation of reaginic antibodies, identified as immunoglobulin E (IgE), which exhibit species and tissue specificity (homocytotropism). IgE fixes itself to selected cells in the skin, gut, and respiratory mucosa, where it can be identified by immunofluorescence techniques attached to epithelial cells, basement membrane, mast cells, and leukocytes. Although serum IgE has a very low concentration, passive sensitization is readily induced in vivo by intradermal injection of serum from a sensitized donor (passive cutaneous anaphylaxis or Prausnitz-Küstner reaction). Similarly lung tissue or leukocytes can be sensitized by contact with serum from an allergic patient. In contrast the success of in vitro leukocyte sensitization is partly dependent upon properties of the donor's cells; leukocytes from allergic patients, not clinically responsive to the antigen, release histamine in response to passive sensitization and allergenic challenge, whereas only 20 percent of nonallergic donors have reactive leukocytes in these conditions. This observation suggests that the host factor in

allergic disease is concerned with the responsiveness of target cells as well as the humoral immune response to environmental antigens. Indeed, nonallergic individuals have been shown to synthesize IgE after exposure to allergenic substances and yet to remain asymptomatic.

In patients subsequent exposure to the antigen probably results in the formation of a bridge between two neighboring IgE molecules attached to the membrane of sensitized cells. The sequence of events thereafter includes the fall of intracellular concentration of cyclic adenosine monophosphate (cAMP) and the release of mediators normally contained within lysosomes. The essential step between antigen fixation and mediator release involves the inactivation of adenylcyclase, necessary to the formation of cAMP and located near or within the cell membrane; the processes associated with this inactivation at the molecular level are as yet unknown.

Histamine and slow-reacting substances of anaphylaxis (SRS-A) are the major mediators whose release by this mechanism has been identified. Both act upon smooth muscle and exocrine glands by inactivating adenylcyclase at the membrane of these effector cells. There follows a decrease of cAMP concentrations, decreased membrane polarization, and finally contraction of bronchial smooth muscle and secretion by mucous glands.

Bronchial Hypersensitivity to Mediators

Bronchial hypersensitivity to acetylcholine distinguishes asthmatics among other allergic patients. Acetylcholine administered by aerosol inhalation causes little reaction in normal persons but induces bronchospasm in asthmatics. The response can be elicited by a minute dose of the mediator.

Asthmatics exhibit increased bronchial sensitivity to other natural mediators (histamine, SRS-A) and to β_2 blocking agents (propanolol but not practolol). Such observations have suggested that partial β_2 blockade is the basic alteration underlying the allergic state (β_2 blockade theory). The exaggerated response to mediators is due to depressed adenylcyclase activity and cAMP levels in the effector cells (smooth muscle and mucous glands). Indeed, the concept that adenylcyclase itself is the beta receptor, or the essential element in the beta receptor, has gained increasing acceptance in recent years. Considerable support for this concept is derived from the fact that β-adrenergic drugs raise intracellular levels of cAMP by increasing the activity of adenylcyclase. The xanthines produce similar effects by decreasing the activity of phosphodiesterase, the enzyme responsible for the hydrolysis of cAMP.

Asthmatic attacks may be triggered by clearly identifiable stimuli that seem totally unrelated to immunologic release of mediators, such as the inhalation of clean, cold air, of inert dust (chalk), or of industrial or domestic fumes and tobacco smoke. These, however, are likely to stimulate irritant receptors in the respiratory passages and induce a vagal response. The appearance of symptomatic bronchial obstruction is attributable to bronchial hypersensitivity to acetylcholine, although the duration of the reaction remains unexplained. Various endogenous factors are also capable of triggering asthmatic attacks in susceptible individuals, notably exercise, cough, hypocapnia, and emotional stress. Administration of atropine in the usual therapeutic dosage can prevent or relieve the bronchial obstruction induced by nonantigenic stimuli, and β-adrenergic substances have the same property.

Clinical Presentation

Asthmatic attacks begin with a feeling of chest tightness and congestion, the latter word used by many patients to describe the sensations associated with the presence of increased bronchial secretions. Aware of his breathing, the patient becomes apprehensive: within the next hours the symptoms will either subside (spontaneously or with the help of some usual medication) or progress to dyspnea at rest with loud wheezing and cough. Examination at that point reveals labored breathing without distress, normal temperature and blood pressure, and increased respiratory rate. The chest is in inspiratory position. Inspiratory retraction of supraclavicular, intercostal, and epigastric areas is manifest. Prolonged expiration is accompanied by contraction of the abdominal muscles and grunting or pursing of the lips. The percussion note is resonant. Breath sounds are well heard at inspiration and through the long expiration. There are a few basal rales but mostly wheezes. Examination of the heart is normal except for mild tachycardia.

Severe attacks present with intense respiratory distress, anxiety, agitation, pallor, and cyanosis. Temperature is normal or elevated, blood pressure slightly high. Tachycardia and tachypnea are often marked. The chest is hyperinflated, tight as a drum and grossly hyperresonant. Breath sounds are diminished and partly covered by diffuse rales. Expiration is prolonged and obviously labored. Wheezing is often loud but not invariably so, since wheezes tend to decrease or disappear with extreme airway obstruction. Heart sounds may be heard with difficulty because of extreme hyperinflation, or a hyperkinetic state may be apparent, resulting from previous use of catecholamines and xanthines, with loud, normally split P2, and occasionally with a third sound heard over the xyphoid area (right ventricular gallop). The abdomen, which tenses with every expiration, may be resonant, and bowel sounds are often absent. Cough is frequent and productive of viscid, thick sputum, whitish or purulent, often with recognizable bronchial casts.

Diagnosis

The clinical picture is characteristic of airway obstruction. A history of previous attacks is usually obtained. Pharyngolaryngeal disease is ruled out by a benign throat examination and the expiratory character of dyspnea. Pulmonary edema is excluded for lack of clinical evidence of left heart disease. However, asthma and pulmonary edema may be hard to differentiate on the basis of clinical findings alone, particularly in older patients with underlying chronic bronchitis and coronary heart disease. Awareness of this difficulty is important, since a wrong diagnostic impression leads to wrong treatment, which is not only ineffective but also deleterious; epinephrine is poorly tolerated in the presence of heart disease and morphine in asthma precipitates CO_2 retention. When in doubt, immediate management should be limited to supportive measures (oxygen, aminophylline) until the diagnosis is ascertained by sputum examination, chest roentgenography, and electrocardiogram.

On microscopic examination (wet mount or Wright stain) the sputum appears loaded with eosinophils; its purulent parts may contain nothing else; a large proportion of neutrophils indicates bacterial superinfection. The sputum may also contain bronchial casts and clumps of eosinophil granules released from leukocytes. A Gram stain is necessary to appreciate the presence and character of bacteria.

The chest film during an asthmatic attack shows striking hyperinflation. The diaphragms are low and nearly straight, and the mediastinum is elongated with a narrow cardiac silhouette. The clear retrosternal space is widened. The pulmonary artery and its main branches are prominent, and the lung fields are uniformly hyperlucent except for any evidence of pneumonitis or atelectasis that may be present.

The electrocardiogram is often normal, except for tachycardia; but there may be evidence of right ventricular strain, with or without frequent extrasystole. The white-cell count is normal and the eosinophil count is high. However, blood eosinophilia may be absent or unremarkable (below 300/mm^3) because patients have used adrenergic drugs earlier. Leukocytosis may be observed for the same reason or as a result of concomitant bacterial infection. As an aid to the diagnosis of asthma and of respiratory infection, the blood count is less valuable than sputum examination and chest film.

The severity of the attack is evaluated from the clinical condition of the patient when first seen and the duration of symptoms before examination. With moderate distress of recent onset, no further investigation is needed, although repeated tests of forced expiration are helpful to document the effect of treatment. With marked distress having lasted several hours, a determination of arterial blood gases is desirable to recognize CO_2 retention and acidosis and to secure initial data for subsequent evaluation of progress or deterioration. A prompt reponse to treatment is the rule in uncomplicated asthma. A slow or poor response suggests the presence of complication or the association of chronic bronchitis, emphysema, or other cardiopulmonary disorder.

Once the presenting attack is cleared, the task remains of identifying the responsible antigens. A thorough interrogation is the first and most important step. It may reveal a dominant antigen, such as ragweed or TDI. Skin testing (scratch test) helps to recognize the presence of reaginic antibodies to common antigens. Multiple allergies are often observed with such tests and their role with respect to the appearance of symptoms is uncertain in the absence of good evidence from the past history. Interrogation should be directed so as to uncover nonallergic triggering factors.

Comprehensive pulmonary function tests are of greatest value in the intervals between attacks when clinical examination suggests little or no residual abnormality. Only pulmonary function tests can precisely evaluate the quality of the remission or the full effect of maintenance therapy. Incomplete remissions are characterized by persistent small-airway disease or even moderate airway obstruction. Administration of a bronchodilator is followed by marked improvement of expiratory flow rates. Repeated testing at intervals of 1 year or a few years allows detection of long-term changes in pulmonary status.

Clinical Course and Complications

One-half of asthmatic patients suffer their first attack before the age of 15 years. Most of these have mild disease, characterized by clearly separated attacks occurring in seasonal clusters and promptly responsive to therapy; these young patients enjoy a good long-term prognosis with a high probability that they will be free of symptoms in adult life.

With onset in late adolescence or in adulthood the probability that the disease will subside spontaneously decreases, but again a majority of patients have a mild disease, controllable with good management. However, lack of medical attention or of patient cooperation when the disease is active results in retention of secretions, widespread bronchial inflammation, and the formation of mucus plugs; a severe attack occurring in such circumstances immediately poses a threat to life.

Regardless of age at onset and quality of care, a small group of patients develop chronic asthma. For these the remissions are brief and incomplete; symptoms persist despite comprehensive therapy, and complications arise from the severity of the disease and the hazards of drugs. In children growth retardation and chest deformity (pectus carinatum) reveal the relentless severity of the disease. In adults continual disability results in lost employment opportunities and in familial conflicts. There is no solid evidence that behavioral or personality disorders are more frequent in asthmatics than in any other sufferers of chronic illness. At all ages chronic bronchitis is the constant companion of chronic asthma and with the passage of time the association becomes a distinct entity diversely referred to as infectious asthma, asthmatic bronchitis, or COLD.

Each asthmatic attack carries a small risk of pneumothorax or pneumomediastinum. Atelectasis is frequent in young children and uncommon in adults.

Status asthmaticus, the end point of prolonged asthmatic attacks, is characterized by dehydration, hypoxemia, CO_2 retention, and metabolic acidosis. Lack of response to catecholamines, common in this circumstance, is attributable in part to the presence of acidosis and in part to mechanical obstruction of airways by solid plugs that can be eliminated only with prolonged treatment. The use of mechanical ventilation and corticosteroids has transformed the management and the prognosis of status asthmaticus, so that the mortality has fallen to less than 10 percent, higher in elderly patients, lower in children.

The numerous side effects and complications of drug therapy encountered in the management of asthma are mentioned below.

Treatment

Long-term management consists of environmental control, desensitization, expectorants, and chest physiotherapy. Bronchodilators, oxygen, rehydration and corticosteroids are needed for treatment of severe attacks, and tracheal intubation and mechanical ventilation are needed when respiratory failure develops in spite of aggressive drug therapy.

Environmental control aims at eliminating exposure to antigens incriminated by clinical history or skin testing. Appropriate recommendations are easily made for pets, foods, and tobacco. Woolen clothes and down pillows are replaced by synthetic fabrics and foam rubber, regardless of expense. A nonallergenic bedroom should be provided, without rugs and with few draperies, made of cotton or fiberglass, and should undergo weekly washings with an antiseptic solution to destroy molds and mites. Air conditioning is helpful to keep out pollens and air pollution. These measures are particularly efficient for asthmatic children whose parents are usually willing to comply but may need help to overcome financial hardship or inadequate housing. When asthma is triggered by occupational exposure, a change of job is indicated, and suitable plans must be made to make this possible without undue economic loss. A change of residence is occasionally helpful to avoid local pockets of air pollution, but moving to another climate is generally useless, except in the case of hyperreactivity to cold.

Desensitization aims at curing the asthmatic patient by inducing the formation of circulating antibodies of the IgG class, capable of binding and neutralizing the offending antigen before it can reach the target cells. Antibody formation is promoted by weekly or biweekly subcutaneous injections of antigen in minute doses that are carefully increased over a period of months. The efficiency of the method amply compensates for its tediousness in the case of hay fever and in rare cases of asthma where a single well-defined antigen is the dominant troublemaker. Continued treatment with less frequent injections is needed for sustained effect.

Expectorants are used in the hope of liquefying bronchial secretion and facilitating their expectoration. Short courses of iodide may be used to this effect; long-term use of iodide is discouraged for it creates a risk of goiter or nasal polyposis. Glycerol guaiacolate has been shown to be ineffective. Acetylcysteine reduces sputum viscosity and dissolves mucus plugs by breaking down mucopolysaccharides; given in aerosols it is irritant to the respiratory mucosa and produces cough and bronchorrhea, both of which promote expectoration; but it also causes bronchospasm, which in asthmatics may be severe. Thus acetylcysteine aerosols have no place in the management of asthma. The safest approach is to prevent the formation of mucus plugs by providing humidified air at night, prescribing effective maintenance medications, using chest physiotherapy as soon as symptoms recur, and starting intravenous rehydration early in the management of severe attacks.

The major bronchodilators are catecholamines, xanthines, and glucocorticoids. The first two groups of drugs act by raising cAMP levels in the immunologic target cell and in the physiologic effector cell. True potentiation has been demonstrated for the association of catecholamines and xanthines, a finding consistent with their acting on different enzyme systems. Glucocorticoids act by a different mechanism. They are synergistic with β-adrenergic catecholamines and possess additional favorable effects such as depression of the immune system and of inflammatory reaction.

Epinephrine and ephedrine have α- and β-adrenergic properties, but their β effects are dominant with respect to bronchial smooth muscle. With epinephrine increased heart rate and blood pressure indicate the intensity of undesirable cardiovascular side effects. With ephedrine excessive CNS stimulation is a frequent problem, which may require the addition of a mild sedative. Epinephrine, given subcutaneously or in aerosol, is preferred for prompt relief; longer acting ephedrine is given orally for maintenance therapy.

Isoproterenol, predominantly β-adrenergic, is effective and safe when given by inhalation in moderate daily doses. Because of its potency and easy use, it has become a popular self-administered medication. Since convenient pocket-size sprayers have become available, abuses have been common, particularly in Great Britain where at first these preparations were available without prescription. When taken alone isoproterenol was insufficient for relief of severe attacks; dosage was then increased without benefit but with increasing side effects, among which arrhythmia was particularly hazardous in the presence of hypoxemia and acidosis. There followed an epidemic of sudden death among asthmatics throughout Great Britain that subsided only after the sale of isoproterenol dispensers was regulated. In spite of legal limitations on the availability of the drug, patients are to be warned of the dangers associated with increased daily dosage of isoproterenol and instructed to report any change in their symptoms so that the physician can adjust their maintenance therapy in a safe way.

In a small number of patients isoproterenol causes drug-induced bronchospasm, attributable to the formation of a methyl derivative that exhibits β blocking properties. This uncommon complication may be recognized by observation during a trial period off the drug or in the laboratory by repeated tests of forced expiration for at least 1 hr after administration of isoproterenol. Affected patients should be informed and instructed to avoid the drug.

As bronchodilators, the xanthines have a potency comparable to that of β-adrenergic drugs. The long established practice of prescribing xanthines and adrenergic medications in association has been vindicated by the re-

cent demonstration that their effects are mutually potentiating rather than simply additive. This property is taken advantage of both in maintenance therapy (theophylline-ephedrine compound) and in the management of acute attacks (epinephrine s.c. or isoproterenol in aerosol with aminophylline i.v.). Aminophylline toxicity, manifested by gastrointestinal and cardiovascular symptoms (nausea, vomiting, arrhythmia, hypotension) is avoided by respecting the limit of 6 mg/kg every 6 hr as a maximal dose and using the intravenous route for immediate and complete absorption. When normal gastrointestinal function is restored, oral administration can be resumed with good effect, even though absorption is likely to be incomplete unless the drug is taken in the fasting state. In mildly affected patients aminophylline alone in four daily doses p.o. may suffice to provide adequate maintenance therapy.

Glucocorticoids are effective and are indicated for acute care and maintenance therapy in patients whose disease cannot be controlled by the measures and medications listed so far. Hydrocortisol hemisuccinate (Solu-Cortef) is the preferred form for intravenous administration in the management of severe attacks or status asthmaticus. Doses of 2–5 mg/kg every 6 hr are given at first while other bronchodilators are continued, since the mode of action of corticoids is distinct from that of β-adrenergic drugs and xanthines. Full effect is usually obtained within 24 hr, and the dose is then reduced to 1–2 mg/kg every 6 hr, later to be replaced by oral medication.

Prednisone is the drug of choice for maintenance because of its rapid absorption and short half-life (4–8 hr), which allows the adjustment of blood level to varying nyctohemeral patterns. Initial treatment usually requires round-the-clock administration at moderate or high dosage (0.5–1 mg/kg/day in four doses). Whenever possible, and preferably at the end of the first week, treatment is changed to one daily dose taken in the early morning. This schedule, which mimics the normal nyctohemeral cycle of cortisol secretion while producing a high peak concentration, has been shown to considerably reduce the incidence and severity of adrenal gland suppression and iatrogenic hypercorticism. Long-term therapy can be adjusted with the same schedule while dosage is reduced to 0.25 mg/kg/day. More effective prevention of hypercorticism is achieved with alternate-day therapy, whereby a larger dose (0.5–0.7 mg/kg) is given every other morning. In a minority of patients, however, the disease cannot be controlled in this manner and daily administration must be continued for prolonged periods of time. Repeated trials of alternate-day therapy are attempted at intervals, in an effort to prevent complications or as an intermediate step before weaning. In the favorable case where prednisone can be discontinued, resumption of therapy may be needed at a later date when recrudescence of symptoms is observed. Often a seasonal schedule is determined whereby maximal benefits may be derived from therapy with minimal hazards.

Adrenal suppression results from round-the-clock administration of corticosteroids. It becomes clinically manifest with sudden discontinuation of the drug (which should be avoided) or with intercurrent illnesses, during which a higher dosage is often required. Adrenal suppression is largely prevented by the use of single daily doses or an alternate-day regimen.

The major hazard of long-term corticoid therapy is iatrogenic hypercorticism, whose multiple manifestations are described elsewhere. To avoid these in severe chronic asthma, all other therapeutic means are used to maximal effect, and repeated attempts are made to institute an alternate-day regimen. In spite of such efforts some patients remain dependent on high or frequent doses of corticoids for relief of their symptoms, and they remain at risk for complications such as gastric ulcer, hypertension, diabetes, osteoporosis, and, in childhood, stunted growth. Decreased requirement in such steroid-dependent patients is often used as a test of effectiveness in the study of new drugs, among which cromoglycate is at present the most promising.

Oxygen and rehydration are a most important element in the management of severe attacks. Their modalities of administration and the indications and methods of mechanical ventilation are reviewed in the chapter on acute respiratory care.

REFERENCES

Aas K: The biochemical and immunological basis of bronchial asthma. Springfield, Ill, Charles C. Thomas, 1972

De La Mata RC, Penna M, Aviado DM: Reversal of sympathomimetic bronchodilation by dichloro-isoproterenol. J Pharmacol Exp Ther 135:197, 1962

Greenert S, Bernstein L, Michael JG: Immune responses of nonatopic individuals to prolonged immunization with ragweed extract. Lancet 2:1121, 1971

Harter HG, Reddy WJ, Thorn GW: Studies on an intermittent corticosteroid dosage regimen. N Engl J Med 269:591, 1963

Hubscher T, Eisen AH: Allergen binding to human peripheral leukocytes. Int Arch Allergy Appl Immunol 41:689, 1971

Ishizaka K, Ishizaka T: Identification of gamma-E-antibodies as a carrier of reaginic activity. J Immunol 99:1187, 1967

Ishizaka K, Tominoka H, Ishizaka T: Mechanism of passive sensitization in the presence of IgE and IgG molecules on human leukocytes. J Immunol 105:1459, 1970

Kerr JW, Govindazaj M, Patel KR: Effect of alpha-receptor blocking drugs and di-sodium-cromoglycate on histamine hypersensitivity in bronchial asthma. Br Med J 2:139, 1970

Lowell FC, Franklin W: A double blind study of the effectiveness and specificity of the injection therapy in ragweed hay fever. N Engl J Med 273:675, 1965

MacDonald AG, Ingram CG, McNeill RS: The effect of propanolol on airway resistance. Br J Anesthesiol 39:919, 1967

Mithoefer JC, Runser RH, Karetzky MS: The use of sodium bicarbonate in the treatment of acute bronchial asthma. N Engl J Med 272:1200, 1965

Orange RP, Kaliner MA, Laraia PJ, Austen KF: Immunological release of histamine and slow reacting substance of anaphylaxis from human lung. II. Influence of cellular levels of cyclic AMP. Fed Proc 30:1725, 1971

Sheffer AL, Valentine MD: The treatment of bronchial asthma. Med Clin North Am 53:239, 1969

Wells RE, Walker JEC, Hickler RB: Effects of cold on respiratory airflow resistance in patients with respiratory tract disease. N Engl J Med 263:268, 1960

BRONCHIECTASIS
Definition

Bronchiectasis is a disease of children and young adults that results from severe infection of the bronchial wall and destruction of its structure. The disease owes its name to the dilatation of large intrapulmonary bronchi, but the associated obstruction and destruction of the small bronchi account for many of its manifestations. Infection is both cause and consequence of the disease. The clinical course varies primarily with the extent of the lesions and the quality of the host's defense mechanisms.

Pathology

The trachea and mainstem bronchi, i.e., the extrapulmonary airways, are normal in size. Dilatation involves segmental and subsegmental bronchi and their branches of division, from the third to the sixth or ninth generations. Affected bronchi are widened, crowded together and misshapen by outpocketings of the walls (varicose bronchiectasis) or ballooning of their blind ends (saccular bronchiectasis). On the cut surface of the lung the dilated bronchi appear as large thin-walled cavities found not only near the hilum but also all the way to the periphery of the lung, many filled with pus (Fig. 10). The intervening parenchyma shows areas of pneumonitis, atelectasis, fibrosis and overinflation, and some normal-appearing alveoli. The more advanced forms, in which no recognizable alveolar tissue remains, are of course limited in their extent, often to one lobe.

Microscopically the extrapulmonary bronchi show changes of chronic bronchitis and an otherwise normal structure. In the wall of affected bronchi, only remnants

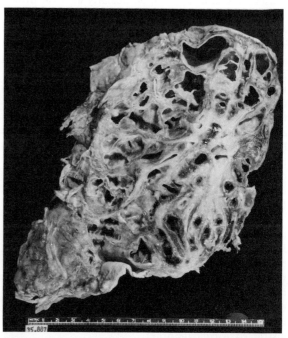

Fig. 10. Severe widespread bronchiectasis with large cystic cavities occupying most of the lungs. This patient, whose x-ray films are shown in Fig. 12, had undergone a left lower lobectomy 15 years before his death at age 52. (Courtesy of Dr. Gerald Nash, Massachusetts General Hospital.)

of cartilage, elastic lamina, smooth muscle, and mucous glands are found. On many sections these normal components of the bronchial wall are completely replaced by fibrosis and granulation tissue. No ciliary epithelium can be recognized. The bronchial sacs are lined with metaplastic squamous epithelium, or they are ulcerated and coated with fibrin and pus. Multiple small abscesses are noted. The surrounding parenchyma is the site of chronic and acute inflammation with fibrotic scarring involving small airways and alveoli.

There are associated vascular changes. Hypertrophy of the right ventricle and dilatation of the large pulmonary arteries result from longstanding pulmonary hypertension. Small pulmonary arteries are narrowed by medial hypertrophy or occluded by organized thrombi, secondary to focal inflammation. The bronchial arteries are grossly increased in number and size.

Pathogenesis

Severe and protracted infection is common to all forms of bronchiectasis. The organisms involved are mouth flora, *Staphylococcus aureus* and *Pseudomonas aeruginosa,* all capable of causing necrotizing bronchitis and pneumonitis. Infection becomes established in parts or in all of the bronchial tree because of a localized lesion or a systemic defect of defense mechanisms.

Prolonged obstruction of a main-stem, lobar, or segmental bronchus is a common cause of bronchiectasis. This may be due to foreign body, fibrous scarring (healed bronchial tuberculosis), tumor, or compression by enlarged lymph nodes. The right middle-lobe bronchus is particularly susceptible to extrinsic compression by lymphadenopathy; the bronchus is relatively long and narrow and is surrounded by lymph nodes draining not only the right middle lobe itself but also the right lower lobe and occasionally the right upper lobe. Thus recurrent atelectasis and chronic inflammation are observed more frequently in the right middle lobe than in any other region of the lung, particularly in young children in whom lobar collapse is facilitated by absent or insufficient collateral ventilation. Today only a small number of children with right middle-lobe syndrome seem to go on to develop right middle-lobe bronchiectasis, but accurate figures are not available. Atelectasis without bronchial obstruction, even if persistent for years, does not cause bronchiectasis.

Localized bronchiectasis may also follow an episode of pneumonia, unusually severe or slowly resolving. In this respect the role of infectious diseases of childhood (measles, pertussis) and bacterial superinfection, emphasized by earlier authors, has been confirmed by the decreased incidence of the disease where antibiotics and immunization have come into general use. Socioeconomic factors remain important: in U.S. populations plagued by poverty, crowding and lack of health care, bronchiectasis is found with much higher incidence than in the general population.

Congenital malformations in which pulmonary arterial blood supply to one lung or one lobe is absent also lead to the development of localized bronchiectasis, particularly agenesis of one pulmonary artery and lobar sequestration.

Generalized bronchiectasis is usually traceable to a specific deficiency of bacterial clearance in the lungs, itself part of a systemic disease. In acquired hypogammaglobulinemia, with low or absent IgA and IgG, respiratory infections may be the dominant clinical manifestation. Severe chronic bronchitis and recurrent pneumonia mark the course of the disease. Generalized bronchiectasis develops insidiously even in carefully treated patients. IgA deficiency alone is not associated with chronic lung disease. In other severe immune deficiencies, often congenital, pulmonary infections may be prominent, but the rapid course does not lead to the development of bronchiectasis.

Cystic fibrosis is an inherited autosomal-recessive disorder with an incidence of 1 in 2500 live births. Affecting all exocrine glands, the disease is manifested by high electrolyte concentration in sweat and high viscosity of mucous secretions in the gastrointestinal, respiratory, and genital tracts. The clinical course reflects the severity of intestinal, pancreatic, and respiratory involvements (Table 4), variable in individual cases. The chronic gastrointestinal manifestations are usually well controlled by pancreatic opotherapy and increased fluid intake, such that a satisfactory nutritional state is preserved. The chronic obstructive lung disease, although responsive to treatment, is relentlessly progressive and leads to the development of widespread bronchiectasis. Acute bronchitis and recurrent bronchopneumonia are due to various common organisms, but as the disease advances *S. aureus* and *P. aeruginosa* become established, and

Table 4
Clinical Manifestations of Cystic Fibrosis

Gastrointestinal	Respiratory	Others
Neonatal meconium ileus	Recurrent pneumonia	Elevated sweat Na and Cl
Rectal prolapse	Atelectasis	Heat strokes
Pancreatic insufficiency	Sinusitis	Sterility in males
Intestinal obstruction	Nasal polyposis	
Cirrhosis of the liver	Chronic bronchitis	
Diabetes	Bronchiectasis	
	Lung abscess	
	Hemoptysis	
	Pneumothorax	
	Cor pulmonale	

persistent infection is the rule in spite of aggressive therapy. Immune competence is normal. The diagnosis, suspected on clinical evidence (Table 4), is proven by the elevation of sweat sodium and chloride concentrations (sweat test). The disease exhibits great genetic variability, and the mean survival age is rising with improved management, so that cystic fibrosis in adults is not exceptional.

Kartagener's syndrome, comprising situs inversus, sinusitis, and bronchiectasis, shows familial clustering without a clear pattern of inheritance. Nearly one-half of affected patients present with IgA deficiency. The clinical course is marked by chronic and recurrent respiratory infections beginning in infancy, and bronchiectasis develops progressively.

Chagas' disease, a parasitic infestation due to *Trypanosoma cruzi*, is prevalent in large areas of Latin America, particularly in southeast Brazil. It is rare for humans to acquire the disease in the U.S., but animal infestation has been identified in Southern and Southwestern states. The acute febrile illness that marks the onset is usually self-limited and is followed by chronic disease. The clinical course is determined by the possible occurrence of myocarditis, myositis, or meningoencephalitis. Destruction of parasympathetic ganglia has been documented in the gastrointestinal tract, where it is associated with achalasia and megacolon, and in the respiratory tract, where it is associated with bronchiectasis in as many as 5 percent of infested patients. This observation suggests that impaired vagal innervation due to peribronchial inflammation may contribute to the development of bronchiectasis.

Clinical Presentation

Chronic cough and production of purulent sputum are the major symptoms of bronchiectasis. Cough is frequent, through day and night. It is triggered by exertion or a change of body position and at times occurs in long exhausting spells. The sputum is almost always purulent and so abundant that even young children learn to expectorate. The foul odor that once was characteristic of bronchiectatic sputum is rarely noted nowadays, as the responsible flora are usually eradicated by medication. Fatigue and exertional dyspnea are common complaints during exacerbations or with advanced disease.

On examination, temperature is normal except during exacerbations, but respiratory rate is increased. Examination of the head and neck may be normal or may reveal purulent rhinitis, nasal polyposis, and tenderness over the paranasal sinuses. Auscultation reveals ronchi and rales over the affected lobes or segment. In diffuse disease, hyperresonance, decreased diaphragmatic motion, and prolonged expiration with wheezing are common. Clubbing of the fingers is always prominent; it occurs long before cyanosis and in advanced cases becomes as marked as in congenital cyanotic heart disease. The remainder of the examination varies with the underlying disorder (cystic fibrosis, Kartagener's syndrome, and with the severity of the disease (emaciation) or its complications (pneumonia, hemoptysis, cor pulmonale).

The chronic abundant expectoration, the persistent presence of rales, and the clubbing suggest a diagnosis of bronchiectasis. A plain chest film usually suffices to confirm or rule out the clinical impression of localized versus generalized disease. The most common sites for localized disease are the posterior segment of either lower lobe or both, the right middle lobe, and the lingula of the left upper lobe. Saccular dilatations are readily visible as cystic radiolucencies with or without fluid level (Figs. 11 and 12). In less advanced disease the bronchi are thickwalled and widened and are often crowded because of loss of volume in the affected areas.

The sputum, on microscopic examination, contains neutrophil polymorphonuclears, bacteria, and mostly amorphous debris. Macrophages and ciliated epithelial cells are few or absent, but red blood cells may be present. Abundance of eosinophils suggests associated hypersensitivity (asthma, aspergillosis, drug reaction). Sputum culture guides the choice of appropriate antibiotic therapy. Hemoglobin and hematocrit may be low because of deficient diet, chronic infection, or significant blood loss from hemoptysis, or they may be elevated in response to chronic hypoxia. The white count is moderately elevated, with marked predominance of mature neutrophils.

After initial treatment pulmonary function tests are helpful to evaluate the overall performance of the lungs. Lobar bronchiectasis usually causes mild airway obstruction because of secondary diffuse chronic bronchitis and hypoxemia because of uneven distribution and right-to-left shunt. Diffuse disease causes airway obstruction, hyperinflation, and severe hypoxemia. Tests are repeated at intervals of 1 or 2 years either to document stabilization or progress of the disease or as a part of preoperative evaluation. In the latter instance radiospirometry is helpful to confirm adequate ventilation and perfusion in those areas of the lungs that are thought to be entirely or relatively free of disease.

Bronchography is indicated when the disease appears to be severe, localized, and unresponsive to medical treatment, so that surgical resection is considered. The procedure aims at demonstrating the extent of the lesions to be resected and the preservation of bronchial structure elsewhere. Thus the whole bronchial tree must be visualized, although preferably by selective bronchography, one or two lobes at a time. Bronchographic studies in the past have established the fact that mild cylindrical dilatation of the bronchi, as observed with incomplete resolution of pneumonia or atelectasis, is a reversible process, although the return of a normal bronchial morphology may be delayed as long as 1 to 3 years. Therefore it is best to reserve the name of bronchiectasis for cases in which bronchograms show varicose or saccular deformation of the bronchi as well as dilatation.

Management

Effective treatment of acute respiratory diseases and prevention of chronic airway infection in childhood have produced a drastic reduction in the incidence of bronchiectasis through the last 30 years. Credit for this

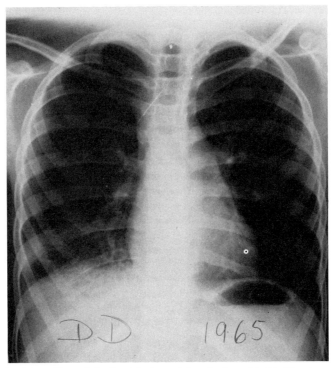

Fig. 11.   Localized bronchiectasis in the right lower lobe of a 6-yr-old girl. (Courtesy of Dr. G. C. B. Harris, Children's Hospital Medical Center, Boston, Mass.

accomplishment goes to immunization against the infectious diseases of childhood and to antibiotic therapy of bacterial infections. Children and young adults who nevertheless develop chronic or recurrent bacterial infections of the lower respiratory tract remain at risk to develop bronchiectasis. Treatment begins with institution of a pulmonary regimen, including postural drainage, chest physiotherapy, and p.r.n. antibiotics. Bronchodilators are

often helpful. This program is to be continued for life in patients with agammaglobulinemia, cystic fibrosis, or Kartagener's syndrome. When no specific host factor can be identified, the program is continued until the patient remains free of disease for a number of months, but it is immediately resumed in the case of another recurrence of pneumonia, atelectasis, or persistent bronchitis.

Surgical   resection   is   indicated   for   localized

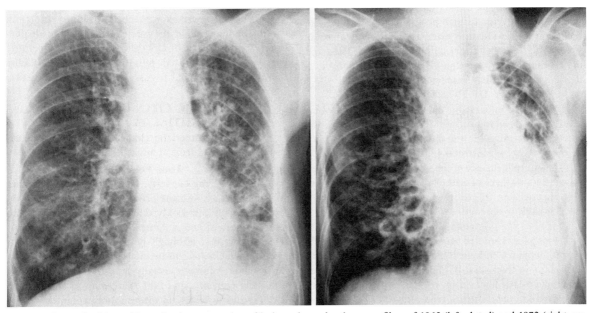

Fig. 12.   Generalized bronchiectasis: the progression of lesions shown by the x-ray films of 1965 (left, dated) and 1972 (right, undated) was reflected in marked clinical deterioration. Same patient as in Fig. 10.

bronchiectasis when a local cause is identified and the remainder of the bronchial tree is essentially intact. Resection of an area of advanced bronchiectasis in the presence of diffuse disease is occasionally helpful, even in patients with agammaglobulinemia or cystic fibrosis, provided that pulmonary function is adequate.

REFERENCES

Nemir RL: Bronchiectasis, in Disorders of the Respiratory Tract in Children, vol 1: Pulmonary Disorders (ed 2). Philadelphia, WB Saunders, 1972, p 268

Shwachman H: Cystic fibrosis, in Disorders of the Respiratory Tract in Children, vol 1: Pulmonary Disorders (ed 2). Philadelphia, WB Saunders, 1972, p 524

INTERSTITIAL LUNG DISEASE

Barry W. Levine

Interstitial lung disease results from injury to one or more of the components of the alveolar–capillary membrane. Immunologic disorders, radiation, chemicals, dusts, circulatory disturbances, allergens, and malignancy can cause such an injury. Although there are over 150 known causes of interstitial lung disease, the majority of cases remain idiopathic. In those instances in which a specific etiology can be found, specific therapy may be available.

Certain clinical characteristics are common to all forms of interstitial lung disease regardless of the specific etiology. The onset of symptoms is insidious. A dry persistent cough is a frequent finding before other clinical signs become apparent. Exertional dyspnea often heralds the advent of interstitial involvement. An early clinical sign is the presence of fine, dry, end-inspiratory, crackling rales. With further pulmonary involvement resting hypoxemia develops, and cyanosis and clubbing of the digits may be noted. With further progression tachypnea becomes a prominent feature, often associated with alveolar hyperventilation. Significant pulmonary hypertension and cor pulmonale may develop. Hypercapnia usually is a later and often terminal manifestation.

ANATOMY OF INTERSTITIAL SPACE

In order to understand the pathologic processes involved in the development of interstitial lung disease, the structure of the alveolar wall must be appreciated.

Alveolar Lining

The internal surface of the alveolar wall is composed of a continuous layer of epithelial cells situated on a basement membrane. The delicate nature of this structure makes it liable to damage.

Interstitial Space

This space is located between the alveolar lining cells and the capillary endothelium. It normally varies from 0.2 to 2.5 μ in thickness. Within this area are located reticular and elastic fibers. They form interstices containing the alveolar interstitial cells (alveolar cells and histiocytes), small lymphatics, and arterioles.

Capillaries

The alveolar capillary is composed of endothelial cells that rest on a basement membrane. The interstitial space is bordered by this membrane and the epithelial basement membrane.

PATHOLOGY IN INTERSTITIAL LUNG DISEASE

The anatomic structure of the lung limits the pathologic response to the following reactions, which may be single or combined (Fig. 1):

Alveolar Lining Cell Injury

When injury to the alveolar lining cell occurs there may be an altered permeability. This will lead to fibrinous intraalveolar exudation. Although the reaction is often reversible, if resolution fails the exudated fibrin will contract and a regenerating cuboid layer of alveolar epithelium will rapidly cover it incorporating the fibrin into the alveolar wall. Fibroblasts will then appear, proliferate, and lay down a layer of interstitial collagen. In addition to fibrin depositions, alveolar lining injury can cause hyaline membrane formation as well as the deposition of hemosiderin or various cells within the intraalveolar space.

Interstitial Infiltrates

The interstitial space can be invaded by a variety of cell types. These are predominantly mononuclear cells, but neutrophils are also common infiltrators. Occasionally the infiltrate may be predominantly eosinophils or giant cells.

Capillary Damage

Rarely does the vascular bed of the lung remain intact following the destruction of the alveolar wall or obliteration of the alveolar airspace. The result of capillary damage is increased permeability and edema formation within the interstitial space, a pathologic finding common to many interstitial diseases.

Chronic Lymph Edema

Whenever there is excessive formation of lymph within the lung, either by overproduction or inadequate drainage, deposition of collagen and reticular fibers occurs causing interstitial pulmonary fibrosis, although there are no lymphatic vessels within the interstitial space.

PHYSIOLOGIC CHANGES IN CHRONIC INTERSTITIAL LUNG DISEASE

Certain characteristic changes in lung function are common to most forms of interstitial lung disease.

Lung Volumes

The total lung capacity, vital capacity, and residual volume decrease with the progression of interstitial lung disease. This is commonly referred to as a restrictive defect. The loss of lung volumes is best correlated with interstitial fibrosis, although it can be quite dramatic in alveolar proteinosis and toxic alveolitis. The reduction in the residual volume is usually less marked than that in total lung capacity, and thus there may be an increased RV/TLC ratio. Early in disease, lung volumes may be normal.

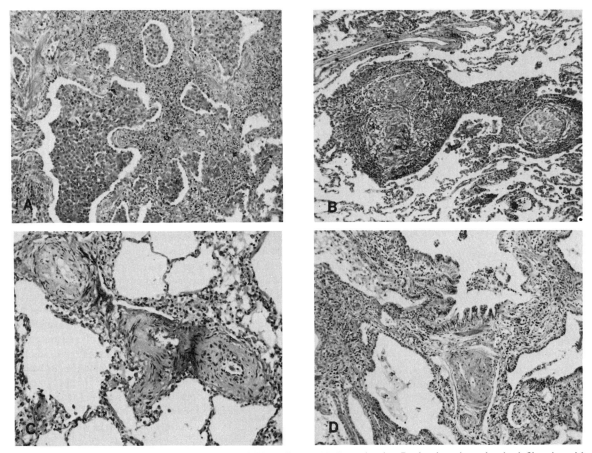

Fig. 1. Histologic changes in various types of interstitial lung disease. (A) Intraalveolar. Predominent intraalveolar infiltration with desquamated alveolar cells from a case of desquamative interstitial pneumonia (H&E, × 130). (B) Granulomatous. Interstitial granuloma formation in sarcoidosis (H&E, × 125). (C) Vascular. Predominant vascular involvement with little fibrosis in a case of scleroderma (H&E, × 170). (D) Diffuse. Diffuse interstitial fibrosis in a case of idiopathic pulmonary fibrosis (H&E, × 130).

Pulmonary Mechanics

The air-flow rates are usually normal in interstitial lung disease until late in the course of illness, when marked reduction in lung volumes may be associated with reduced flow rates. Static compliance is diminished in interstitial lung disease, but airway resistance remains normal. The resultant "stiff" lung will increase the work of breathing and contribute to the sensation of breathlessness.

Gas Exchange

The earliest changes in lung function in interstitial lung disease occur in pulmonary gas exchange. Hypoxemia on exercise is probably the first change, followed by hypoxemia at rest and a fall in the lung diffusing capacity. Classically, the arterial blood in patients with interstitial lung disease has a diminished P_{O_2}, a normal or low P_{CO_2}, and a normal or alkaline pH. These abnormalities may precede any other change in lung function. A combination of pathologic alterations in compliance, lung volume, diffusing surface, and vascular compartments of gas-exchanging units may lead to abnormalities in ventilation perfusion ratios, which accounts for most of the gas-exchange abnormalities in interstitial disease.

Patients with interstitial lung disease will often have Pa_{O_2} less than 80 mm Hg and increases in the alveolar–arterial O_2 gradient ($A–aD_{O_2}$) on room air and 14 percent oxygen breathing despite normal lung volumes. In addition to hypoxemia, hyperventilation with resulting respiratory alkalosis is common in patients with interstitial lung disease. The hyperventilation is partly due to hypoxemia, with increased hypoxic drive to ventilation through stimulation of the peripheral chemoreceptors, but is mainly due to pathologic alterations in the lung interstitium. The stretch receptors in the lung parenchyma are stimulated by the interstitial process leading to sustained hyperventilation even when O_2 is given to abolish the hypoxic drive. As interstitial lung disease progresses the maldistribution of perfusion and ventilation becomes more apparent. Areas of the lung develop infinitely high or low $\dot{V}/\dot{Q}$ ratios, which ultimately ends in either increases in dead space or right-to-left shunting.

The diffusing capacity of the lung for oxygen ($D_{L_{O_2}}$) or carbon monoxide ($D_{L_{CO}}$) is diminished in interstitial lung disease. This reduction in diffusing capacity has been interpreted to indicate the presence of a barrier to passage of oxygen through the alveolar–capillary membrane because of increased thickness of the membrane leading to development of hypoxemia. The term alveolar–capillary block was coined to describe the basic pathophysiologic process. Recent evidence suggests that this concept is probably incorrect and that a block to diffusion of oxygen is not the cause of hypoxemia in most instances of interstitial lung disease. This can be appreciated by considering the equation relating the diffusing capacity of the lung for oxygen ($D_{L_{O_2}}$) to its two components, the membrane diffusing capacity (D_M) and the pulmonary capillary red-cell volume (V_c), and the reaction rate between oxygen and hemoglobin (θ):

$$\frac{1}{D_{L_{O_2}}} = \frac{1}{D_M} + \frac{1}{\theta V_c}$$

The effect of increasing the membrane thickness on the diffusion of oxygen can be calculated. Membrane thickness can be increased six to eight times its normal, and therefore D_M can be reduced to one-sixth to one-eighth of its normal value before a measurable 1-mm Hg increase in the alveolar–arterial O_2 gradient due to impaired diffusion occurs. Therefore an increase in membrane thickness itself plays a minor role in the pathogenesis of hypoxemia in interstitial lung disease. By increasing the thickness of the membrane from 1 μ to 8 μ, smaller alveoli would be reduced 60 percent in volume, and middle-range alveoli by 20 percent. Uneven thickening of alveolar–capillary membranes would have an important effect on the distribution of ventilation by diminishing the compliance of the alveolar walls. Because of the stiffening and reduced volume, ventilation to the affected alveoli would be reduced. If the perfusion of these affected alveoli was not reduced proportionately, hypoxemia would occur from the uneven ventilation/perfusion relationship. In patients with interstitial lung disease, therefore, resting hypoxemia is presently felt to be due to the unequal distribution of ventilation and perfusion.

A feature common to interstitial lung disease is development of hypoxemia on exercise, which may antedate the onset of resting hypoxemia. During exercise cardiac output and oxygen consumption increase. As a result of the increased cardiac output, the red-blood-cell transit time through the pulmonary capillary bed is decreased. Since the size of the capillary bed is reduced in interstitial lung disease, the decreased transit time of the red blood cell does not permit adequate equilibration of mixed venous blood with alveolar oxygen, resulting in hypoxemia.

A later additional mechanism of hypoxemia in interstitial lung disease is through the development of increased right-to-left shunting (venous admixture), secondary to progressive destruction of alveoli and obliteration of ventilated areas whose pulmonary perfusion is maintained to a varying degree. Marked increase in venous admixture is a late manifestation of interstitial lung disease. Increase in dead space is also seen late in the disease and signifies disproportionate destruction of the vascular bed in relation to alveolar loss.

Summary of Physiologic Changes

The physiologic abnormalities in interstitial lung disease may antedate any clinical or chest x-ray abnormalities. Rest and exercise hypoxemia and reduction in the diffusing capacity are early physiologic findings. Variable degrees of right-to-left shunting and increases in the physiologic dead space can be present. Mild respiratory alkalosis is a frequent finding. Reduction in total lung capacity and vital capacity is common, although early in the disease these volumes can be normal. Reduction in compliance is common.

DIAGNOSIS OF INTERSTITIAL LUNG DISEASE

Interstitial lung disease can be classified under pathologic abnormalities or associated systemic disease, and in specific instances it is based on environmental factors. In all instances a thorough historical review, including all occupational and environmental exposures, a family history, and a complete review of systems, are needed. Any physical abnormality must be viewed as a possible associated manifestation of a systemic disorder causing interstitial lung disease. The diagnostic evaluation should also include both biochemical and radiologic evaluation of the patient. In those instances in which a clear etiology of the lung disease is not found, a percutaneous or open lung biopsy should be performed. Table 1 classifies the more common forms of interstitial lung disease. Two categories emerge that enable the clinician to differentiate the various causes of interstitial lung disease on the basis of either clinical or histologic findings. It is important to realize that the lung biopsy will not only delineate the pathologic process within the lung, but will also help in defining the natural history of the disorder and an appropriate mode of therapy. Table 2 summarizes the histologic findings on biopsy and the related diagnoses and therapeutic modalities.

DIFFERENTIATION ON PATHOLOGIC CLASSIFICATION

Idiopathic Pulmonary Fibrosis (Hamman-Rich Syndrome)

Hamman-Rich syndrome is a progressive form of interstitial fibrosis, often with a fatal outcome. The etiology of this disorder is unknown. It may appear 1 to 2 years following a severe virallike respiratory illness. On rare occasion it has been noted to occur in families without any demonstrable mode of inheritance. A positive rheumatoid factor may be found in the serum of as many as 40 percent of cases. This association is particularly frequent among patients in their seventh and eighth decades of life. Although there are excessively high titers of serum rheumatoid factor in the serum of these patients, there may be no clinical evidence of rheumatoid arthritis, and the course of the pulmonary fibrosis tends to be indolent. These high titers are felt to be responsible for an excessive reactivity of the pulmonary interstitium to presently unknown exogenous or endogenous insults.

Idiopathic pulmonary fibrosis usually appears in the fourth and fifth decades with a slight male pre-

Table 1
Classification of Chronic Interstitial Lung Disease

Pathologic Classification	Etiologic Classification
Diagnosis established by lung biopsy	Diagnosis established by history and clinical findings
Idiopathic pulmonary fibrosis (Hamman-Rich syndrome)	Drug-induced
Desquamative interstitial pneumonia	Inherited
Histiocytosis X	Radiation-induced
Chronic eosinophilic pneumonia	Collagen-vascular disease
Alveolar proteinosis	Rheumatoid arthritis
Sarcoidosis	Lupus erythematosus
Hypersensitivity pneumonitis	Systemic sclerosis
	Periarteritis nodosa
	Wegener's granulomatosis
	Vascular
	Goodpasture's syndrome
	Idiopathic pulmonary hemosiderosis
	Idiopathic pulmonary hypertension
	Hypersensitivity lung disease
	Cardiac disease—"mitral lung"
	Pneumoconioses
	Noxious gases

ponderance. The course can be variable. Death has been known to occur from 4 to 34 weeks after the onset of symptoms. However, the course tends to become more chronic as the age of onset increases. Survival for 20 or more years is not uncommon.

When considering all types of interstitial pneumonia, between 40 percent and 50 percent of such patients are classified into the category of idiopathic pulmonary fibrosis.

Pathology. The lungs from such patients are heavy, firm, and rubbery. On microscopic section there is structural distortion and the alveolar lining cells are enlarged, appearing cuboid or low columnar. Foci of organizing hemorrhage and fibroblastic proliferation are seen within the alveolar walls. The alveolar lumina are often filled with alveolar cells and an exudate composed of histiocytes and eosinophils. Fibroblasts often obliterate the alveolar spaces, and occasionally there is organization of intraalveolar exudate. The interstitial space is edematous and infiltrated with monocytes and lymphocytes. There are also small numbers of plasma cells and eosinophils. The regeneration of alveolar epithelium covers the exudated alveolar cells incorporating them into the interstitium. Elongated fibroblasts are also found within the interstitium. Within these areas collagen fibers are prominent. In other areas of the interstitium there is very little cellular activity and complete replacement by fibrous tissue.

Table 2
Value of Lung Biopsy as to Etiology and Treatment

Lung Biopsy Findings	Disease	Treatment
Predominantly granulomas	Sarcoidosis	Likely steroid-responsive if not infectious
	Fungal-tuberculosis	Appropriate chemotherapy
Predominantly intraalveolar desquamation	DIP	Likely steroid-responsive
Intraalveolar exudation (PAS+)	Alveolar proteinosis	Pulmonary lavage; steroids contra-indicated
Interstitial histiocytes, eosinophils, and granulomas	Histiocytosis X	Likely steroid-responsive
	Chronic eosinophilic pneumonia	
Intense monocytic, lymphocytic, interstitial infiltration (alveolitis)	Collagen-vascular; idiopathic fibrosis	Definite trial of steroids ± responsive
Vasculitis		Trial of antimetabolite if negative steroid response
Histiocytes, interstitial foam cells, eosinophils, occasional granuloma	Hypersensitivity; pneumonitis	Check exposure, steroid-responsive; remove from offending allergen
Predominantly fibrosis, little or no cellular reaction	Hamman-Rich	Unlikely steroid-responsive
	Collagen disease; drug-induced; radiation	Unlikely antimetabolite-responsive
Vasculitis	Collagen-vascular	Trial of steroid ± responsive; trial of antimetabolites if negative steroid response

Clinical findings. The majority of patients present with dyspnea and a sensation of restricted breathing. Fatigue and weakness may accompany these complaints. Less than 25 percent of patients complain of a nonproductive cough and, less frequently, hemoptysis. If cor pulmonale is present, the primary complaint may be substernal exertional chest pain.

On physical examination the patient breathes shallowly and rapidly. Diffuse fine crackling rales are usually present. The rales have a characteristic fine, dry quality similar to the crackling of cellophane. Clubbing of the fingers and toes with or without clinically apparent cyanosis is a frequent finding. Signs of right heart failure and cor pulmonale are late and denote the terminal stages of the disease.

Chest x-ray. The appearance of the chest x-ray is nonspecific and occasionally normal. Miliary, reticular, nodular, or coalescent infiltrates are present. These changes may antedate the onset of symptoms by many years. Rarely, pleural thickening, plaques, calcifications, and effusions can be associated with idiopathic pulmonary fibrosis. Over the course of the disease, repeated chest x-rays show progressive reduction of lung volume.

Treatment. In chronic idiopathic pulmonary fibrosis corticosteroids are rarely of benefit, but in acute fulminant cases they have been associated with some improvement and in a few well-documented cases they have been of long-term value. Therefore a clinical trial is indicated. Oxygen, continuously used at low flow rates, has enabled patients to return to their normal activities. Right-heart failure should be treated appropriately with digitalis and diuretics. Of utmost importance is the rigorous therapy of any superimposed pulmonary infection, since this is one of the most common causes of death. In general the prognosis is poor, with death occurring from several months to years after the onset of the disease. Recently the use of antimetabolites such as cytoxin and methotrexate has resulted in clinical improvement.

Desquamative Interstitial Pneumonia (DIP)

DIP is a pathologic entity differing from idiopathic pulmonary fibrosis on the basis of histologic findings and responsiveness to steroids.

Pathology. Desquamative interstitial pneumonia is characterized by the striking finding on histologic examination of the lungs of large alveolar cells within the alveolar lumen. These larger than normal cells have an eosinophilic cytoplasm containing PAS-positive yellow-brown granules. The alveoli are lined with hypertrophic cells similar to those within the lumen. The cells have a stratified configuration suggesting a desquamative process. The alveolar wall is often edematous. The bronchiole walls also show edema as well as fibroblast and smooth-muscle proliferation. The bronchi and bronchioles can be filled with desquamated cells. The pathologic process is usually uniform throughout the entire biopsy specimen.

Clinical findings. Desquamative interstitial pneu-

monia usually occurs in the fourth decade of life and is equally distributed among the sexes. Most often dyspnea is the presenting complaint associated with a paroxysmal nonproductive cough. In many instances the rapid progression of dyspnea follows an acute upper respiratory infection. Clubbing is found in 50 percent of the cases. The disease is commonly complicated by either recurrent spontaneous pneumothorax or pleural effusion. Infrequently, cor pulmonale is found. The course of the disease is variable. In some patients there is only a slow progression of dyspnea with the appearance of a restrictive defect and hypoxemia on lung function testing over several years. In others severe pulmonary fibrosis and hypoxemia progress rapidly over a period of several months.

Chest x-ray. The chest x-ray can be unique in DIP. In 75 percent of cases there is a slight triangular haziness radiating from the hilus along the heart borders toward both bases, but not extending to the costophrenic angles. The vascular markings at the bases appear increased and ill-defined. The characteristic x-ray appearance may remain unchanged up to 10 years after the onset of symptoms.

Therapy. In many patients with DIP long-term steroid therapy has abated or controlled progression of the disease. Steroids in large doses (60 mg/day prednisone) have resulted in dramatic clinical improvement with reduction of dyspnea and clubbing and an improvement in exercise tolerance. This steroid response appears unique for the DIP form of idiopathic pulmonary fibrosis.

Alveolar Proteinosis

Alveolar proteinosis is a disorder in which amorphous proteinaceous material rich in lipids fills the alveoli and bronchioles.

Pathology. Grossly, numerous yellow-grey or grey nodules are seen beneath the pleura. Large portions of these lungs are consolidated, oozing yellow fluid from the cut surface. On light microscopy, finely granular acidophilic material fills groups of alveoli. There are only minimal septal changes, and alveoli adjacent to the involved zones are often normal. Small bronchioles are also filled with this material. The acidophilic, amorphous substance is strongly PAS-positive.

Clinical findings. The majority of patients have a cough (with or without sputum production), dyspnea, fatigue, and malaise. Other symptoms include weight loss, chest pain, and hemoptysis. A low-grade fever, which is often present, is thought to be secondary to associated infection. Rarely there are no symptoms and the disease is first noted on a routine chest x-ray. Physical findings include clubbing, cyanosis, and rales. The course of the disease is variable. Some patients have spontaneous improvement; in others death occurs from respiratory failure or superimposed infection. Associated fungal infections are frequent with nocardiosis the most common. The diagnosis is made either by lung biopsy or at autopsy.

Chest x-ray. The chest x-ray is often characteristic. Very fine coalescent nodules radiating from the perihilar region give a symmetric alveolar pattern, the so-called butterfly distribution.

Therapy. Various forms of therapy have been proposed including tracheal instillation of heparin and proteolytic agents or the inhalation of acetylcysteine and pancreatic dornase. However, none is uniformly effective. Recently, lavage of each lung with copious amounts of normal saline containing heparin and acetylcysteine administered with positive pressure through a Carlens tube has been effective in controlling alveolar proteinosis. Steroids are contraindicated in this disease.

Histiocytosis X

This generic name encompasses a group of diseases that affect the reticuloendothelial system. Under the heading of histiocytosis X are grouped Letterer-Siwe disease, Hand-Schüller-Christian disease, and eosinophilic granuloma. All of these diseases have similar histologic findings and therefore overlap. They differ only in the extent of involvement. age of onset, and primary organs involved. The lung can be affected in any of them with often the same result. Therefore, only eosinophilic granuloma will be discussed, as it predominantly involves the lung.

Eosinophilic Granuloma of the Lung

Pulmonary eosinophilic granuloma is a rare disorder of unknown etiology. As a variant of histiocytosis X it is often associated with other systemic manifestations such as diabetes insipidus and cystic bone lesions.

Pathology. On gross inspection the lungs have single or multiple nodules located beneath the pleura. Their distribution may be lobar or diffuse. Often localized areas of fibrosis and honeycombing are seen. Microscopic examination reveals nodules ranging from several millimeters to centimeters in diameter. The nodules are composed of histiocytes located within both the interstitium and alveoli. Numerous eosinophils are also present. Reticulum stains of the lung show increased interstitial collagen and elastic tissue. In advanced cases severe fibrosis and honeycombing are present.

Clinical findings. About 20 percent of patients with pulmonary eosinophilic granuloma are diagnosed from an incidental finding on an abnormal chest x-ray. Others have an insidious onset with a low-grade fever and malaise, dyspnea not being a common feature. In addition to pulmonary involvement, 20 percent have diabetes insipidus and 20 percent have single or multiple granulomas involving the long bones. Peripheral eosinophilia is not a feature of this disorder. The course of the disease is variable, with spontaneous remission frequently occurring. Progression may occur and result in severe pulmonary fibrosis, cystic degeneration of the lung, cor pulmonale, respiratory failure, and death. Although pulmonary involvement may not be extensive, at least 20 percent of patients with this disorder have recurrent spontaneous pneumothorax. The diagnosis is established by histologic examination of lung tissue.

Chest x-ray. There are no characteristic x-ray findings. The most consistent findings are small, ill-defined nodules varying in size and located peripherally in the up-per lung fields. Occasionally a single cyst or an area of honeycombing may be the only abnormality.

Therapy. The efficacy of steroid therapy in this disease is questionable. However, because of the possibility that the process may progress to pulmonary fibrosis, a course of steroid therapy should be given.

Chronic Eosinophilic Pneumonia

Chronic eosinophilic pneumonia is a debilitating illness characterized by high fever, weight loss, night sweats, and progressive massive pulmonary infiltrates.

Pathology. Histologic examination of lung reveals gross consolidation due to interstitial and small-airspace leukocytic infiltration. The majority of these cells are mature eosinophils, with small numbers of histiocytes and lymphocytes also present within the interstitium. A consistent finding is the presence of multinucleated histiocytic giant cells within the airspaces. Some of these giant cells contain eosinophilic granules and minute Charcot-Leyden crystals. There may be a mild angiitis affecting a few small vessels, predominantly venules. Fibroblast proliferation and deposition of collagen within the interstitium is infrequently found. Occasionally there are a few scattered epithelioid granulomas.

Clinical findings. The disease almost invariably affects females. An evening fever, nearly normal morning temperature, and drenching night sweats are common features. There is also a moderate cough, productive of a variable amount of mucoid sputum and progressive, often severe, dyspnea. Hemoptysis can also occur. Significant weight loss is common. Peripheral eosinophilia is present in only about 30 percent of cases.

Chest x-ray. There are three roentgenographic features unique for chronic eosinophilic pneumonia. Pulmonary infiltrates are noted at the periphery of the lungs without segmental or lobar distribution. These lesions are often in apposition to the chest wall and have the appearance of small pockets of pleural fluid. A second feature is that these lesions disappear rapidly on steroid therapy; third, during relapse they occur in the same locations and are nearly of the same size and shape as the initial lesions.

Therapy. Corticosteroid therapy results in dramatic improvement with often a complete disappearance of the syndrome. Recent experience has shown that prolonged steroid administration for upward of 1 year must be used in the more chronic forms of the illness.

Pulmonary Myomatosis

Pulmonary myomatosis is a rare disorder in which there is smooth-muscle proliferation within the pulmonary interstitium. The disease usually occurs in young females, who often have had an antecedent viral infection. Although as with other interstitial diseases hypoxia and loss of lung volume are common, the distinguishing feature of this disease is that lung elastic recoil and pulmonary compliance are increased. The course of the disease is complicated by cystic degeneration of the lung, with respiratory failure and death. There is no effective therapy.

CLASSIFICATION OF INTERSTITIAL LUNG DISEASE BASED ON KNOWN OR SPECIFIC ETIOLOGY

Although the majority of cases of pulmonary fibrosis fall into idiopathic categories, many forms may be classified into inherited, drug- or radiation-induced, autoimmune, or hypersensitivity disorders.

Inherited or Familial Forms

A genetic basis for pulmonary fibrosis is suggested by the reported cases of familial clustering of pulmonary fibrosis. In addition, pulmonary fibrosis has been associated with such hereditary diseases as tuberous sclerosis and neurofibromatosis. These forms tend to be mild and self-limited in character.

Drug-induced Forms

Systemically administered drugs such as hexamethonium, busulfan, methysergide, nitrofurantoin, methotrexate, penicillin, and Bleomycin have been associated with the development of pulmonary fibrosis. The period between the onset of signs and symptoms of pulmonary fibrosis and the administration of these drugs is variable. Most often either mild dyspnea or an abnormal chest x-ray are the initial clinical findings. The pulmonary involvement is self-limited provided that the offending drug is discontinued. Steroid therapy is of questionable value. At present it is not known why these drugs have fibrogenic properties in the lungs. A variety of industrial agents also cause interstitial lung disease, and these are discussed in the chapter on industrial lung disease.

Radiation Fibrosis

Radiation therapy to the thoracic cavity can injure the pulmonary interstitium. The severity of the radiation reaction is related to the dose and portal size. The threshold dose is 2500–3000 rads given over 3 weeks. Pneumonitis can occur within 3 to 12 weeks. Increasing age is associated with increased severity of the radiation reaction in the lung. Radiation pneumonitis is heralded by the onset of a dry persistent cough, dyspnea, fever, and malaise. Fine rales are often heard over the involved area, and the chest x-ray demonstrates an infiltrative type of interstitial process. Within several weeks the clinical and x-ray findings may clear, or in some cases persist with contraction and fibrosis of the involved area. Cavitation is extremely rare. If radiation to the lung is extensive, severe fibrosis and death may ensue. Often a superimposed infection will occur in the involved area. Steroid administration has been beneficial in alleviating the symptoms of radiation pneumonitis and occasionally in reducing the occurrence of subsequent pulmonary fibrosis.

Collagen Diseases

Pulmonary disease associated with rheumatoid arthritis. Five distinct lesions in the lung are associated with rheumatoid arthritis. They are pleuritis, pleural effusions, necrotizing alveolitis, interstitial fibrosis, and pulmonary nodules. Although such patients are usually seropositive for rheumatoid arthritis, their lung pathology may be the first manifestation of their disease.

The most common pulmonary lesion in rheumatoid arthritis is pleuritis. This may be asymptomatic or may be accompanied by chest pain. A pleural effusion is frequently found and characteristically contains little or no glucose. The reason for this is unclear. Episodes of pleuritis tend to be mild and often go unnoticed. Pleural biospy may reveal typical rheumatoid granuloma or nonspecific inflammation.

Necrotizing alveolitis is the most life-threatening form of pulmonary involvement. Clinically these patients have a fulminant course hallmarked by severe dyspnea, a dry cough, malaise, and hypoxemia. Death may occur within several months after the onset of symptoms. Pathologic examination reveals interstitial infiltration with lymphocytes, edema formation, and fibrosis. The chest x-ray demonstrates a diffuse reticular-nodular pattern. Some patients have improved after steroid therapy, and therefore a trial of steroids is indicated. Most, however, are steroid-resistant. Antimetabolites may be of value in some instances.

The overall incidence of pulmonary fibrosis associated with clinical rheumatoid arthritis is about 3 percent. Such patients have a prevalence of subcutaneous nodules located about the elbows and wrists. The interval between the onset of arthritis and the pulmonary lesions ranges from 2 to 10 years. Unusually high serum titers for rheumatoid factor are found and may exceed a dilution factor of 1:5280. The clinical features include the early appearance of dyspnea, recurrent bronchitis with sputum production, persistent cough, and clubbing. The pathologic changes in the lung include lymphocytic infiltration, edema, and fibrosis within the alveolar septum. The alveolar epithelium may become cuboid, and foci of lymphocytes resembling germinal follicles may be prominent. Death from respiratory insufficiency is not uncommon.

The nodular form of rheumatoid lung disease was first recognized in Welsh coal miners with coalworkers' pneumoconiosis (Caplan's syndrome). Clinically these patients are usually asymptomatic. However, excavation of the nodules can occur and may result in either a spontaneous pneumothorax or bronchopleural fistula. Histologically the nodules show palisading of epithelial cells and fibrinoid degeneration typical of rheumatoid nodules found elsewhere.

These pulmonary rheumatoid nodules are known to make rheumatoid factor, but their etiology is unclear. As in the extremities, cells capable of making rheumatoid factor may sequester around areas of irritation. In the lung these irritated areas may be scars or pneumoconiotic nodules.

Systemic sclerosis. In progressive systemic sclerosis (scleroderma) atrophy and sclerotic changes occur in the skin and internal organs. The sclerotic changes are usually preceded by Raynaud's phenomenon. This disorder affects women more frequently than men and is associated with some form of pulmonary disease. The lung interstitium can be fibrotic, the pulmonary arterioles often sclerosed, and the intercostal muscles infiltrated with sclerotic connective tissue. It is estimated that up to 90 percent of patients with scleroderma have some form of pulmonary involvement.

Pathology. There is diffuse interstitial fibrosis with obliteration of the alveolar spaces and distortion of the airways. Multiple cysts and honeycombing are prominent features. The pulmonary arterioles demonstrate hypertrophy of the media and perivascular infiltration by polymorphonucleocytes and lymphocytes. The intima is often disrupted, and atherosclerotic plaques are common. Often there may be only vascular involvement without significant interstitial fibrosis. On the other hand, diffuse interstitial fibrosis may be the only pathology in the lung in systemic sclerosis.

Clinical findings. The majority of patients first present with coldness of the fingers and shortness of breath associated with a dry cough. These findings may be present without x-ray evidence of pulmonary involvement. The physical examination may reveal sclerosis and ulceration of the digits, telangiectasis, and subcutaneous calcifications. Fine rales are often present in the lower lung fields. Clinical evidence of pulmonary hypertension, such as an increased pulmonic component of the second heart sound and a right ventricular heave, is also common. Pulmonary hypertension may be present even in the absence of any parenchymal lesions. Although involvement of the chest wall with sclerosis of the intercostal muscles is common, impairment of thoracic wall mechanics is not felt to cause respiratory symptoms. The diagnosis can be made by skin biopsy or the demonstration of altered esophageal, small-bowel, or colonic function.

Chest x-ray. Despite the presence of pulmonary hypertension and dyspnea, the chest x-ray may be surprisingly normal. The earliest radiographic change is a diffuse reticular shadowing in the lower two-thirds of the lung fields. Small cysts are common and give rise to a honeycomb appearance.

Therapy. Steroid therapy is of limited value in pulmonary scleroderma, but may result in improvement of the pulmonary hypertension. Penicillamine may have limited therapeutic value in scleroderma by its effect on collagen metabolism.

Systemic Lupus Erythematosus (SLE). SLE can affect the lung in several ways, causing either pleuritis, pleural effusions, pleural thickening, pulmonary fibrosis, pneumonitis, or discoid atelectasis. In some instances there may be only some abnormality of lung function and pulmonary gas exchange without any apparent or radiologically shown involvement of the lung.

Pathology. Various pulmonary pathologic changes have been described in SLE. Fibrinoid degeneration, necrosis, and lymphocytic infiltration of the pulmonary interstitium are often observed. Destruction of the alveolar walls and endothelial lining can also be seen. Plasma and lymphocytic cell infiltrations around capillaries are common, as are fibrin thrombi within the arterioles and capillaries, and vasculitis.

Clinical findings. The most common respiratory complaint in SLE is pleuritic chest pain, although dyspnea at rest is also frequent. In the majority of patients with SLE and clinically apparent lung involvement, total lung capacity is reduced. The greatest degree of restriction is found in those patients with pleural involvement. In all cases with lung involvement, whether clinically apparent or not, reduction of the carbon monoxide diffusing capacity can be found. Correlations between clinical and x-ray evidence of pulmonary involvement and the physiologic and pathologic abnormalities of the lung in SLE are poor. Some 80 percent of patients with SLE, despite lack of clinical evidence, show significant abnormalities in lung function.

Therapy. Steroid therapy will usually abate respiratory symptoms and signs in SLE. Some of the acute forms of pulmonary involvement can be treated with a course of Atabrine. Despite the poor overall prognosis in SLE, the pulmonary involvement has very little effect on the disease process.

Periarteritis Nodosa. This is a rare disease characterized by foci of necrotizing arteritis. The pulmonary involvement can take four forms: (1) necrotic, caseating lesions resembling tuberculosis, varying from miliary foci to massive lobar involvement; (2) areas of infarction; (3) bronchiectasis; (4) asthma.

Pathology. Microscopic examination reveals necrotic lesions surrounded by giant cells, lymphocytes, plasma cells, and neutrophils. Diffuse or local eosinophilic infiltration can be seen. The pulmonary vasculature shows proliferation of the internal connective tissue, with neutrophilic and eosinophilic infiltration. Fibrinoid degeneration with occasional giant cell infiltration of the arterial media is seen.

Clinical findings. In 30 percent of patients with periarteritis nodosa the lung is involved. Fifty percent of such patients have peripheral eosinophilia. Most patients with pulmonary involvement give a history of an antecedent respiratory illness. Wheezing or chronic cough are often the presenting complaints. The course of pulmonary involvement in polyarteritis is complicated by recurrent pneumonia, hemoptysis, and pleurisy. Superimposed infection of the necrotic pulmonary lesions or actual breakdown of these lesions results in the pneumonitis. Occasionally abscesses form in these areas. Pleural effusion can occur, the character being either lymphocytic or seropurulent. In 25 percent of cases with polyarteritis, hemolytic streptococci are found in the sputum. Death in this disease can occur from respiratory failure, hemoptysis, or rupture of an abscess. The etiology is unknown, although there is a relationship between serum sickness, sulfonamide and thiouracil therapy, and an antecedent hemolytic streptococcal infection.

Chest x-ray. Either segmental or lobar consolidation on chest x-ray is the most common finding. These infiltrates are often transient and are not limited by anatomic boundaries. The appearance of the infiltrates varies over 2 to 12 weeks. On occasion there is a miliary pattern on the chest film or a large homogeneous round density that may cavitate.

Therapy. Steroid therapy can be effective in large doses (40–60 mg/day prednisone). Complete suppression of symptoms can occur, and this is the desired effect. After remission is achieved, the steroid dose can be appropriately tapered. Despite remissions, 70 percent of patients with pulmonary involvement are dead within 1 year.

Wegener's granulomatosis. This disease is a necrotizing granulomatous disorder of the upper air passage, the lower respiratory tract, or both, as well as other internal organs.

Pathology. Grossly, large nodular pulmonary lesions, often with cavities, are frequent. Microscopically, these lesions show necrosis, caseation, granuloma formation, and foreign-body giant cells. Vasculitis is also present.

Clinical findings. In Wegener's granulomatosis there is usually evidence for presence of generalized arteritis, glomerulonephritis, midline granuloma of the tracheobronchial tree, and pulmonary involvement. Death is due to respiratory insufficiency in 20 percent of patients; the remainder die of renal failure. The disease is heralded by a septic type of fever and persistent purulent rhinorrhea. The distribution is equal in both sexes, commonly occurring in the fourth and fifth decades of life.

Chest x-ray. In 50 percent of the cases with Wegener's granulomatosis the chest x-ray shows round densities, multiple or solitary, and often cavitated. Rarely there are diffuse miliary densities, bronchopneumonia, or pleural effusions.

Therapy. The initial drug of choice is steroids. In steroid-refractory cases, however, cyclophosphamide has been shown to be effective.

INTERSTITIAL LUNG DISEASE INVOLVING THE PULMONARY BED

There are several diseases involving the lung that appear to originate in the pulmonary vascular bed as a result of actual damage or altered permeability.

Primary Pulmonary Hypertension

Idiopathic pulmonary hypertension is a progressive, often fatal, disease affecting young females. The diagnosis is made only after the known causes of pulmonary hypertension have been excluded.

Pathology. The pathology is confined to the heart and lungs. Characteristically there is right ventricular dilatation and hypertrophy. The lung lesions involve the pulmonary arteries and arterioles. Bronchioles, bronchial vessels, and pulmonary veins are normal. Interstitial pulmonary fibrosis is absent. The pulmonary artery trunk is dilated, with arteriosclerotic plaques extending into the primary and secondary branches. Mild to moderate medial muscular hypertrophy is common. There are also degenerative medial changes consisting of hyalinization, thinning of the muscular walls, and disruption of the internal elastic lamina. Intimal proliferation is a common feature, and asteroid bodies may be found in the arterial wall. Occasionally there is arteritis. Gross and microscopic pulmonary thromboemboli are also common.

Clinical findings. The disease affects females in a 5:1 ratio as compared to males. The median age of onset is in the fourth decade; however, it often appears in the teens. Dyspnea, the most common presenting symptom, has an insidious onset, and about one-third of cases have Raynaud's phenomenon. Syncope, also a common complaint, is thought to be secondary to diminished cerebral blood flow. Arthralgias and sometimes arthritis may be noted. Anginal chest pain is also a prominent feature. The characteristic physical findings are an increased pulmonic component of the second heart sound, an ejection systolic murmur, heard along the lower left sternal border, and in about 20 percent of patients an early diastolic murmur along the left sternal border consistent with pulmonic insufficiency. Right ventricular failure is a frequent finding. Electrocardiographic evidence of right ventricular hypertrophy is present in 90 percent of cases. In addition to congestive heart failure, pulmonary emboli and thrombi frequently complicate this disease. Median survival from the onset of symptoms is 2–3 years.

Chest x-ray. Prominence of the central pulmonary artery is a consistent finding. Decrease in the peripheral pulmonary vascular markings is usual. Generalized cardiac enlargement and right ventricular prominence are also frequent findings.

Physiologic findings. Pulmonary artery pressure and pulmonary vascular resistance are increased. Cardiac catheterization is hazardous in these patients because of cardiac arrhythmias. Hypoxemia and a diminished carbon monoxide diffusing capacity are common features in this disorder.

Therapy. The therapy is limited and mostly symptomatic. It includes the usual measures for congestive heart failure. Anticoagulant therapy with Coumadin should be considered as prophylaxis of pulmonary thromboembolization.

Goodpasture's syndrome

Goodpasture's syndrome is a disorder where pulmonary hemorrhage and glomerulonephritis occur in the same patient, although both may not be apparent initially.

Pathology. Grossly, the lungs are usually large and bulky, with diffuse hemorrhage on the surface. Cut section reveals edema and recent and old hemorrhage. Microscopically there are intraalveolar hemorrhages and hemosiderin-laden macrophages. These macrophages are usually found within the alveolar lumen and infrequently in the interstitial space. Alveolar necrosis is absent, as is vasculitis and pulmonary arteritis. Focal areas of alveolar fibrosis are often seen. Electron microscope studies show alterations in the alveolar septal basement membrane. Fluorescent staining techniques show these to be deposition of antigen–antibody complexes. The pulmonary capillary endothelium appears normal.

Clinical findings. The usual age of onset is in the second and third decades of life, with a male-to-female ratio of approximately 4:1. The mean duration of survival is 41 weeks. The clinical features of Goodpasture's syndrome include hemoptysis, anemia, hematuria, and pulmonary infiltration. The pulmonary lesions usually precede the renal disease. The etiology of this syndrome is unknown. There is a suggestion that an antibody directed against glomerular basement membrane may be responsible. This disease is rapidly fatal, with death occurring secondary to either pulmonary hemorrhage, respiratory failure, or uremia.

Chest x-ray. There are diffuse, often fleeting, granular infiltrates. These infiltrates radiate from the hilar areas, spreading outward into the lung fields and sparing the extreme bases and apices.

Therapy. Steroid therapy in this syndrome appears to have an overall benefit through lessening the pulmonary hemorrhage. Improvement in the pulmonary lesions has occurred following total nephrectomy and subsequent renal transplantation. It is felt that nephrectomy removes a renal antigen that forms an antibody complex injurious to the lung. Methotrexate therapy has also been beneficial.

Idiopathic Pulmonary Hemosiderosis

This is a disease associated with severe hemoptysis and no other systemic finding except for iron-deficiency anemia.

Pathology. Grossly, the lungs are heavy. On cross section there is a diffuse deposition of brownish pigment. Microscopically, hemosiderin-laden macrophages are present within the alveoli and interstitium. In chronic cases there is extensive loss of elastic fibers. The degree of elastic tissue damage is proportional to the duration of the disease. On light microscopy the capillary endothelium and basement membrane appear normal, but electron microscopy shows disruption of the vascular endothelium.

Clinical findings. Idiopathic pulmonary hemosiderosis frequently occurs in children. The disease is characterized by recurrent acute episodes of dyspnea, cyanosis, and cough with hemoptysis. A persistent cough is one of the major features of this disorder.

In children there is a very slight female preponderance. The youngest patient reported was 10 years old. In the majority of patients the diagnosis is established in the second and third decades. In the adult population there is a 2:1 male preponderance. Acute symptoms may last several hours to several days, subsiding slowly. Between exacerbations the patient is usually symptom-free for several weeks or months, except for pallor and generalized weakness. Findings on physical examination are minimal with reference to the chest. Cyanosis can be prominent provided that the anemia is not severe, and in more advanced cases cor pulmonale and clubbing are found. In chronic cases hepatosplenomegaly may appear.

Unlike Goodpasture's syndrome, idiopathic pulmonary hemosiderosis is chronic, and sometimes the course may last for up to 18 years or more. Occasionally, massive pulmonary hemorrhage occurs and death ensues shortly after the onset of the disease. Diagnosis is made only after ruling out other systemic diseases associated with pulmonary hemorrhage or structural abnormalities in the lung such as vascular malformations, tumors, and bronchiectasis.

Chest x-ray. Initially the chest roentgenogram may show no abnormality. Pulmonary infiltrates have appeared as early as 2 weeks after the onset of hemoptysis and as late as 5 years. Rarely, hilar lymphadenopathy is seen associated with diffuse pulmonary infiltrates. The infrequency of hilar adenopathy appears to be an important differential diagnostic consideration, especially with regard to miliary tuberculosis in children and sarcoidosis in adults.

The infiltrates are characteristically bilateral, very small nodules giving a ground-glass appearance. This appearance is found in the perihilar and lower lung fields. During an acute attack there is intensification of these densities, and clearing occurs following remission. Rarely, in adults, the infiltrates appear as large confluent densities. Unilateral densities have also been reported.

Therapy. During acute exacerbation steroids can frequently control the hemorrhage. However, their chronic use has not been found to be beneficial. Chronic oral iron supplementation will control the anemia.

Hypersensitivity Lung Disease Due to Fungi and Organic Dusts

Extrinsic allergic alveolitis is a pneumonitis precipitated by an environmental allergen and associated with high levels of precipitating antibody in the serum. The list of such diseases is rapidly expanding and includes farmer's lung, maple-bark-stripper's lung, sequoiosis, and pigeon-breeder's disease.

Although this group of diseases is associated with high titers of precipitating antibodies, the histologic alveolar reaction is not that seen in the Arthus Type III response, which is presumably mediated by precipitating antibodies. Thus far it is not clear whether the pathologic findings in the lung are due to circulating precipitin Type III antibodies or cell-mediated (Type IV) antibodies. The systemic manifestations consisting of fever, chills, malaise, and weight loss may be attributed to a Type III reaction. Therefore perhaps the combination of a Type III Arthus reaction and a Type IV tissue-mediated hypersensitivity results in extrinsic allergic alveolitis. To further complicate the issue, the intensity of the systemic Type III reaction after exposure to allergens is thought to be proportional to the intensity of the Type I acute hypersensitivity reaction precipitated by that allergen. These allergens include thermophilic spores, avian proteins, and several fungi and are listed in Table 1 of the chapter Occupational Respiratory Disease.

Clinical findings. Exposure to the offending allergen can cause acute dyspnea, malaise, and cough in patients with hypersensitivity lung disease. However, dyspnea, cough, and weight loss can develop gradually over several months. Severe respiratory distress and hypoxia can also result. The chest x-ray will show a diffuse, fine infiltrate. Serologic evaluation is of utmost importance in that there will be precipitating antibodies to the offending allergen. Precipitating antibodies are frequent findings in normal individuals, and therefore their presence in the serum does not necessarily indicate hypersensitivity pneumonitis. The diagnosis can be made by the demonstration of an improvement in lung function following removal of the patient from exposure to the allergen, or by precipitation of symptoms after the controlled inhalation of the allergen. The lung biopsy is characteristic but not diagnostic.

Pathology. The pulmonary pathology in extrinsic allergic alveolitis reveals submucosal infiltration by plasma cells, lymphocytes, and histiocytes. Eosinophils are scarce. Smooth-muscle hypertrophy causing marked narrowing of bronchiolar lumen is also seen. Interstitial changes consist of dense focal infiltration with plasma cells, lymphocytes, and histiocytes, as well as fibrosis. There is granuloma formation. Electron microscopy demonstrates extensive sheets of interstitial collagen and focal basement membrane thickening.

Clinical course and therapy. The course in this group of interstitial lung diseases is self-limited provided that the offending allergen is removed from the environment. There is usually physiologic improvement and disappearance of precipitating antibodies when such a therapeutic procedure is taken. A 2- to 3-month course of steroids should be given to lessen the possibility of developing pulmonary fibrosis.

REFERENCES

Austrian R, McClement JH, Renzetti AD Jr, et al: The syndrome of "alveolar capillary block." Am J Med 11:667, 1951

Caplan A: Rheumatoid disease and pneumoconiosis (Caplan's syndrome). Thorax 10:9, 1955

Carrington CB, Addington WW, Goff AM: Chronic eosinophilic pneumonia. N Engl J Med 280:787, 1967

Cruickshank JG, Parker RA: Pulmonary hemosiderosis with severe renal lesions (Goodpasture's syndrome). Thorax 16:22, 1961

Finley TN, Swenson EQ, Comroe JH: The cause of arterial hypoxemia at rest in patients with "alveolar-capillary block syndrome." J Clin Invest 41:618, 1962

Liebow AA, Steer A, Bilingsley JG: Desquamative interstitial pneumonia. Am J Med 39:369, 1965

McCombs RP: Diseases due to immunologic reactions in the lung. N Engl J Med 286:1245, 1972

Marks A: Diffuse interstitial pulmonary fibrosis. Med Clin North Am 51:439, 1967

Oliver H, Schwartz R, Rubio R Jr, Dameshak W: Interstitial pulmonary fibrosis following busulfon therapy. Am J Med 31:134, 1961

Opie LH: The pulmonary manifestations of generalized scleroderma (progressive systemic sclerosis). Dis Chest 28:655, 1955

Rosen SH, Castleman B, Liebow AA: Pulmonary alveolar proteinosis. N Engl J Med 258:1123, 1958

Scadding JG, Hinson KFW: Diffuse fibrosing alveolitis (diffuse interstitial fibrosis of the lungs). Correlation of histology at biopsy with progenosis. Thorax 22:29, 1967

Smith JC; Radiation pneumonitis. A review. Am Rev Respir Dis 87:647, 1963

Soergel RH, Sommers SC: Idiopathic pulmonary hemosiderosis and related syndromes. Am J Med 32:499, 1962

Tomasi RB Jr, Fudenberg HH, Finley N: Possible relation of rheumatoid factors and pulmonary disease. Am J Med 33:243, 1962

Weese WC, Levine BW, Kazemi H: Interstitial lung disease resistant to corticosteroid therapy: Report of three cases treated with azathioprine or cyclophosphamide. Chest 67:57, 1975

OCCUPATIONAL RESPIRATORY DISEASE

John D. Stoeckle

Occupational respiratory diseases are but special instances of pulmonary inflammation, fibrosis, and neoplasia in which the etiologic agents are manmade, produced as a result of industrial or agricultural work.

Despite the inhalation and deposition of airborne contaminants from industrial and agricultural processes, these three pulmonary reactions do not always occur. The lung may simply be a storage site with little or no inflammation or fibrosis. Of the many occupational respiratory disease agents, three important categories are mineral dusts, toxic chemicals, and organic dusts.

MINERAL DUSTS: FIBROGENIC AND NONFIBROGENIC

Some inert nonfibrogenic mineral dusts are iron, tin, barium, calcium, and coal. Among the fibrogenic dusts are asbestos, silica, talc, and diatomaceous earths. Despite their retention in the lungs (pneumoconiosis) and the appearance of diffuse nodular opacities on chest x-rays, the nonfibrogenic dusts produce little or no pulmonary reaction, and only if the bulk of such retained dust is very great does functional abnormality result. Two disorders from these two categories of mineral dusts are described: coalworkers' pneumoconiosis and asbestosis. Coalworkers' pneumoconiosis (CWP) is an example of a nonfibrogenic dust disease, but in its complicated form, progressive massive fibrosis (PMF), it is also an exception to the lack of fibrogenic reaction to coal dust. Asbestosis is a pneumoconiosis due to a fibrogenic dust in which fibrosis with x-ray and functional abnormalities can occur at low dose exposure.

Coalworkers' Pneumoconiosis (CWP)

The definition of this disorder is based on a specific pathologic picture, deposition of coal dust in peribronchial tissues (the coal macule) and the distension of terminal bronchioles (focal emphysema), first described by Gough among Welsh coal trimmers. A carbon dust with small amounts of silica (1–4 percent), coal produces little or no fibrogenic reaction. However, if deposited in sufficient amounts in the peribronchial tissues of the terminal respiratory bronchioles the retained coal dust can produce distension of these structures (focal emphysema). The tissue deposits of dust can be recognized from nodular-reticular opacities seen on the chest x-ray.

Diagnosis is based on a history of exposure to coal dust and on diffuse nodular-reticular opacities on the chest x-ray. If lung biopsy or autopsy tissue is available, the typical pathologic picture is an additional but not necessary diagnostic confirmation. Usually 10 years of exposure is required for the x-ray nodulation to first appear (Category 1), but intense exposures may produce such changes even earlier. With continued or more intense dust exposure the size of nodular densities increases. Three categories of CWP can be distinguished from classification of the size of x-ray opacities, using the modified International Labor Organization scheme (U.I.C.C., Cincinnati). Thus, categories 1, 2, and 3, termed simple CWP, describe x-ray opacities of increasing size that represent increasing amounts of retained dust.

Complicated CWP: Progressive Massive Fibrosis

A fibrotic complication, progressive massive fibrosis (PMF), to the retained coal dust of the simple pneumoconiosis occurs in about 2–3 percent of cases. PMF is characterized by dense fibrotic masses, most often in the upper lobes. The development of PMF following Category 2 or 3 is thought to depend on more extensive coal dust deposition and on infection, in many instances tuberculosis. Others have related the PMF development to larger amounts of silica in the coal mine dust, to autoimmune factors, or to vascular obliteration.

Caplan's Syndrome

A clinical variant of CWP is Caplan's syndrome. In the CWP of coal miners who also have rheumatoid arthritis, large collagenous nodular fibrosis may develop in the lung, a reaction thought to be dependent on host factors and unrelated to increasing dust deposition alone. Clinical signs of rheumatoid arthritis and often high titers of rheumatoid factor are present.

Clinical findings. CWP is often asymptomatic. With more advanced Categories 2 and 3 of simple CWP, breathlessness may be the only symptom. Interpretation of lung function studies is often difficult because miners with CWP may also have pulmonary reactions to mine dusts other than coal, e.g., silica, or they may develop bronchitis as a result of their work exposures, smoking, atmospheric air pollution, and respiratory infections contracted outside the mine. Among asymptomatic miners with simple CWP, only an increase in residual volume may occur. Among symptomatic miners with simple CWP, reduced vital capacity and diffusing capacity occur, particularly if bronchitis is also present. When PMF develops, reduced lung volumes are found along with low diffusing capacities and abnormal gas exchange, reflecting uneven ventilation and perfusion distribution. In advanced, PMF, pulmonary hypertension and cor pulmonale are present.

Prevalence studies suggest that CWP, among the current 140,000 active and 200,000 retired miners, is dependent not only on the dustiness of the mine but on the rank of the coal. For example, anthracite miners have a higher prevalence of CWP than do bituminous miners. The "hard coal," anthracite, is of the highest rank, having the most carbon and the least volatile matter compared to the bituminous soft coal, and to lignite, a still softer coal. Such factors appear to explain these regional differences. Results of the 1969 ongoing National Coal Study indicate some 30 percent of active miners in Appalachia have either simple CWP or CWP complicated by PMF. Because retired miners with CWP are not included, this percentage cannot be an accurate view of the overall prevalence.

REFERENCES

Caplan A, Payne RB, Withey JL: A broader concept of Caplan's syndrome related to rheumatoid factors. Thorax 17:205, 1962

Gough J: Pneumoconiosis in coal trimmers. J Pathol Bacteriol 51:277, 1940

Key MM, Kerr LE, Bundy M (eds): Pulmonary Reactions to Coal Dust. New York, Academic Press, 1971

Morgan WKC: Coal worker's pneumoconiosis. Am Indus Hyg Assoc 32:39, 1971

Stoeckle JD, Hardy HL, King WB, Nemiah JC: Respiratory disease in U.S. soft coal miners: Clinical and etiologic considerations. J Chron Dis 15:887, 1962

Asbestosis

Asbestos is among the mineral dusts such as silica that are fibrogenic. This silicate fiber has well-known uses for heat- and fire-resistant insulation in homes and industry, but also has extensive uses in such diverse products as textiles, cement, rubber tires, vinyl plastics, graphite, and resins. Asbestos varies in its chemical and physical properties. In the U.S. the fiber chrysotile is the most widely used (93 percent), while crocidolite (3–4 percent) and amosite (2–3 percent) make up small percentages. Exposures may occur in mining asbestos, in the various manufacturing processes, in insulation work, and even by residing near asbestos mines.

Five clinical disorders have been produced by asbestos exposures: (1) pulmonary fibrosis (asbestosis), (2) pleural fibrosis and/or calcification, (3) bronchogenic carcinoma, (4) mesothelioma, and (5) pleural effusion. Pulmonary fibrosis is the most common. It is estimated that 3.5 million workers are exposed to asbestos, but the number of cases of disease that result is not known.

Clinical findings. Asbestosis: The pulmonary fibrosis of asbestosis is chiefly of the lower lobes, since asbestos fibers some 50 μ in length locate in lower-lobe bronchioles; they are too large to enter alveoli throughout the lung. The fibrosis is diffuse rather than focal, as in silicosis. The severity and latency in the development of the disease are related to dose and duration of exposure. Even at low-dose exposures for 10–20 years some 40 percent of exposed workers will develop asbestosis; further low-dose exposure up to 30 years will produce detectable disease in 70 percent. The major symptom is dyspnea. The x-ray shows linear densities with reduction in the volume of the lower lobes. Lung function studies show a restrictive pattern and reduced diffusing capacity. The latter, attributable to ventilation/perfusion inequality, may even occur before radiologic changes can be detected.

The clinical diagnosis is based on a history of exposure, the x-ray picture, and a restrictive pattern of reduced lung function. Lung biopsy or postmortem examination is not necessary for diagnosis; the interstitial fibrosis with asbestos bodies in the tissues is an additional confirmation. Looking for asbestos bodies in the sputum may be neither useful nor productive. Often the patient comes for medical evaluation years after active exposure, with little likelihood of daily excretion of inhaled fibers. Also, such "bodies" are not asbestos fibers per se, but ferruginous bodies, protein-iron complexes that may be encasing asbestos fibers but also may encase other inhaled and retained fibers such as cotton. In widely separate cities, such ferruginous bodies have been found in 20–40 percent of postmortem lungs. When the core is asbestos fiber, it may reflect atmospheric exposure and the potential for health hazards in the community.

Pleural plaques and calcifications: A second clinical effect of asbestosis is the development of pleural plaques and calcification. These may occur separately or together in scattered locations over the lung, but especially in the diaphragmic pleura. Pulmonary asbestosis may or may not be present. Plaques occur in high frequency in the population around asbestos mines in Finland where still another fiber type, anthophyllite, is found. Asbestos fibers are difficult to identify in plaques and have been reported in but 25–50 percent of cases.

Carcinoma of the lung: As a cause of death lung cancer occurs among asbestos workers with reported frequences up to 26 percent. It is not certain that asbestos alone is an etiologic agent or that the carcinogenic potential resides in the oils associated with asbestos fibers or in the iron the fiber contains. Very likely asbestos acts as a co-carcinogen along with smoking and pulmonary inflammation. The risk for lung cancer in asbestos workers is 7 times that in the general population; the risk among workers who smoke is 90 times.

Mesothelioma: This connective-tissue tumor may occur in the pleura or peritoneum. Two-thirds of reported cases have had exposure to asbestos, an exposure that antedates the development of the tumor by some 30–35 years. Dose does not appear to be related to tumor development. Sometimes the tumor may coexist with pulmonary asbestosis. It may present as recurrent effusion or as a gradually enlarging pleural plaque. The symptoms are chest pain and breathlessness, the latter from reduced lung volumes due to effusion or to the encasement of the lung by the extensive pleural growth. Hyaluronic acid may be elevated in the pleural or peritoneal fluid. Because the pleural biopsy often appears not unlike ordinary connective tissue, the diagnosis will often depend not on the biopsy per se but on the progressive clinical course of the pleural disorder. While local invasion of ribs is frequent, less frequent are hematogenous metastases to other bony sites and liver.

Pleural effusion: Among some asbestos workers a benign pleural effusion may occur without recurrence or the development of mesothelioma. However, before this diagnostic label is used the patient should be observed long enough to be sure that other causes of effusion and mesothelioma are not present.

Treatment. There is no treatment of the disorders due to asbestos, although the disease can be prevented through limitation in atmospheric concentrations, limited duration of industrial employment, personal protective devices, and substitute materials.

REFERENCES

Gaensler EA, Addington WW: Asbestos or ferruginous bodies. N Engl J Med 280:488, 1969

Gaensler E, Kaplan AI: Asbestos pleural effusion. Ann Intern Med 74:178, 1971

Selikoff IJ, Hammond EC, Churg J: Asbestos exposure, smoking and neoplasms. JAMA 204:104, 1968

Whipple HE: Biological effects of asbestos. Ann NY Acad Med 132:765, 1965

TOXIC CHEMICALS

A wide variety of chemicals are bronchopulmonary irritants or injurious sensitizing agents. These include metals (beryllium, cadmium oxide, manganese dioxide, cobalt), gases and fumes such as phosgene, oxides of nitrogen, toluene diisocyanate, and acid and brass fumes. Three examples, beryllium disease, silo-filler's disease, and toluene diisocyanate toxicity are described.

Beryllium Disease

Beryllium is a light heat-resistant metal with widespread uses in nuclear reactors, space vehicles and fuels, metal alloys for aircraft, electronic equipment, ceramics, and formerly in fluorescent lamps and neon signs. Toxic forms are the metal, its salts, and beryllium oxide. The ore, beryl, from which beryllium is extracted is itself nontoxic. Toxic exposures occur both in the extraction of the ore and in the many industrial uses of the metal and its compounds; reactions are both acute and chronic. The acute disease is generally a self-limited reaction if exposure ceases; the chronic disease may last many years, with a mortality of 30 percent; 860 cases of beryllium disease were recorded in 1975 in the Beryllium Case Registry; 649 of these are chronic, 211 are acute.

Acute Beryllium Disease

The acute disease, related to high atmospheric concentrations of beryllium, may present as dermatitis of the contact type, as conjunctivitis, as upper respiratory tract irritation, or in severe cases as acute pneumonitis. This acute chemical pneumonitis may result in death (13 percent), resolution (82 percent), or progress to chronic disease (15 percent). Death is due to respiratory-circulatory failure from extensive beryllium-induced pulmonary edema and pneumonitis.

Chronic Beryllium Disease

Although chronic beryllium disease presents as an interstitial noncaseating granulomatous inflammation of the lung, other organs such as lymph nodes, skin, liver, spleen, and kidneys may be similarly involved, since inhaled beryllium is widely distributed. This chronic pneumonitis and systemic disease occurs with low concentrations of beryllium; it often develops many years after exposure has ceased (0–23 years) and may remain active with exacerbations and remissions or eventually heal by fibrosis.

Clinical findings. Clinical findings in chronic beryllium disease commonly include dyspnea, cough, fatigue, and weight loss; a few patients are asymptomatic but have x-ray and lung function changes. The physical examination is commonly normal; however, in advanced cases fingers may be clubbed and scattered dry rales heard throughout the chest. Papular skin lesions may be seen in a few (5 percent). Chest x-ray shows diffuse nodular opacities. With extensive fibrosis the nodular opacities may disappear, so that only contracted upperlobe and compensatory emphysema of lower lobes remain. Hilar nodes are often enlarged (45 percent), but very rarely alone as in sarcoidosis, and nearly always in association with pulmonary densities. Calcification of lymph nodes and pulmonary nodules (13 percent) develops late. Hepatic or splenic enlargement is infrequent (5 percent). Laboratory findings are variable. With active disease, the sedimentation rate and serum globulins may be elevated; with hepatomegaly, the BSP may be elevated also. Hypercalcemia (4 percent), hypercalciuria (20 percent), and hyperuricemia (8 percent) occur. Urine beryllium assays are not helpful in diagnosis, since even if positive they indicate only exposure to beryllium, not disease. Even with exposure, assays may be negative by the time the patient comes for medical study many years later. Despite nonspecificity of Kveim tests, so far such tests have been negative in beryllium disease patients. Skin tests with beryllium salts may be positive, but are not recommended as a routine because these salts are potent sensitizing agents and may exacerbate the disease. Lung function tests show three patterns: most commonly a restrictive pattern, sometimes only a reduced diffusing capacity, and in some late cases also an obstructive pattern. Lung biopsy and postmortem specimens show two patterns of reaction: one a widely decimated cellular reaction with few granulomas, a second with well-formed granulomas and cellular inflammation that is focal and mild. The major complications of the chronic disease are (1) renal stones, in part due to the hypercalcemia and/or hypercalciuria found in the disorder, (2) pneumothorax, due to ruptured cysts produced by extensive lung necrosis, and fibrosis, and (3) cor pulmonale from extensive pulmonary fibrosis.

As with other occupational diseases the diagnosis is based on both epidemiologic and clinical criteria. The epidemiologic criterion is a significant exposure to beryllium or its toxic compounds, and one that has produced disease in others. The clinical criteria are diffuse densities on x-ray with or without symptoms, typical patterns of respiratory insufficiency determined on lung function tests, interstitial granulomatous pneumonitis on lung biopsy or postmortem specimens, beryllium found in such tissues, and evidence of disease in other organ systems besides the lung.

Treatment. Prevention is critical and must be through control of beryllium in the environment. Steroids are helpful in modifying symptoms and signs, but their effect on mortality is uncertain.

REFERENCES

Andrews JL, Kazemi H, Hardy HL: Patterns of lung dysfunction in chronic beryllium disease. Am Rev Respir Dis 100:791, 1969

Freiman D, Hardy HL: Beryllium disease. The relation of pulmonary pathology to clinical course and prognosis based on a study of 130 cases from the U.S. Beryllium Case Registry. Hum Pathol 1:25, 1970

Stoeckle JD, Hardy HL, Weber AL: Chronic beryllium disease, report of 60 cases and selective review of the literature. Am J Med 46:545, 1969

Weber AL, Stoeckle JD, Hardy HL: Roentgenologic patterns in longstanding beryllium disease. Am J Roentgenol 93:879, 1965

Nitrogen Dioxide Toxicity (Silo-Filler's Disease)

This is a bronchiolitis-pneumonitis and, in severe cases, a pulmonary edema produced by the inhalation of nitrogen dioxide. Nitrogen dioxide is a reddish-brown gas with a pungent odor. Dissolving in water in the lower respiratory tract it releases nitric and nitrous acids, both very corrosive to mucus membranes. Oxides of nitrogen (NO, NO_2) are important factors in the air pollution constantly being generated by cars, power plants, and industrial boilers. Thus exposures may be atmospheric, in-dustrial, and in the case of silo-filler's disease agricultural. In silo-filler's disease the NO_2 exposure results from the fermentation of fresh silage. Plant nitrates are fermented into nitrites and oxygen. As nitrites combine with organic acid in plants, nitrous acid is formed; with increasing temperatures of the stored silage, nitrogen dioxide is released.

Clinical findings. Shortness of breath, cough, fever, wheezing and sputa may all occur following exposure and persist for days to weeks. Diffuse rales may be heard throughout. Chest films show patchy infiltrates that may clear slowly along with symptoms and signs. In some patients residual x-ray changes, nodulation, and linear markings may persist. Lung biopsy and postmortem specimens have shown an obliterative bronchiolitis and interstitial cellular infiltration. There are a few studies of lung function in acute exposures. Despite symptomatic recovery, reduced diffusing capacity may persist for weeks to months. Death from pulmonary edema may occur with severe exposures.

Treatment. Supportive care to manage the respiratory insufficiency is critical, and steroids may be beneficial.

Toluene Diisocyanate Toxicity

Toluene diisocyanate (TDI), a highly volatile liquid polymerizing agent, reacts with resins to produce polyurethanes. Urethanes are widely used in lacquers, adhesives, wire coatings, cushions, and shielding. TDI exposure occurs in the manufacturing process of polyurethane; it may produce three clinical effects: (1) conjunctivitis and upper respiratory irritation, (2) bronchospasm, or (3) bronchiolitis-pneumonitis.

Clinical findings. Symptoms are itchy eyes, nasal congestion, and sore throat. Respiratory distress may present as "asthma," dry cough, wheezing, sometimes with chest pain or tightness. The physical examination may be normal, but often rhonchi or rales are heard. If intense, exposures produce a severe chemical bronchiolitis-pneumonitis; the usual normal chest x-ray may then show scattered infiltrates. The four patterns of impaired respiratory function are dependent on duration, severity of exposure, and the type of host response: (1) among asymptomatic exposed workers, a gradual 8-hr decrease in FEV_1 at work will be noted; tests are normal by the following morning; (2) those with severe bronchiolitis will have reduced vital capacity, FEV_1, and hypoxemia; (3) continued low-dose exposure may result in a chronically depressed FEV_1; (4) some with recurrent asthmalike patterns will have abnormal tests only during these acute episodes. This latter pattern occurs especially in those with histories or findings suggesting an allergic background.

Diagnosis of TDI toxicity is based on a combination of facts: exposure, clinical symptoms and signs, and functional abnormalities.

Treatment. Steroids may be helpful along with other measures to relieve bronchospasm, but prevention through control of concentration in air should be the major effort. It is estimated that 40,000–100,000 workers are exposed to the isocyanates.

REFERENCES

Brugsch HG, Elkins HB: Toluene di-isocyanate (TDI) toxicity. N Engl J Med 268:353, 1963

Peters JM, Murphy RLH, Pagnotto LD, Whittenberger JL: Respiratory impairment in workers exposed to "safe" levels of toluene di-isocyanate (TDI). Arch Environ Health 20:364, 1970

ORGANIC DUSTS

Dusts such as sugar cane, moldy hay, *Bacillus subtilis* enzyme detergents, pituitary snuff, maple bark, mushrooms, malt, sequoia bark, pigeon litter, coffee beans, and cheese washings are but some known examples of organic occupational dusts that may produce an allergic lung disease. These dusts are discussed in general because of the similarities of the signs, symptoms, and pulmonary reactions and because the mechanisms by which they produce disease are very likely similar. Byssinosis from cotton dust has a different mechanism of injury.

These allergic pulmonary reactions appear to be mediated by precipitation of antigen–antibody complexes that produce cellular and vascular injury. The antigens may be molds associated with plants, animal matter, bacteria, and organic material. Two examples of such pulmonary reactions are bagassosis from sugar cane and farmer's lung from moldy hay. Table 1 lists some other exposures and organic dusts producing hypersensitivity pneumonitis.

In general, one or more of four types of clinical disorders may occur: (1) allergic rhinitis, (2) asthma or recurrent bronchitis, (3) acute or (4) chronic interstitial pneumonitis. Pulmonary hypersensitivity reactions to organic dusts may be the most appropriate term for these disorders.

Clinical findings. These will depend on the site of reaction within the respiratory tract. With allergic rhinitis there may be conjunctivitis as well as nasal stuffiness and discharge. This is often overlooked, as the pulmonary symptoms and signs are more dramatic. With acute asthma or bronchitis, symptoms and signs will be chest tightness and wheezing. Even in the absence of symptoms, lung function tests may show a diminished FEV_1. With interstitial pneumonitis, acute or chronic, there may be fever, chills, dyspnea, and rales, depending on the degree of involvement. Lung volumes are restricted and impairment of gas exchange is found. Chest x-ray may show nodular and linear infiltrates. Diagnosis is based on exposure history, onset of symptoms and exacerbation with exposure, and typical clinical picture, including lung function tests. In addition, serum precipitins to offending antigens and recurrence of symptoms and signs on provocative exposure to the dust or antigen may be used as confirmatory measures. Of the many organic dusts, farmer's lung, a hypersensitivity pneumonitis, and byssinosis, an airway constriction from cotton dust, are described in more detail.

Farmer's Lung

This disorder is an acute bronchitis-pneumonitis and/or chronic pneumonitis due to exposure to the dust of moldy hay or grain, whether oats, barley, or wheat. Mold forms on such crops when lying wet in fields after cutting; when these are handled, spore-bearing dust is inhaled. Thermophilic *Actinomycetes* in the moldy hay have been incriminated as the sensitizing agents.

Clinical findings. In the acute disease, cough, chest tightness, dyspnea, and sometimes chills and fever develop 2–6 hr after working with moldy hay. Basal rales may be noted. Chest films may be clear or show transient infiltrates. Lung function studies show an obstructive pattern with diminished FEV_1. Eosinophilia may be present. Recurrent exposure may lead to the chronic disease, a granulomatous pneumonitis that may be difficult to distinguish from the pathologic findings in sarcoidosis and beryllium disease. Shortness of breath and cough are major symptoms. Chest films show diffuse linear and nodular opacities. Lung function studies are variable, revealing airway obstruction and a restrictive pattern with impaired diffusion and reduced vital capacity. Immunoglobulins IgG, IgA, and IgM are often elevated in the serum of sensitive patients. IgE is normal unless the patient also has allergic rhinitis or asthma. Diagnosis is based on exposure and clinical findings. Precipitins to these molds can be found in the serum; bronchoconstriction can occur with provocative inhalation tests as a diagnostic measure.

Treatment. Symptoms may be relieved by removal from exposure and by the use of steroids and bronchodilators.

Byssinosis

Byssinosis is an airway constriction producing chest tightness, cough, wheezing, and sometimes dyspnea as a result of exposure to textile dusts of cotton, flax, or hemp. These asthmalike symptoms occur primarily among card-room workers. The mechanism of the disease is incompletely understood. These textile dusts release histamine in vitro and may act similarly in vivo, producing the bronchoconstriction.

Clinical features. In the acute form the symptoms occur on coming to work on Mondays and are reversible. Physical examination may reveal rhonchi. Lung function studies show an obstructive pattern with reduced FEV_1. Some workers develop chronic obstructive lung disease in which repeated exposures to the dust may be responsible.

Treatment. Removal from exposure is the only realistic treatment.

NONOCCUPATIONAL EXPOSURES

Exposures to occupational disease agents are not invariably at work. In the case of asbestos, beryllium, cadmium and possibly toluene diisocyanate, *Bacillus subtilis* enzymes, and sensitizing molds, neighborhood and household exposures may occur. From neighborhood contamination near plants and mines or from household contacts with working husbands, cases of beryllium disease and asbestos-related disorders, plaques and mesothelioma, have developed. Home use of products such as *Bacillus subtilis* enzyme detergents may be a potential household exposure, as are kits for the home-making of polyurethanes with toluene diisocyante. Likewise, typical farmer's lung has been noted from molds contaminating home air conditioners, and pigeon-

Table 1
Pulmonary Hypersensitivity Disorders

Antigen	Exposure	Dust	Disorder
Thermoactinomyces vulgaris *Thermoactinomyces saccharii* *Micropolyspora faeni*	Moldy vegetable compost	Sugar cane	Bagassosis
Thermoactinomyces vulgaris *Thermoactmomyces saccharii* *Micropolyspora faeni*	Dairy farming	Moldy hay	Farmer's lung
Cryptostroma corticale	Saw mills	Wood dust	Maple bark pneumonitis
proteins	Pigeon breeding, parakeets, etc.	Bird droppings, serum proteins	Bird-breeder's lung
Bacillus subtilis enzymes	Detergent manufacture	Detergent dust	Enzyme-detergent pneumonitis
Aspergillus clavatus	Handling barley	Barley dust	Malt-worker's lung

breeder's lung occurs in those whose hobby is bird-raising. Thus the research for etiologic explanations of respiratory disease must look to neighborhood and home environment as well as to the patient's place of work.

REFERENCES

Barbee, RA, Callies O, Dickie HA: The long-term prognosis in farmer's lung. Am Rev Respir Dis 97:223, 1968

Bouyhuys A, Heapty LJ, Schilling RSF, Welborn LW: Byssinosis in U.S. N Engl J Med 227:170, 1967

Dickie HA, Rankin J: Farmer's lung. JAMA 167:1069, 1957

Hapke EJ, Seal RME, Thomas GO: Farmer's lung. Thorax 23:451, 1968

Patterson R, Fink JN, Pruzansky JJ, Reed C, Roberts M, Slavin R, Zeiss CR: Immunoglobulin levels in pulmonary allergic aspergillosis and certain other lung diseases with special reference to immunoglobulin E. Am J Med 54:16, 1973

Pepys J: Hypersensitivity Diseases of the Lung Due to Fungi and Organic Dusts. Basel, Karger, 1969

SARCOIDOSIS

Russell C. Klein

Sarcoidosis is a disease of unknown etiology characterized by the presence of noncaseating granulomas in many organs of the body. It was first described by Jonathan Huchinson in 1869. Boeck supplied the name sarcoid because he believed this was a benign sarcoma. Most early workers felt that sarcoidosis was a skin condition until Schaumann noted its multisystem involvement in 1914. The lungs are involved at some time in over 90 percent of recognized cases. This disease is worldwide in distribution but is more often recognized in those countries where mass x-ray screening is commonplace, such as Scandinavia and the United Kingdom.

The true prevalence of sarcoidosis in the U.S. is unknown, since many patients are asymptomatic and are discovered accidentally. Statistics from Denmark indicate that asymptomatic accidentally discovered disease is four times as common as symptomatic disease. Estimates for asymptomatic disease in this country are lower.

The disease appears to be 10 to 20 times as common in the American black as in the white, but is rare among American Indians, Eskimos, and Chinese living in Hawaii. It is most often recognized during ages 20 to 40 but has been diagnosed from the first to eighth decades of life. Females are affected slightly more often than males.

ETIOLOGY AND PATHOLOGY

Many diseases (e.g., histoplasmosis and berylliosis) show noncaseating granulomas in tissue sections that may be indistinguishable from those of sarcoidosis, but most workers believe sarcoidosis to be a specific entity rather than a nonspecific reaction to multiple inciting agents. This belief is based largely on the observation that a similar clinical course is noted among many diverse races and over widely scattered geographic areas.

Tubercle bacilli, atypical mycobacteria, viruses, and other organisms have been suggested as possible causes. Many nonliving substances, most notably pine pollen, have also been suggested as inciting agents, but there is no unequivocal evidence to accept any as the etiologic agent. Because sarcoidosis often manifests abnormalities of serum proteins, changes in delayed hypersensitivity, and biologic false positive tests for syphilis (to name a few), it is considered to be an immunologically based problem by many workers.

The typical histologic lesion in sarcoidosis is the noncaseating granuloma, which does not differ significantly in appearance no matter what organ is involved. The granuloma of sarcoidosis may remain "active" for indefinite periods, or healing may take place either by resolution or by hyalinization with ultimate replacement by fibrosis.

CLINICAL PICTURE
Pulmonary Manifestations

Pulmonary involvement (Fig. 1), at least if judged by roentgen abnormalities, is present at some time in well over 90 percent of patients with sarcoidosis. The earliest stage is characterized by the presence of hilar and possibly paratracheal adenopathy. When erythema nodosum and fever accompany hilar and paratracheal adenopathy, the condition is called Lofgren's syndrome. Arthritic symptoms may also be present in this syndrome, which seems to carry an especially good prognosis.

Stage two consists of hilar adenopathy associated with pulmonary infiltrate that may take the form of fine or coarse miliary densities or larger fluffy opacities that may appear to coalesce. The amount of parenchymal in-

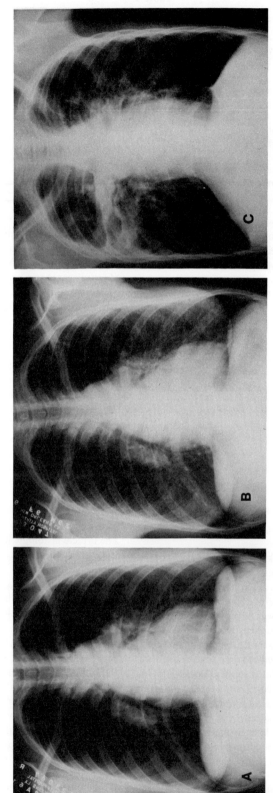

Fig. 1. *A.* Stage I bilateral hilar and right paratracheal adenopathy. *B.* Stage II hilar adenopathy and fluffy bilateral parenchymal densities. *C.* State III advanced fibrosis with hilar distortion and bullae formation. Several of the bullae contain fluid.

volvement is variable. In stage three adenopathy disappears altogether but infiltrates remain or worsen. With advanced pulmonary involvement, fibrosis may lead to considerable distortion of the hilar areas. Similarly, fibrosis and distortion may cause partial obstruction of airways, and formation of bullae may follow. Parenchymal calcifications can be noted occasionally, and cor pulmonale may develop at this stage secondary to restriction of the lungs and obliteration of the vascular bed. Pleural effusions are uncommon at any time in the course of sarcoidosis. If one develops another cause should be sought.

Principal pulmonary symptoms are shortness of breath, especially with exertion, and nonproductive cough. Hemoptysis may occur, but since large endobronchial lesions are rare, this is likely due to coughing. Substernal chest pain may occur especially in those with considerable hilar node enlargement. There may be no pulmonary or constitutional symptoms despite considerable x-ray abnormality.

Pulmonary function studies may be normal, but reduction in vital capacity and lowered diffusing capacity are common. Mild hypoxemia is frequent and may worsen as the disease progresses. Carbon dioxide retention is a late and ominous development. Evidence of airway obstruction is not a common manifestation, but it may be present.

Physical findings are often absent. Signs of restriction may include increase in respiratory rate, decrease in chest expansion, and use of accessory muscles of respiration. Evidence of right-sided cardiac enlargement and increased intensity of the pulmonary second sound can be present. Dry, end-inspiratory rales may be heard, but wet rales and wheezes are uncommon.

Other Manifestations of Sarcoidosis

Constitutional symptoms. In all patients with sarcoidosis constitutional symptoms may be present, but they often vary in severity. The most common are fatigue, weakness, weight loss, and fever. The latter two complaints may be found in up to 25 percent of patients.

Lymph nodes, spleen, and liver. In Mayock's large combined series clinically enlarged lymph nodes were present in three-quarters of sarcoid patients. In all but a few instances the enlargement did not give rise to symptoms and was considered unimportant. Both the liver and spleen may be enlarged in sarcoidosis, but massive enlargement of either organ is rare. Microscopic involvement of these organs is extremely common. The most frequent manifestation of abnormal liver function is elevation of the alkaline phosphatase. Thrombocytopenia is a rare but potentially devastating manifestation of sarcoidosis. It is not always related to hypersplenism, since it may not remit either with steroids or after splenectomy.

Skin. Again in Mayock's series skin manifestations were observed in approximately one-third of patients. Maculopapular lesions were the most common. Many of the lesions have a violaceous cast and slightly depressed centers. The face, extremities, and shoulders are common sites.

Eyes. Ocular involvement may occur in as many as 25 percent of patients, with the cornea, sclera, conjunctiva, or uveal tract being involved. While eye involvement is not always serious, careful search must be made, as it can lead to blindness. When uveitis is accompanied by salivary gland swelling and fever, Heerfordt's syndrome is said to be present. Cranial nerve palsies may also be part of this syndrome.

Nervous system. In 10 series neurologic involvement occurred in from 1 percent to 16 percent of patients. Cranial nerve palsies (especially N VII) was the most common manifestation and when present was secondary to basilar meningeal involvement. Peripheral nerve involvement with muscle weakness may occur, as may signs of cerebritis (headache, vomiting, visual disturbances), but these problems are often transient and may require no treatment. A far more serious state exists when sarcoidosis involves the hypothalamic-pituitary area with development of one or more hormonal deficiency states. Diabetes insipidus has been most frequently noted, followed by deficiency of gonadotropin, thyroid-stimulating hormone, and ACTH.

Other organs. Hypercalcemia, thought to be related to increased sensitivity to vitamin D, is rare but may give rise to symptoms or lead to nephrocalcinosis. Direct involvement of the kidney by sarcoid granuloma rarely gives rise to serious disease. Bone involvement characterized especially by punched-out lesions in the phalanges is variably present. X-rays of bones are occasionally useful in substantiating the diagnosis but rarely have other clinical significance. Transient arthritic and periarthritic symptoms are sometimes seen in sarcoid patients, especially those manifesting erythema nodosum. Myositis is very rare.

Sarcoidosis may involve either the myocardium or the conducting system of the heart, giving rise to congestive failure or rhythm abnormalities; but cardiac failure, if present, is more likely to be right-sided and secondary to pulmonary parenchymal disease. Sarcoid involvement of the gastrointestinal tract, pancreas, adrenal, parathyroid, or ovary is virtually nonexistent.

LABORATORY STUDIES

Mild anemia and mild leukopenia may be present but are rarely significant. Eosinophilia of 5 percent or more has been noted in approximately 25 percent of patients. Serum protein abnormalities, most often hyperglobulinemia, will be found in over half of patients. Biologic false positive tests for syphilis may be present. Loss of cutaneous hypersensitivity to tuberculin has long been noted to occur in most sarcoid patients who were tuberculin positive before sarcoidosis developed. This loss is not limited to tuberculin, however, since delayed hypersensitivity reactions to many antigens (e.g., mumps) may be abolished during "active" disease. Immediate hypersensitivity of the wheal and flare type is not affected, and responses of circulating antibodies are normal. Hypercalcemia is a rare but important finding. Hypercalciuria is more common. Elevations of alkaline phosphatase can occur in the absence of other evidence of hepatic abnormality.

If an extract of lymph node or spleen involved by sarcoid is injected into a patient with sarcoidosis, a typical noncaseating granuloma will often develop several weeks later at the injection site. This test, the Kveim reaction, has been known for years and has become so accepted by some physicians that the diagnosis of sarcoid is often made when a compatible clinical picture and a positive Kveim test are found without other organ tissue biopsy. The antigen is not generally available, and its use should probably be limited to experienced workers using carefully made standardized preparations.

DIAGNOSIS AND DIFFERENTIAL DIAGNOSIS

The diagnosis of sarcoidosis can be made with some certainty if a satisfactory tissue biopsy is available in a patient with a compatible clinical picture. Ideally tissue material should be cultured for acid-fast bacilli and fungi, as these diseases may give similar x-ray or histopathologic appearances. The choice of biopsy site is important. Skin lesions or accessible enlarged lymph nodes should be the first choice. Transbronchial lung biopsy through the fiberoptic bronchoscope is a safe method of confirming the diagnosis in the vast majority of patients. Medistinal lymph node biopsy also gives a very high yield but is more dangerous. Liver biopsy is often positive, but interpretation is hazardous since many conditions can give rise to hepatic granulomas. Biopsy of the scalene lymph nodes is positive in three-quarters of the cases where the patient has sarcoid but transbronchial biopsy has reduced its usefulness. Biopsy of the lung parenchyma must be considered where a diagnosis is imperative and more simple methods have failed. Appropriate x-rays of the extremities may give confirmatory evidence of boney involvement. Skin tests with mumps antigen, or some similar substance, will help determine if the patient's delayed hypersensitivity mechanism is intact.

The differential diagnosis depends largely upon whether one is presented with an abnormal chest x-ray or a histopathologic diagnosis of noncaseating granuloma. Hodgkin's disease or other malignancy may be suggested by the presence of hilar adenopathy or adenopathy with parenchymal involvement. When only parenchymal involvement is noted, tuberculosis and fibrotic lung problems, especially those of industrial origin, should be considered.

When noncaseating granulomas are found on tissue examination, tuberculosis, histoplasmosis, coccidioidomycosis, beryllium disease, or foreign-body reaction should be considered. It should be noted that lymph nodes draining visceral malignancies and chalazions sometimes contain sarcoidlike granulomas.

One should consider the possibility of sarcoid in patients with fever of unknown origin or unusual neurologic findings or endocrine deficiency states with no obvious explanation.

CLINICAL COURSE AND PROGNOSIS

From clinical observation sarcoid has been divided into subacute and chronic stages. When manifestations of disease are present for 2 years or less subacute disease is said to be present, and chronic disease when manifesta-

tions are present for longer than 2 years. In general the subacute stage is characterized by involvement of lymph nodes, lungs, eyes, and salivary glands. Clinical involvement of bone, liver, and kidney usually indicates chronic disease. Spontaneous remission or worsening may be noted at any stage, or the patient may remain relatively static if untreated. Sarcoid may involve few or many organs, but it should be considered as chronic when it has been present for 2 years no matter what organs are involved. In most patients the disease seems to "burn out" after a variable period, although there may be considerable residual organ dysfunction.

Some idea of prognosis can be gained from the chest x-ray appearance at time of initial diagnosis. If only adenopathy is present, complete resolution can be expected in approximately half. The majority of the remainder will either remain stable or improve somewhat. In only about 10 percent will the lesions progress. Exacerbation after complete remission is rare, but complete remission may require several years. When hilar adenopathy and parenchymal involvement are both present, spontaneous complete remission is rare, but substantial improvement may be expected in one-third. A variable number will worsen, but the majority will remain relatively stable. When there is considerable parenchymal involvement without adenopathy, complete resolution is quite rare. Spontaneous improvement can sometimes be seen, but the majority of sarcoid-associated deaths occur among these patients. Fortunately they are not common. Clinical involvement of several organ systems indicates a poorer prognosis, as does nephrocalcinosis.

MANAGEMENT

Patients with sarcoidosis are treated to improve or preserve organ function or to help relieve disabling systemic manifestations of disease. It is unrealistic to hope that advanced fibrosis will remit, and only "active" disease can be expected to improve.

Many drugs have been used to treat sarcoidosis. Antimalarials were once popular but have been generally abandoned because of eye toxicity. Steroids are the only compounds commonly used today. Their mode of action is unknown, but they may aid in lysing the granulomas and/or in altering any immunologic aspects of the disease. Since these are potentially dangerous drugs, one must always consider whether the risks of treatment are worth the potential benefit.

In patients with only hilar adenopathy, treatment is normally withheld. In Stage II disease (adenopathy and parenchymal infiltrates) treatment can be withheld if the degree of symptoms or physiologic (not roentgenologic) abnormality is small. If Stage II disease is progressing significantly, treatment should be considered strongly. Stage III disease seldom responds, but treatment should be considered if there is significant dysfunction.

Major neurologic involvement demands treatment, especially if it has given rise to an endocrine deficiency state. These do not always respond, and specific hormone supplementation may be necessary. Disfiguring skin lesions may need treatment for cosmetic purposes. Serious eye involvement, persistent hypercalcemia, hypercalcuria, and nephrocalcinosis demand treatment, as may cardiac involvement. Cor pulmonale will not normally improve on steroids.

It should be noted that while most authorities accept the efficacy of steroids in such situations as ocular or neurologic involvement, many believe that steroids have no significant or lasting effect on pulmonary sarcoidosis. Thus while one should always have objective means of measuring improvement in cases of sarcoid, it is especially important in those treated for lung involvement. X-rays are not sufficient; ventilatory studies and blood gases are much more useful. In treating patients with sarcoidosis, prednisone 30–40 mg given once daily in the morning is recommended. Remissions, if they are to occur, begin promptly, usually within 2 weeks. Remission beginning after 8 weeks on steroids is extremely rare. At 6–8 weeks the dose is tapered slowly to 15 mg or less daily if treatment appears successful and is discontinued if significant objective improvement has not taken place. Total treatment should be continued for up to 1 year. Should relapse occur, treatment may be reinstituted, although it may not be as successful as it was initially.

Sarcoid-associated deaths are usually due to cor pulmonale, ventilatory failure, or complicating infection. Tuberculosis may be a problem, especially in those receiving steroid therapy. INH prophylaxis should be considered in such cases. Pregnancy does not usually exacerbate sarcoidosis, and decisions about pregnancy should be based on the patient's general health.

REFERENCES

1. Becker K, Katz S, Winnacker J: Endocrine aspects of sarcoidosis. N Engl J Med 278:427, 1968
2. Lofgren S (ed): Third International Conference on Sarcoidosis. Stockholm, Scandinavian University Books, 1964
3. Longcope W, Freiman D: A study of sarcoidosis. Baltimore, Williams & Wilkins, 1964
4. Mayock RL, Bertrand P, Morrison CE, Scott JH: Manifestations of sarcoidosis. Am J Med 35:67, 1963
5. Mitchell D, Scadding J: Sarcoidosis. Am Rev Respir Dis 110:774, 1974
6. Second International Conference on Sarcoidosis. Am Rev Respir Dis 84 (Suppl), 1961 (Part 2)
7. Siltzbach L: Current thoughts on the epidemiology and etiology of sarcoidosis. Am J Med 39:361, 1965
8. Siltzbach L: Sarcoidosis: Clinical features and management. Med Clin North Am 51:483, 1967

RESPIRATORY FAILURE

Neil S. Shore

Respiratory failure should be defined at the tissue or cellular level, i.e., inadequate gas exchange for the metabolic demands of that tissue or cell. Tissue or cellular respiratory failure could result from alterations in the air breathed (e.g., reduced inspired oxygen tension, as at altitude, or low oxygen concentration at sea level), impaired gas exchange in the lung, inadequate circulation, or failure of the gas transport system. Since we cannot readily measure gas exchange for tissue or cells,

the usual definitions of respiratory failure concern themselves with the failure of the lungs to add oxygen and remove carbon dioxide from the blood brought to them. Thus one can set values for the P_{O_2} and P_{CO_2} in arterial blood that define respiratory failure. Since $P_{a_{O_2}}$ falls normally with age, the significance of a given $P_{a_{O_2}}$ will vary with age. However, by defining respiratory failure by an arterial oxygen tension ($P_{a_{O_2}}$) or carbon dioxide tension ($P_{a_{CO_2}}$) well outside the normal range, one has a practical working definition that can be used until tissue or cellular gas exchange can be measured easily. In this context, a $P_{a_{O_2}}$ below 60 mm Hg or $P_{a_{CO_2}}$ above 49 mm Hg for a patient at rest and at sea level signifies respiratory failure.

CAUSES OF RESPIRATORY FAILURE

By definition, any phenomenon that will lower $P_{a_{O_2}}$ or raise $P_{a_{CO_2}}$ can lead to respiratory failure. Arterial carbon dioxide tension ($P_{a_{CO_2}}$) is inversely related to alveolar ventilation $\dot{V}_A$ and directly to CO_2 output ($\dot{V}_{CO_2}$). This relationship is defined by the equation

$$P_{a_{CO_2}} = K \frac{\dot{V}_{CO_2}}{\dot{V}_A}$$

Since in this equation CO_2 output ($\dot{V}_{CO_2}$) is relatively constant and does not vary from minute to minute, reduction in alveolar ventilation $\dot{V}_A$ will raise $P_{a_{CO_2}}$. In fact, reduced alveolar ventilation is a most important cause of respiratory failure. Such reduction in ventilation may result from weakness of the skeletal muscles of the chest wall, diaphragm, abdomen, or neck, resulting in a thoracic bellows unable to move adequate air. Table 1 lists some common causes of this type of extrapulmonary respiratory failure.

Ventilation can also be reduced as a result of al-

Table 1
Conditions Leading to Ventilatory Respiratory Failure

Neuromuscular defects
  Polio, Guillain-Barré syndrome, multiple sclerosis, brain and spinal cord injuries, myasthenia gravis, drugs or toxic agents (e.g., curare, polymycin, karamycin, streptomycin, neomycin)
Restrictive defects
  Limited thorax expansion
    Scoliosis, spinal arthritis
  Decreased lung expansion
    Pleural effusion, fibrothorax, interstitial fibrosis
  Decreased diaphragmatic movement
    Peritonitis, ascites, obesity, high abdominal surgery
Airway obstruction
  Asthma, bronchitis, emphysema
Respiratory center depression
  Drugs (narcotics, barbiturates, tranquilizers)
  Cerebral trauma or infarction
  High cervical cordotomy
  Ondine's curse

tered respiratory drive by changes occurring in the respiratory integratory neurons in the medulla. Respiratory rate and rhythm as well as tidal volume may be affected. Table 1 lists the possible causes of this so-called central ventilatory failure. It is important to note that decreased central drive is more pronounced in sleep, perhaps due to decreased activity in the reticular activating system. Thus patients with altered central respiratory drive are more likely to show alveolar hypoventilation during sleep and are susceptible to the depressant effect of sedatives or hypnotics.

While extrapulmonary causes of respiratory failure are important, the pulmonary causes are even more so. Even with adequate minute ventilation at the mouth, alveolar ventilation may be reduced because of a large dead-space ventilation, since $\dot{V}_A = \dot{V}_E - \dot{V}_D$, where $\dot{V}_A$ is alveolar ventilation, $\dot{V}_E$ is minute ventilation, and $\dot{V}_D$ is dead-space ventilation. This type of ventilatory failure is almost always due to abnormalities in the lung leading to markedly increased dead space. A common example is overwhelming pneumonia.

Failure of oxygenation, as well as of carbon dioxide elimination, results from alveolar hypoventilation, since $P_{a_{O_2}}$ falls pari passu with the rise in $P_{a_{CO_2}}$. In fact, with an exchange ratio of 1, every 1-mm Hg rise in $P_{a_{CO_2}}$ results in a 1-mm Hg fall in $P_{a_{O_2}}$ (see section on Gas Exchange). Thus alveolar hypoventilation causes hypoxemia in addition to hypercapnia. In addition to alveolar hypoventilation, right-to-left shunts and ventilation/perfusion imbalance are other significant physiologic causes of hypoxemia. Right-to-left shunts occur in congenital or acquired cardiac disease. Intrapulmonary right-to-left shunting occurs when blood passes through the lung but is not exposed to alveolar air with atelectasis or alveolar consolidation. In normal individuals, 3 to 5 percent of the cardiac output is shunted from the right to the left side of the circulation. This shunting increases abnormally in the presence of edema fluid in the lung, such as occurs in cardiogenic pulmonary edema, or in those conditions that cause edema without evidence of left ventricular failure, such as high-altitude pulmonary edema, uremic pneumonia, central neurogenic pulmonary edema, heroin-induced pulmonary edema, and most probably the "shock lung" or large group of disorders that have been called the "wet lung syndrome" or "respiratory distress syndrome of the adult." It appears that altered capillary permeability may be the initiating mechanism for edema formation in these latter states. In addition, one rarely finds direct pulmonary arterial-to-pulmonary venous anastomoses accounting for pulmonary right-to-left shunts. Complete lack of ventilation to an area while perfusion persists, as might occur with complete airway obstruction, is another cause of intrapulmonary right-to-left shunting. Statistically, mismatch of ventilation and perfusion is by far the most common physiologic cause of hypoxemia. It accounts for most of the hypoxemia in chronic obstructive lung disease and a significant por-

tion of the hypoxemia in other disease states affecting the cardiac and respiratory systems. It is important to realize that the contributions of areas of low ventilation/perfusion ratios result in a lowered saturation of blood for oxygen that cannot be overcome by increased saturation of blood for oxygen by areas of high ventilation/perfusion ratios, due to the sigmoid shape of the oxyhemoglobin dissociation curve (see chapter on Oxygen and Carbon Dioxide Transport). It is for this reason that one sees the effect of ventilation/perfusion imbalance more with oxygen than with carbon dioxide, whose dissociation curve is linear in the physiologic range, and areas of high $\dot{V}/\dot{Q}$ can blow off more CO_2 to compensate for areas of low $\dot{V}/\dot{Q}$ with less CO_2 elimination.

SYMPTOMS AND SIGNS OF RESPIRATORY FAILURE

Respiratory failure results in clinical changes primarily involving the neurologic system. While tachypnea and dyspnea may indicate respiratory failure, this is not always the case, nor does a patient with respiratory failure necessarily have an increased respiratory rate or complain of dyspnea. Hypercapnia (increased P_{CO_2}) results in cerebral vasodilation and increased cerebral blood flow. The resultant headache, worse on awakening in the morning after the $P_{a_{CO_2}}$ has increased slightly during the sleep of the night before, is characteristic. As $P_{a_{CO_2}}$ continues to rise it has more of a narcotic effect, and the patient's family and acquaintances may note increased drowsiness, decreased alertness and memory, and irritability. Indications of increased intracranial pressure due to increased cerebral blood flow and vasodilation may be noted in the retina with papilledema or just as increased systemic blood pressure. An acute rise in $P_{a_{CO_2}}$ may result in coma and respiratory failure and must be considered in the differential diagnosis of any comatose patient. Hypoxemia also manifests itself primarily through its neurologic effects. Irritability, drowsiness, and decreased intellectual function are all nonspecific symptoms of lowered cerebral oxygenation.

Hypoxemia may result in cyanosis, but this sign may be absent in severe hypoxemia, since at least 5–7 g/100 ml unsaturated hemoglobin must be present before it is noted and the skin color and thickness will affect the ability to detect it. Cyanosis, when present, is helpful in pointing to hypoxemia. The other signs of hypoxemia are nonspecific and include at first tachycardia and hypertension and later hypotension and bradycardia. Either hypercapnia or hypoxemia may result in asterixis.

DIAGNOSIS OF RESPIRATORY FAILURE

It is impossible to accurately assess $P_{a_{CO_2}}$ or $P_{a_{O_2}}$ by clinical means. One must obtain arterial blood gases to make the diagnosis of respiratory failure. This point cannot be overemphasized. It is important to have a high degree of suspicion for such inpatients in whom respiratory failure could occur and obtain arterial blood gases whenever there is a possibility that respiratory failure may be present. It is easy to ignore the "sleeping" patient so as not to disturb him, when in reality the patient has severe undiagnosed respiratory failure. Similarly, the agitated elderly patient requiring sedatives may need arterial blood gases and treatment of his respiratory failure.

ASSESSMENT OF RESPIRATORY FUNCTION

Measurement of respiratory function is indispensable for the provision of adequate respiratory care at all stages: diagnosis, estimation of the efficacy of preventative or therapeutic measures, and criteria for the institution of artificial ventilation as well as its discontinuance (weaning). To be useful, a measurement must lend itself to easy performance in an acutely ill patient; it must be reproducible in order to guide care.

When one is concerned with ventilatory failure, measurements of ventilation are most important. With the aid of portable spirometers one may measure a patient's tidal volume and vital capacity at the bedside. The vital capacity indicates the ventilatory reserve. Empirically, from retrospective review of a number of patients with ventilatory respiratory failure, it has been found that a vital capacity less than 10–15 ml/kg of lean body weight does not provide enough reserve for adequate ventilation. For a 70-kg man this corresponds to a vital capacity of approximately 1050 ml. Thus when following a patient with possible ventilatory failure from extrapulmonary causes, it is most important to obtain serial vital capacity measurements as frequently as the possibility of change dictates. Since arterial blood gases may not deteriorate in such a setting until severe ventilatory failure occurs, one can use the vital capacity alone as an indicator of the need for respiratory support. Thus a patient with myasthenia gravis is best monitored by frequent measurements of vital capacity, which can easily be done at the bedside. Plotting the results against time will indicate trends and allow one to plan on respiratory support in an orderly manner.

In the case of obstructive airways disease, both the vital capacity and the first-second expired volume (FEV_1) or peak flow rate (PFR) are useful in assessing the ventilatory reserve as well as the efficacy of measures to overcome the airway obstruction. When following a patient with bronchial asthma, serial measurements of FEV_1 and vital capacity are excellent indicators of functional status. In the case of ventilatory failure because of primary pulmonary disease it is useful to measure the ratio of dead space to tidal volume (V_D/V_T). Again from retrospective review of patients in respiratory failure, it has been found that spontaneous respiration cannot long be supported when V_D/V_T ratio is greater than 0.6.

Whenever one is assessing hypoxemia, it is helpful to determine the alveolar-to-arterial oxygen gradient ($A-aD_{O_2}$) on 100 percent oxygen. This can be done at the bedside by having the patient breathe 100 percent oxygen for a time sufficient to wash the nitrogen out of the lung. Even with severe maldistribution of inspired air this can be accomplished in 30 min. One can obtain the alveolar oxygen tension $P_{A_{O_2}}$ either by direct sampling or calculate it by the alveolar air equation. Arterial oxygen tension $P_{a_{O_2}}$ is obtained by direct sampling, and the $A-aD_{O_2}$ is determined. The right-to-left shunt can then be approximated, since an $A-aD_{O_2}$ on 100 percent oxygen of 16 mm Hg corresponds to approximately 1 percent right-to-left shunt (see section on Oxygen and Carbon Dioxide Transport). With a decreased cardiac output this number overestimates the right-to-left shunt, while with an increased cardiac output it underestimates the shunt. From retrospective review of patients with failure of oxygenation it has been found that an $A-aD_{O_2}$ greater than 400 mm Hg on 100 percent oxygen indicates inadequate oxygenation reserve and the need for respiratory support. It is not unreasonable to follow the $P_{a_{O_2}}$ on a given $F_{I_{O_2}}$, however, when evaluating the response to treatment; or one may follow the $P_{a_{O_2}}$ on 100 percent oxygen for comparison.

In the assessment of failure of carbon dioxide elimination the absolute value of the $P_{a_{CO_2}}$ is helpful in the patient with no previous CO_2 retention. $P_{a_{CO_2}}$ greater than 60 mm Hg has been found to be the cutoff point where reserve is inadequate and respiratory support is needed to provide adequate ventilation. In the patient with chronic CO_2 retention, however, it is more useful to follow the trend rather than use a given number to assess the need for respiratory support; and one may have patients with $P_{a_{CO_2}}$ of 80 mm Hg or more. In these patients the hydrogen-ion rise from respiratory acidosis rather than the $P_{a_{CO_2}}$ may be used as a helpful adjunct in making the decision for respiratory support. Arterial pH less than 7.20 represents acidemia severe enough to require prompt correction, and if this cannot be accomplished effectively and definitively without respiratory support, then this is an indication for such.

Simple measurements of respiratory rate give overall indication of respiratory distress. In patients with respiratory failure it has been found that a respiratory rate greater than 35 may signal a need for early respiratory support, but since there are many causes of tachypnea, one must use the measurements of blood gases to make the definitive decision as to the need for respiratory assistance.

THERAPY OF RESPIRATORY FAILURE

Acute respiratory failure is a common medical emergency. It occurs whenever the respiratory apparatus fails to provide adequate tissue oxygenation and carbon dioxide removal. Thus respiratory failure may occur in many clinical situations including disorders affecting the lungs, such as chronic obstructive lung disease, but

Table 2
Criteria for Respiratory Support

	Acceptable Range	Close-Monitoring Range	Artificial Ventilation
Ventilation			
Respiratory rate	12–25	25–35	>35
Vital capacity (ml/kg)	70–30	30–15	<15
V_D/V_T ratio	<0.35	0.4–0.6	>0.6
P_{aCO_2} (mm Hg)	35–45	45–60	>60*
Oxygenation			
P_{aO_2} (mm Hg)	100–70 (air)	200–70 (on mask O_2)	<70 (on mask O_2)
A–aD_{O_2} (mm Hg) (on 100% O_2)	50–200	200–350	>350

*Except in chronic hypercapnia.

also in acute neurologic emergencies, poisoning, surgical states, and a variety of less common clinical problems. The proper management of patients with acute respiratory failure involves, first, identification or diagnosis; second, respiratory support; third, management of the underlying precipitating cause; and fourth, prevention and control of complications. Chronic respiratory failure occurs whenever the respiratory apparatus fails more gradually and certain compensatory adjustments are brought forth by the system. Proper management of patients with chronic respiratory failure involves identification or diagnosis, respiratory support (although it may be different than that for acute respiratory failure), and prevention and control of complications. Certain general principles may be stated: First, hypoventilation cannot be very well corrected by any respiratory stimulants. Their usefulness is markedly limited by their short-lived effects. Severe alveolar hypoventilation requires artificial ventilation. Second, hypoxemia can be managed to a large extent by increasing the concentration of the inspired oxygen. The problems with this method of management are that one may still have an inadequate $P_{a_{O_2}}$ despite the added oxygen and/or oxygen toxicity may result from prolonged use of higher concentrations of inspired oxygen. Artificial ventilation can be used to minimize both these problems. Third, respiratory acidosis, when severe, must be corrected promptly, and this usually means the use of intravenous buffers such as sodium bicarbonate. Fourth, in the case of acute respiratory failure, precipitating factors such as emboli, bronchospasm, infection, and excess fluid in the lungs from any cause must be successfully treated for the patient to recover. Except for its probable beneficial effect on pulmonary edema, positive-pressure ventilation does not affect the disease process that leads to respiratory failure and only enables life support during the time it is used to allow the patient to live while recuperative processes are taking place.

ASSISTED VENTILATION

Artificial ventilation plays a central role in the management of acute respiratory failure. It is an effective means of providing adequate ventilation when this otherwise cannot be done. Moreover, it can result in improved oxygenation.

The patients in whom one considers use of assisted ventilation are (1) those with acute respiratory failure in whom the failure is severe enough to require support as shown by the empiric criteria presented above and summarized in Table 2 and (2) those in whom respiratory failure is inevitable even with optimal management. For the most part this preventative use of assisted ventilation applies to surgical patients. Included in this group are patients in shock and patients in whom recovery from major surgery or body trauma is complicated by obesity, severe chronic obstructive lung disease, heart disease, muscle weakness, or general debility. In both groups physiologic assessment of respiratory status guides the initiation, use, and discontinuance of the artificial ventilation.

There are many positive-pressure ventilators available. Most important in their proper use is a genuine familiarity with their characteristics. This is more important than any special feature that a given ventilator may have.

VENTILATOR PATTERNS

The ventilator pattern is defined by: (1) the tidal volume; (2) the duration of inspiration and expiration, which then determines the frequency; (3) the inspiratory and expiratory flow rates and pressures; and (4) the frequency and magnitude of passive hyperinflation.

The optimal pattern for artificial ventilation is not known, but varies with the nature of the underlying disease.

Optimal tidal volume appears to be relatively large, in the range of 10–15 ml/kg of lean body mass. Tidal volumes of approximately 7 ml/kg even with frequent intermittent hyperinflation have been shown to be associated with a larger A–aD_{O_2} on 100 percent oxygen than the larger tidal volumes. In addition, patients with nonpulmonary respiratory failure, e.g., myasthenia, accept ventilation better with larger tidal volumes. Since the V_D/V_T ratio falls with larger tidal volumes, carbon dioxide elimination is more efficient with larger tidal volumes as well.

Once tidal volume is set, one uses a frequency adequate to provide a sufficient minute ventilation for CO_2 removal. What this is will depend upon the V_D/V_T ratio. Thus a standard pattern for assisted ventilation is a tidal volume of 12 ml/kg of lean body mass, an inspiratory duration of 1.5 to 3 sec, and a rate sufficient to provide adequate minute ventilation for CO_2 removal. The most effective ratio of inspiration to expiration time is approximately 1:2 to 1:3. Inspiratory pressure depends upon the lung and chest compliance and the tidal volume used. Inspiratory pressures need be high when lungs are stiff, as in pulmonary edema. Above 50 to 60 cm H_2O the incidence of pneumothorax markedly increases.

VENTILATORY PATTERN AND CIRCULATION

Ventilatory assistance with positive pressure influences the systemic circulation and thus oxygen delivery to the tissues. The systemic circulatory response to positive-pressure ventilation is not easily predictable in a given patient. Patients with acute nonemphysematous pulmonary disease tolerate positive pressure well as a rule, including the use of large tidal volumes and high mean airway pressures. A transient reduction in cardiac output may be expected when mechanical ventilation is first begun and a rise when terminated. Once circulatory adjustment has occurred, variations in ventilatory pattern are generally well tolerated. A reduction in cardiac output may be expected with the use of large tidal volumes in patients with severe emphysema, probably due to a more marked tourniquet effect on the systemic circulation than in the case with patients with more normal elastic recoil. Similarly, patients with diminished blood volume or in frank shock will be expected to have a fall in cardiac output with positive-pressure ventilation. Also, patients with impaired sympathetic activity (e.g., idiopathic polyneuritis, cervical cord transection, chronic intake of antihypertensive drugs) may be expected to show a fall in cardiac output with positive-pressure ventilation. In such patients administration of volume helps restore adequate venous filling pressure and thereby cardiac output.

USE OF POSITIVE END-EXPIRATORY PRESSURE DURING ASSISTED AND SPONTANEOUS VENTILATION

Use of continuous positive end-expiratory pressure has been advocated as an effective supplement to oxygen therapy in patients with acute pulmonary edema. This was not widely used, however, until recently. It has now been demonstrated to be of value to the patient with severe hypoxemia, the patient on mechanical ventilation, or the patient breathing spontaneously. The use of positive end-expiratory pressure (PEEP) can result in a rise in $P_{a_{O_2}}$. Many patients with severe hypoxemia and large right-to-left intrapulmonary shunts can be protected somewhat from the toxic effects of a high $F_{I_{O_2}}$ by this means.

There is generally a linear increase in $P_{a_{O_2}}$ with increasing amounts of PEEP up to approximately 15 cm H_2O, although in any given patient the response is unpredictable. Moreover, any given patient's response to PEEP will vary over a period of time. One needs to continually reevaluate the patient's response for this reason.

The means by which PEEP relieves hypoxemia have not been clearly established. It is clear that most patients with respiratory failure have low lung volumes and low functional residual capacities. It is known that $P_{a_{O_2}}$ will increase in these patients with increase in their functional residual capacity (FRC), and PEEP increases FRC. One may argue, then, that PEEP exerts its effect by increasing the FRC in these patients with respiratory failure and preexisting low lung volumes. While at the present time there are no predictors of the patient who will respond well to PEEP, if one could easily measure the FRC at the bedside this might well be a good predictor. It is possible that for those patients who do not respond to PEEP, their lung volume is at or near normal, and that the increase in lung volume produced by PEEP is not beneficial to their gas exchange.

Use of PEEP may be associated with an increase in rate of complications, such as subcutaneous or mediastinal emphysema and pneumothorax, when compared with intermittent positive-pressure breathing. However, data on the frequency of these complications are not clear, and it is possible that the incidence is more closely related to the type and degree of underlying disease than to the ventilatory pattern.

The value of PEEP lies in the ability to improve the $P_{a_{O_2}}$ so that a lower inspired oxygen concentration can be used and thereby provide respiratory support with a lessened chance of oxygen toxicity while the basic recuperative processes are underway. There is no evidence to suggest it favorably influences the underlying disease.

OXYGEN REQUIREMENTS

Supplemental inspired oxygen is invariably required in the presence of acute respiratory failure except in the case of pure extrapulmonary ventilatory failure, and then only if adequate measures are instituted early to forestall pulmonary complications such as atelectasis, pneumonia, or pulmonary edema.

An optimal arterial oxygen tension is one that will permit full utilization of the oxygen-carrying capacity of arterial blood and result in minimal adverse effects from the inspired oxygen concentration used. The variables here are the fraction of inspired oxygen, $F_{I_{O_2}}$, the arterial oxygen tension, $P_{a_{O_2}}$, the hemoglobin concentration, and the oxyhemoglobin dissociation curve. Key also in considering total oxygen transport is the adequacy of the circulatory system both in terms of cardiac output and individual organ microcirculation. What one is concerned with most is actual oxygen delivery and not just oxygen concentration in arterial blood.

While no positive guidelines can be given as to what

is the lowest $P_{a_{O_2}}$ at which any given patient can safely be kept, there are certain facts and general principles that are helpful in making the decision for each patient on an individual basis. First, with a normal oxyhemoglobin dissociation curve, a $P_{a_{O_2}}$ of 65 mm Hg corresponds to an approximate 90 percent saturation. This saturation should be adequate in most situations. Second, one must maintain an adequate hemoglobin concentration in blood and use red blood cells with a relatively normal oxyhemoglobin dissociation curve when transfusing patients with acute respiratory failure. Third, in the presence of a large right-to-left shunt, i.e., greater than 30 percent of the cardiac output, one produces only small increases in the $P_{a_{O_2}}$ by increasing the $F_{I_{O_2}}$ even up to 1.0, because of the sigmoid shape of the oxyhemoglobin dissociation curve and the marked influence of the mixed venous P_{O_2} in determining the final arterial P_{O_2}. The meaning of this is that the cost of high $F_{I_{O_2}}$, i.e., the oxygen toxicity, is too high when one can only minimally increase the $P_{a_{O_2}}$.

Whenever added oxygen is used, careful titration of the inspired oxygen concentration is especially important. Facilities for doing so differ with the type of equipment available. Prediction of inspired oxygen concentration is difficult with gas-driven pressure-limited machines. Precise regulation of inspired oxygen concentration will become simpler with the use of mixing valves incorporated at compressed oxygen and air outlets. One can measure the $F_{I_{O_2}}$ by equipment now available for use at the bedside, and this measurement should be a routine one for patients receiving added oxygen via ventilators.

SPECIAL SITUATIONS

Treatment of Pulmonary Edema in Acute Respiratory Failure

The most effective immediate treatment for the hypoxemia associated with pulmonary edema is to increase the $F_{I_{O_2}}$ and use the appropriate pattern of ventilation (see above). Success of subsequent measures depends on the etiology of the pulmonary edema. In the absence of pulmonary capillary damage, diuretic therapy and water restriction lead to improvement of respiratory function. In the presence of pulmonary capillary lesions with loss of capillary integrity and loss of protein, Starling's law no longer pertains. Even vigorous dehydrations are often ineffective. There is no convincing evidence that the simultaneous administration of salt-poor albumin and a diuretic agent is of greater value in improving oxygenation than diuresis alone. Unfortunately the pulmonary water is poorly mobilizable, and no benefit can be obtained from overdiuresis and dehydration.

Respiratory Failure in Chronic Obstructive Lung Disease

Indications for intubation and ventilation in this group are more stringent than in patients with other forms of underlying disease, for several reasons. First, patients acclimatized to chronic hypoxemia often tolerate extremely low levels of $P_{a_{O_2}}$ (below 40 mm Hg). Second, mechanical ventilation is not easily managed and is probably associated with a greater frequency of complications such as tension pneumothorax and a fall in cardiac output. In these patients with severe hypoxemia a substantial increase in arterial oxygen content is attainable with a small increase in $P_{a_{O_2}}$ because the oxyhemoglobin dissociation curve is steep in this range. Adequate relief of hypoxemia without attendant suppression of chemoreceptor drive and excessive hypercapnia is the aim of controlled oxygen therapy, which has been reported effective in the majority of patients with acute exacerbations of chronic obstructive lung disease. Known oxygen concentrations are administered either with calibrated Venturi facemasks or accurate oxygen flowmeters delivering low flow (e.g., 1–2 l/min) of oxygen. Careful supervision and frequent measurement of arterial blood gases are necessary to ensure the safety of this method. However, if significant respiratory acidosis occurs despite vigorous treatment of all reversible factors, one is left with no choice but intubation and mechanical ventilation to treat the respiratory failure.

Analeptic drugs may be self-defeating in that they may increase total metabolic rate and carbon dioxide production in excess of the patient's limited ability for CO_2 elimination. Controlled oxygen therapy, chest physiotherapy, adequate bronchial drainage, and careful treatment of infection are the best modes of therapy in the majority of these patients.

Respiratory Failure in Bronchial Asthma

The asthmatic differs from the patient with chronic obstructive lung disease in that the lung parenchyma is relatively normal and airway obstruction is episodic. Patients in acute exacerbation have low levels of $P_{a_{CO_2}}$, and the rise to normal or hypercapnic levels is a late phenomenon signifying fatigue and decompensation. However, hypoxemia is present even in mild exacerbations. Such patients require continuous monitoring. If progressive hypercapnia and exhaustion develop despite treatment with high-humidity oxygen, bronchodilator drugs, corticosteroids, hydration, treatment of infection if present, and correction of acidosis, then intubation and mechanical ventilation are indicated. Heavy sedation and occasional paralysis are usually required to facilitate the mechanical ventilation.

Status asthmatics unresponsive to all the above may be helped by bronchial lavage under general anesthesia to remove mucus plugs, but this procedure requires considerable expertise. General anesthesia alone may provide some bronchodilation, but it does not improve pulmonary mechanics nor gas exchange and is rarely used today.

AIRWAY FOR RESPIRATORY CARE

Intubation and tracheostomy and support of ventilation are now done in a wide range of clinical conditions. Indications for endotracheal intubation and tracheostomy often are overlapping. They are:

1. In upper respiratory tract obstruction the presence of an endotracheal tube that passes through the obstructed area, or a tracheostomy tube that bypasses this region, helps obtain a patent airway.
2. Either an endotracheal or a tracheostomy tube provides a reliable means of efficient delivery of a ventilator's stroke volume directly to the lungs.
3. Where effective coughing and deep breathing are absent, insertion of an endotracheal tube may greatly facilitate chest physiotherapy.
4. Facemasks cannot reliably deliver oxygen concentrations greater than 60 percent. When requirements exceed this, either an especially well-fitting mask or an endotracheal or tracheostomy tube must be resorted to for adequate oxygen delivery.
5. The use of a tube with an inflatable cuff provides a seal that helps protect against aspiration when this is a concern.

Endotracheal intubation can be accomplished speedily and atraumatically in most patients. Emergency tracheostomy is invariably associated with some delay before airway control is achieved; it rarely is more effective than an endotracheal tube and introduces the hazard of hurried surgery. For this reason the only indication for an emergency tracheostomy is upper airway obstruction that cannot be bypassed by an endotracheal tube.

Endotracheal tubes may be passed through the nose or mouth. The nasal tube has the advantage of better fixation and no oral irritation. It carries the added risk of causing sinus infection due to interference with drainage. The disadvantages of both types of endotracheal tubes are as follows: (1) Since they are longer, they will pass more easily into one of the main-stem bronchi; (2) they are softer and are subject to kinking or compression in the upper airway; (3) suboptimal humidification of inspired gases carries the risk of lumen occlusion by dried secretions.

Prolonged use of endotracheal tubes has been made possible by the use of new materials and the use of excellent care, including reduction of movement of the tube by the use of a swivel attachment from the respirator tubing. It is not possible to predict exact periods during which no laryngeal damage will occur; 6 to 10 days in adults under optimal conditions are regarded as a permissible period.

Whenever a direct route to the trachea is required for a prolonged period of time, a tracheostomy is needed, and a tracheostomy tube may be tolerated indefinitely with proper management.

WEANING FROM ARTIFICIAL TO SPONTANEOUS VENTILATION

Every step during management of the patient in acute respiratory failure is directed toward relieving the patient of his dependency on the ventilator. The transition from artificial to spontaneous ventilation can be attempted only when objective evidence indicates that respiratory function is adequate to permit this changeover.

The weaning process must proceed gradually, particularly if the patient has required prolonged artificial ventilation (that is, more than 72 hr) or has residual evidence of chest wall instability such as seen following chest wall trauma. Weaning is contraindicated in the presence of paradoxical chest wall movement, and controlled ventilation must be continued until stabilization of these structures has occurred. The requirement for controlled ventilation depends upon the location and extent of the rib fractures. Presence of a bronchopleural fistula is not an indication per se for premature weaning. Most fistulas will close spontaneously during the course of controlled ventilation. Early weaning is contraindicated in patients with severe tetanus or any clinical situation that requires large doses of muscle relaxants, narcotics, or sedatives.

Sustained spontaneous respiration in patients recovering from respiratory failure requires the ability to generate a minimal vital capacity of 10 ml/kg or a volume essentially twice as large as the normal resting tidal volume. The presence of a large ratio of dead space to tidal volume, i.e., greater than 0.6, indicates that ventilatory reserve is markedly limited and the likelihood of exhaustion and recurrence of respiratory failure is high. A patient usually may become independent of ventilatory support for a total of 24 hr, with the endotracheal or tracheostomy tube being removed whenever the vital capacity exceeds 15–20 ml/kg of lean body mass. In a study of patients weaned from artificial ventilation, the vital capacity was found to be a more reliable index of the ability to breathe spontaneously than either the alveolar–arterial oxygen gradient on 100 percent oxygen or the V_D/V_T ratio. However, weaning from the ventilator when the alveolar–arterial oxygen gradient is greater than 350 mm Hg, or the V_D/V_T ratio is greater than 0.6, is rarely successful. These minimal requirements for oxygenation and ventilation are consistent with those listed earlier as empirical indicators for ventilator support of the patient with incipient respiratory failure.

Difficulty in weaning from ventilatory support may be due to abnormal pulmonary mechanics and blood gas exchange, to low cardiac output, to hypermetabolic state, or to muscle weakness. Patients who have required prolonged ventilation show marked variation in their response to the discomfort of dyspnea associated with the weaning period in the face of abnormal pulmonary and chest wall mechanics. Most are apprehensive and display wide fluctuations in vital signs when first faced with the need to breathe spontaneously. Hypotension and bradycardia are indicative of hypoxemia and occur infrequently, while hypertension, tachycardia, and tachypnea are common. Unless thoroughly documented, their appearance should not be attributed to psychological dependence on the ventilator. There is little or no evidence to justify this diagnosis in the adult. Objective discomfort may arise when pronounced changes in pulmonary and chest wall mechanics give rise to severe dyspnea and marked sympathetic discharge. At this time, arterial blood gas values are frequently in the normal range. Many patients will show transient arrhythmias when being switched from a ventilator to spontaneous respiration. The mechanism of this is not clear, but usually it is not due to new abnormalities in arterial blood gases. It is now clear that several degrees of respiratory discoordination occur in patients who have undergone prolonged assisted ventilation and are of sufficient magnitude to interfere with all attempts to sustain spontaneous respiration. This phenomenon arises from inability to generate a smooth coordinate contraction and relaxation of the diaphragm and chest wall muscles. Return to a normal synchronized pattern of ventilation occurs gradually and may delay weaning from the ventilator.

The need for careful monitoring of blood gas exchange and pulmonary mechanics during the initial phase of weaning cannot be overemphasized. Additional trials of spontaneous respiration must be made under close supervision and must provide adequate concentrations of oxygen to compensate for an anticipated fall in $P_{a_{O_2}}$, which could further decrease ventilatory and gas-exchange reserve.

COMPLICATIONS ASSOCIATED WITH POSITIVE-PRESSURE VENTILATION

The approach to respiratory support of a patient with acute respiratory failure is relatively simple compared to the management of the complications that commonly occur in such patients. Many times the outcome of efforts will depend most on the ability to manage them successfully.

They involve all organ systems. Cardiovascular complications include hypotension, hypertension, congestive heart failure, low cardiac output, cardiac arrhythmias, cardiac arrest, and pulmonary thromboembolism. Fluid and electrolyte abnormalities occur, including acid–base imbalance, hypokalemia, hyponatremia and hyperchloremia, and water retention. Gastrointestinal complications are common, with upper gastrointestinal bleeding secondary to ulcers, obstruction, gastric dilatation, ileus, and fecal impaction. Neurologic complications regularly occur as well and include mental changes, motor changes, and seizures. One may commonly see evidence of malfunction of the renal, hepatic, and hematologic systems. The respiratory system complications, per se, include oxygen toxicity, upper airway obstruction, tracheal and laryngeal injury, pneumothorax and pneumomediastinum, and super-

infection; they will be discussed in somewhat greater detail here.

Oxygen Toxicity

Since ventilators introduce the capability to provide oxygen continuously in high concentration, the problem of oxygen toxicity may be considered a complication of artificial ventilation. A study by Nash and associates of 70 patients who died after prolonged artificial ventilation demonstrated a characteristic pulmonary lesion. The lungs were heavy, "beefy," and edematous. On histologic examination there was an exudative phase characterized by congestion, alveolar edema, intraalveolar hemorrhage, and a fibrinous exudate with formation of prominent hyaline membranes without an associated inflammatory component. A late proliferative phase was characterized by pronounced alveolar and intraalveolar septal edema, fibroblastic proliferation with early fibrosis, and prominent hyperplasia of alveolar lining cells. The morphologic changes were unrelated to the duration of artificial ventilation per se, but they did correlate with the prolonged use of ventilation and high inspired oxygen concentration. Kaplan and associates found similar changes in monkeys exposed to 100 percent oxygen for up to 12 days. Both the exudative and proliferative phase described by Nash and associates could be demonstrated. Since these animals were breathing spontaneously throughout the experiment, the effect of positive-pressure ventilation could be excluded. Formation of interstitial and intraalveolar edema and hyaline membranes are nonspecific responses of the lung to a variety of injuries of which oxygen toxicity is only one. That oxygen can cause such changes alone, however, is clear from these studies.

The limits of what may be considered a safe inspired oxygen concentration have not yet been established. In addition, duration of exposure is of critical importance in the production of changes due to high inspired oxygen concentration. Continuous exposure to oxygen at 1 atm is fatal to all mammals studied. Prospective studies on patients recovering from cardiac surgery demonstrated no physiologic evidence of oxygen toxicity for up to 48 hr of exposure to pure oxygen. Another study on subjects without preexisting cardiopulmonary disease demonstrated unequivocal decrease in $P_{a_{O_2}}$ with pure oxygen ventilation, increased intrapulmonary shunt, and increased V_D/V_T ratio, as well as an increased lung weight on autopsy. The changes were dependent on time of pure oxygen breathing and began to become evident at 40 hr. The most sensitive index of pulmonary involvement was a decreasing $P_{a_{O_2}}$ on 100 percent oxygen. Various factors may influence a person's susceptibility to the adverse pulmonary effects of prolonged exposure to high oxygen concentrations. Tolerance is known to develop in lungs after exposure to a number of different noxious gases, and the development of tolerance to oxygen may influence the individual susceptibility.

Inspired oxygen pressures less than 300–400 mm Hg

can be tolerated for prolonged periods of time with no evidence of significant pulmonary damage in human volunteers.

The available data indicate that concentrations of oxygen equivalent to 0.6 to 1.0 atm are likely to produce clinically significant changes after more than 48 hr of continuous exposure. This is manifest first by a fall in $P_{a_{O_2}}$ on 100 percent oxygen, and also by an increased V_D/V_T ratio and decreased compliance. X-ray changes consisting of diffuse alveolar pattern may be expected to be seen at this time as well. Since absolute guidelines are not available, it is prudent to use the lowest possible fraction of inspired oxygen consistent with adequate oxygenation of the patient.

Water Retention

In 100 patients treated with prolonged positive-pressure ventilation, Sladen and associates described a clinical syndrome characterized by a positive water balance and radiographic changes consistent with pulmonary edema in the absence of recognizable cardiac failure or elevated central venous pressure. The average weight gain at the peak of respiratory insufficiency was 2.6 kg. There was evidence also of decreased compliance and altered gas exchange. The reason for this tendency of patients receiving positive-pressure ventilation to retain fluid is not known. The syndrome may be prevented by keeping total fluid intake low in patients on artificial ventilation. Total fluid administration usually need be no more than 1000 to 1500 ml per 24 hr. The contribution to respiratory water balance of nebulizers must be taken into account in this calculation. Frequently diuretics should be used to prevent a positive fluid balance, however. Since water restriction and diuretic therapy reverse all evidence of pulmonary edema, it is probable that the pulmonary edema fluid is a transudate and its occurrence is related to an indirect effect of positive-pressure ventilation on the body to retain water, resulting in hemodilution and relative hyponatremia.

Postintubation and Tracheostomy Injury

Ulceration of the larynx is the fundamental lesion that follows endotracheal intubation and may develop as early as 6 hr after intubation. Brief intubation is usually associated with superficial erosion that heals readily. The severity of damage is directly related to the duration of intubation and may be manifest by hoarseness, stridor, and difficulty in swallowing shortly after extubation. Sequelae of prolonged intubation occur due to granulation tissue, a consequence of ulcer repair. When the vocal cords are affected, this results in hoarseness and dysphagia. When situated in the subglottic area they may cause airway obstruction. These lesions usually regress spontaneously, and no special treatment is necessary unless obstruction ensues. Healing of laryngeal ulcers may also cause upper airway obstruction by formation of laryngotracheal membranes or vocal cord adhesions. Both adhesions are correctable by surgery. Far more serious are the sequelae that arise from the fibrotic changes that follow healing of deep ulcers. Fibrotic stenosis at the subglottic level or immobilization of one or both vocal cords from fibrosis around the arytenoids can produce upper airway obstruction, correction of which is difficult and complex.

Serious laryngeal sequelae commonly occur when the endotracheal tube fits too tightly within the larynx. This may happen when an excessively large tube is used or if the tracheal lumen is narrowed by edema. The incidence of difficult and traumatic intubation is significantly higher among patients who show evidence of laryngeal damage. It is probable that similar damage may be caused by excessive movements of a tube in the larynx.

Tubes manufactured using chemically abrasive or irritating materials can produce tissue damage. Sterilization of rubber and plastics with ethylene oxide can also make the materials potentially harmful to surrounding tissues. Inadequate airing of tubes sterilized in ethylene oxide results in accumulation of ethylene chlorhydrate and ethylene glycol interphase, both of which are irritating to the tissues. Awareness of these facts is most important in the choice and handling of tubes used for endotracheal intubation.

Serious tracheal complications that demand surgical intervention are still rare following prolonged tracheostomy. However, they may demand special attention because definitive surgical treatment is now available and many times is successful with proper timing and technique. Recent evidence suggests that most, if not all, of such complications are preventable by the use of better materials and cuff design.

Damage to the trachea occurs at three sites: (1) the level of the tip of the tube, (2) the tracheal stoma, and (3) the level of the inflatable cuff.

Erosion of the tracheal wall on a low stoma at the distal end of the tube may lead to acute fatal hemorrhage if a major artery is eroded. It is a rare complication.

The lesions produced at the stoma and at the level of the cuff culminate in delayed tracheal stenosis and tracheal malacia, with functional obstruction to air flow. The symptoms of tracheal stenosis usually appear within 6 weeks of extubation but may take up to 18 months to develop. Dyspnea and diminished effort tolerance are the usual presenting symptoms. A slight cough is common. Stridor is a late manifestation and, to the unsuspecting, will be diagnosed as asthma. Its presence invariably implies a reduction in the tracheal diameter to less than 5 mm at the site of stenosis. Auscultation at the neck over the cervical trachea may help with the diagnosis and locate the lesion. Far more precise information regarding site and size can be obtained with an air tracheogram and laminogram. Tracheal malacia can be detected by fluoroscopy and cineradiography by looking for the flail segment of narrowing of the airway on inspiration. Contrast media are of little help in the diagnosis and are potentially troublesome when added occlusion of an already narrow trachea occurs. Bronchoscopy is essential, and in severely obstructed patients it is best deferred until the time of definitive surgery. The trauma produced by bronchoscopy is potentially hazardous and may cause further edema and increase obstruction sufficient to require hasty surgical intervention. When underlying pathology indicates stomal granulation, this is seldom serious enough to require anything but removal by way of a bronchoscope. Tracheal deformities arising from excessive tissue damage, however, can be extensive and more difficult to correct. The typical lesion is the cuff lesion. The lumen is usually narrowed by a circumferential ring of fibrous tissue and contrasts to the anterior localized scarring that narrows the trachea at the stoma level. Tracheal malacia is seldom the predominant obstructive deformity, but is common in its association with the fibrotic annulus, usually being located above the stenosis. Occasionally the normal tracheal architecture is completely destroyed and the cartilaginous rings are obliterated.

The pathogenesis of these lesions is as follows: the stomal-level lesions are unrelated to the use of artificial ventilation. They are the end result of damage from an excessively large stoma or tracheostomy tube, excessive to and fro movement of the tube, and severe local sepsis. Cuff-site lesions are the result of direct pressure necrosis. Cuffs that have been in standard use have been found to exert pressures of the order of 160–200 mm Hg. The use of "soft" cuffs that allow an airtight seal to be obtained at low intracuff pressures of 20–40 mm Hg and that mold themselves to the inner contour of the trachea allowing occlusion without deformity of the tracheal wall are associated with a much lower incidence of pressure necrosis. Duration of exposure to the inflated cuff is of crucial importance in determining the extent of damage produced. Other factors, such as superimposed infection and inappropriate methods of equipment sterilization, may also contribute to the pathology.

REFERENCES

Bendixen HH, Egbert LB, Hedley-Whyte J, et al: Respiratory Care. St Louis, CV Mosby, 1965

Kaplan HP, Robinson FR, Kapanci Y, et al: Pathogenesis and reversibility of the pulmonary lesions of oxygen toxicity in monkeys. I. Clinical and light microscopy studies. Lab Invest 20:94–100, 1969

Nash G, Blennerhassett JB, Pontoppidan H: Pulmonary Lesions associated with oxygen therapy and artificial ventilation. N Engl J Med 276:368, 1967

Petty TL: Intensive and Rehabilitative Respiratory Care. Philadelphia, Lea & Febiger, 1971

Pontoppidan H, Geffin B, Lowenstein E: Acute respiratory failure in the adult. N Engl J Med 287:690, 743, 799, 1972

Pontoppidan H, Laver MB, Geffin B: Acute respiratory failure in the surgical patient, in Welch CE (ed): Chicago, Year Book Medical Publishers, 1970, p 163

Sladen A, Laver MB, Pontoppidan H: Pulmonary complica-tions and water retention in prolonged mechanical ventilation. N Engl J Med 279:448–453, 1968

Sykes MK, McNichol MW, Campbell EJM: Respiratory Failure. Philadelphia, FA Davis, 1969

RESPIRATORY DISTRESS SYNDROME

Daniel C. Shannon

In order to exit gracefully from intrauterine life, the infant must quickly and smoothly replace those conditions that permitted only 5 percent of cardiac output to perfuse the lung in utero with a new set of conditions that will permit pulmonary gas exchange to support metabolism. If alveolar development has been incomplete, if the infant fails to clear fetal lung fluid, if a variety of other reflex, mechanical, or metabolic alterations occur, resistance to pulmonary blood flow will be high and extrauterine life will begin awkwardly. Many of these factors that increase resistance to pulmonary blood flow are interdependent and result in a commonality of signs and symptoms, regardless of the primary cause. For example, deficiency of surfactant leads to alveolar collapse and low lung volume, which increases resistance to flow and diverts a varying proportion of cardiac output from right to left through a patent foramen ovale and/or ductus arteriosus. The resultant systemic hypoxemia may be severe enough to (1) induce anaerobic glycolysis and increased H^+ concentration and (2) lower mixed venous P_{O_2}. Both of these events can increase pulmonary precapillary arteriolar spasm and increase resistance to flow even further. Expanding the lung from a low volume requires a great effort and greater substrate and thus compounds the problem by demanding increased oxygen uptake and CO_2 elimination from the lung. Adequate alveolar surfactant is probably responsible for maintaining a dry interstitial and alveolar space. Thus lack of surfactant may compound alveolar disability by imposing a fluid barrier between alveolar air and pulmonary capillary blood. This may be even further aggravated by hypoproteinemia, which is commonly seen in the very sick infant with respiratory distress syndrome (RDS).

Thus the RDS is a collage of respiratory and metabolic dysfunctions, each of which can discolor the others. Not surprisingly the signs and symptoms are similar in all infants, and the primary cause may be difficult to discern. Tachypnea, retractions, grunting, tachycardia, and increasing cyanosis are early signs of the syndrome. Each is a reflection of the underlying pathophysiology and may be due to a variety of mechanisms. Tachypnea can initially be explained by stimulation of intrapulmonary vagal receptors by attempts to inflate a stiff lung. Later, increased ventilation may be required to eliminate CO_2 either from increased production or from increased physiologic dead space or in response to stimulation of the carotid body chemoreceptors by increased

H^+ or decreased $P_{a_{O_2}}$. Retractions of the sternum and costal cartilage occur when the lung becomes less compliant than the chest wall, and increasing retractions generally reflect worsening of pulmonary disease. As alveolar collapse progresses the infant responds by expiring forcibly against a partially closed glottis, producing an audible grunt reflecting remarkable intuition since this maneuver tends to prevent alveolar collapse. As pulmonary vascular resistance increases systemic arterial P_{O_2} falls; cyanosis only becomes apparent when a major portion of cardiac output is shunted from right to left. Frequent nonrespiratory complications are hyperbilirubinemia, hypocalcemia, and hypoglycemia.

Laboratory investigations are dictated by the pathophysiology and are useful both diagnostically and as a guide to therapy. Thus the initial evaluation should include chest x-ray, 12-lead electrocardiogram, hematocrit, white-blood-cell count and differential, the concentration in serum of total protein, sodium, potassium, and glucose, arterial blood gas values, and measurement of systemic blood pressure. Although the findings on chest radiography are generally considered to be typical enough (Fig. 1) to make the diagnosis of the RDS, similar findings can be seen with congestive heart failure.

In measuring arterial blood gases it is critical that the inspired oxygen concentration at the infant's nose be analyzed at the same time. Arterialized capillary blood is not satisfactory for determination of P_{O_2}, although it is useful for pH and P_{CO_2}. Thus blood drawn from the arterial circulation is necessary. The technique for catheterization of the umbilical artery is now well standardized, but it is associated with unacceptable complications due mainly to embolization and consequent infarction. Maintenance of a cannula in the radial artery for sampling and pressure monitoring is a safer procedure.

Adequate measurement of systemic blood pressure is necessary since hypovolemia can contribute or even cause respiratory distress. Measurement by Doppler effect has been proved useful in normal premature infants, but may not be as reliable in those critically ill. The most certain method is to connect an electronic transducer to the arterial catheter. The pulse waveform can then be viewed intermittently or continuously on an oscilloscope screen. Therapy can then be directed at aberration of any or all of these measurements. Systemic hypotension can be managed with infusions of red cells and/or plasma, depending on the deficit, until arterial pressure returns to normal. It must be remembered that normal systolic pressure is 65 mm Hg for a 3-kg infant, 45 mm Hg for a 1-kg infant. Hematocrit is best kept above 45 percent and total protein above 4.5 g/100 ml.

Arterial hypoxemia ($P_{a_{O_2}}$ less than 50 mm Hg) should be treated with additional inspired oxygen, but $P_{a_{O_2}}$ should not exceed about 70 mm Hg. If the $F_{I_{O_2}}$ must be greater than 0.40, it is most easily achieved with

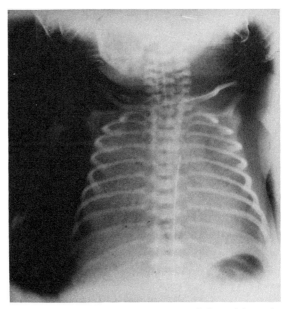

Fig. 1. Typical chest radiograph of 1.7-kg infant with respiratory distress syndrome (IRDS) showing reticulogranular pattern and air bronchogram.

a small hood over the infant's head. The level and duration of $F_{I_{O_2}}$ greater than 0.60 that endangers the lung is not known, but few physicians caring for these infants would feel comfortable with an $F_{I_{O_2}}$ greater than 0.60 for over 48 hr. Since administration of positive end-expiratory pressure is very effective in a large number of these infants, its use is advocated early in the course of the disease so that oxygen toxicity does not become a problem; with early use, rapid and lasting improvement can be anticipated. Early treatment may even prevent progression of the disease.

Dramatic elevation of $P_{a_{O_2}}$ can be best demonstrated while the infant breathes gas at an $F_{I_{O_2}}$ of 1.0 for as little as 10 min (Fig. 2). This improvement then permits reduction of $F_{I_{O_2}}$ to less than 0.6 in a very short time. The major effect of this technique seems to be an increase in resting lung volume toward normal, reducing pulmonary vascular resistance and thus enhancing gas exchange. The risk of pneumothorax is not increased; however, the technique should not be initiated in the presence of a pneumothorax. It should be used with caution when increased vascular resistance and shunting are associated with hypovolemia or lung hyper-inflation.

Arterial pH must be maintained above 7.20 as appropriate with either bicarbonate infusion for metabolic acidosis or increased ventilation for respiratory acidosis. Correction of hypovolemic hypotension generally obviates the need to use sodium bicarbonate. This is fortunate because use of the standard hyperosmolar (1760 mOsm/L) clinical solution is associated with serum hyperosmolality and intracranial hemorrhage in the

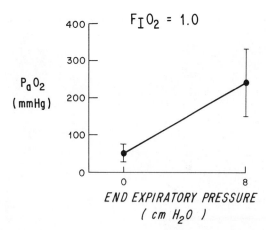

Fig. 2. Arterial P_{O_2} ($P_{a_{O_2}}$) in 30 infants with respiratory distress syndrome (IRDS) at $F_{I_{O_2}}$ = 1.0 when end-expiratory pressure was zero and 10 min later at 8 cm H_2O end-expiratory pressure. Vertical bars = 2 SD.

premature infant. Ventilation can be accomplished transiently with mask-and-bag ventilation. For prolonged periods there are a variety of respirators; although not ideal, they can successfully be used on small infants.

With application of new techniques to the infant with the respiratory distress syndrome, a distinct improvement in the mortality rate is expected. The reported mortality of under 20 percent in a small series of premature infants treated with positive end-expiratory pressure is heartening. Even more important will be evaluation of the effect of such therapy on subsequent psychomotor development.

It is hoped that future investigations will define the pathophysiologic role of the α_1-antitryptic protein, elastase inhibitors, fibrinolysins, serum protein metabolism, and perhaps most important adrenocorticosteroids. These compounds may be the prime stimuli for production of surfactant in utero.

REFERENCES

Avery ME, Mead J: Surface properties in relation to atelectasis and hyalin membrane disease. Am J Dis Child 97:517, 1959

Chu J, Clements JA, Cotton EK, et al: Neonatal pulmonary ischemia. Pediatrics 40:709, 1967

Clements JA: Surface tension of lung extracts. Proc Soc Exp Biol Med 95:170, 1957

Gluck L, Kulovich MV, Borer RC, et al: Diagnosis of the respiratory distress syndrome by amniocentesis. Am J Obstet Gynecol 109:440, 1967

Gluck L, Motoyama EK, Smits HL, Kulovich MV: The biochemical development of surface activity in mammalian lung. I. The surface active phospholipids; the separation and distribution of surface active lecithin in the lung of the developing rabbit fetus. Pediatr Res 1:237, 1967

Gregory GA, Kitterman JA, Phibbs R, et al: Treatment of IRDS with continuous positive airway pressure. N Engl J Med 284:1333, 1971

Scarpelli EM: The surfactant system of the lung. Philadelphia, Lea & Febiger, 1968

THORACIC DEFORMITIES AND LUNG DISEASE

Daniel C. Shannon

Deformity of the thorax would be expected to interfere with efficient function of the respiratory system; yet many patients with chest deformity have no complaints until gross structural alterations occur or until another disease of the respiratory tract supervenes. Parents of children with chest deformity seek medical advice as soon as a problem is recognized, and the physician must be ready to provide or arrange for appropriate medical therapy for each child. Properly done, this involves knowledge of the natural history of each defect as well as functional assessment of the respiratory system.

Any component of the chest wall may be involved primarily, and since the thorax must behave as a unit, involvement of one specific structure affects the function of those adjacent to it or even the entire chest. Table 1 outlines the areas of primary involvement with representative examples.

INVOLVEMENT OF THE THORAX AS A WHOLE

This group of disorders has only one factor in common, an apparent symmetrical alteration in size and shape of the thorax. Acromegaly and pituitary gigantism, both induced by an excess of growth hormone, are associated with large chests. While Brody has suggested that there is a disproportionate increase in lung size in such patients, particularly in males, Bartlett has been unable to substantiate a specific effect of growth hormone on the lung in animals. It is likely that overdistention of already present lung tissue accounts for appearance of new growth. There is no recognized alteration in lung function in these patients.

In Marfan's disease the chest becomes elongated, and at full growth it is increased in vertical height and decreased in its anteroposterior dimension, particularly when pectus excavatum is also associated. Lung function is generally preserved unless there is scoliosis or an intrapulmonary cyst. Apical bullae and an increased incidence of pneumothorax have also been described in these patients. These findings suggest that increased vertical lung height leads to (1) more negative transpulmonary pressure at the apex and (2) diminished apical pulmonary blood flow and that the combination of factors predisposes to development of bullae and pneumothorax. As children, these patients frequently develop scoliosis and kyphosis.

Chest hyperinflation is generally associated with obstructive airway disease. In 1921 Scheuerman described the physical and radiographic appearance of hyperinflation in a number of young patients. These

Table 1
Deformities of the Thorax and Its Parts

Thorax as a whole
  Increased size or shape
    Acromegaly
    Marfan's syndrome
    Scheuerman's disease
  Decreased size or shape
    Asphyxiating thoracic dystrophy
    Arthrogryposis
    Morquio-Ulrich

Sternum
  Failure of fusion
  Abnormal costochondral junction
    Unilateral
    Bilateral
      pectus carinatum
      pectus excavatum

Ribs
  Absence or hypoplasia
  Fusion

Spine
  Congenital
    Vertebral
      fusion
      hemivertebrae
      metabolic
      mucopolysaccharidoses
    Muscle
      dystrophies
    Neural
      Werdnig-Hoffmann
      Neurofibromatosis
    Ligament
      Marfan's
  Traumatic
  Inflammatory
    Vertebral—Pott's
    Neural—poliomyelitis
    Pleural—empyema
  Radiation
  Idiopathic

patients are asymptomatic, have normal pulmonary function, including lung volume, air flow rates, and gas exchange, and probably represent a normal but unusual variation in thoracic structure.

DECREASED SIZE IN THORAX

Several dystrophic conditions are associated with a thorax that is clearly too small in proportion to the body. Fortunately these are rare, for the associated pulmonary disability is responsible for significant morbidity and early mortality.

Asphyxiating thoracic dystrophy was first described by Maroteaux and Savart in 1964 and is manifest at birth by a very small bell-shaped thorax. These infants have large intrapulmonary right-to-left shunts resulting in significant hypoxemia, apparently as a result of impaired alveolar expansion. In these infants atelectasis and pneu-

monia are frequent problems and account for their early deaths. Microscopic examination of rib and costal cartilage reveals dysplasia and is reflected in beading of the costochondral junctions. Reduction in thoracic size is also seen in arthrogryposis and in the Morquio-Ulrich syndrome.

STERNUM: FAILURE OF FUSION

The sternum develops from fusion of six paired segmented cartilaginous structures. When fusion fails completely, or in the more caudad portion gross cardiac defects are also found. With complete failure of fusion, this includes ectopia cordis in which the heart and great vessels may lie outside the chest wall.

Much more frequent abnormalities involve the costochondral junction. Protrusion of adjoining rib cartilage and sternum may occur on one or both sides over varying lengths along the sternum resulting in pectus carinatum. The etiology of these defects is unknown, and their only cause for concern is cosmetic. Pectus excavatum (Fig. 1) is the most frequent of the costochondral abnormalities. Again the cause is uncertain, but some of the most striking depressions occur in Marfan's syndrome, in which a defect in collagen formation is suspected. Retractions of the lower sternum and costochondral junction occur frequently in infants with respiratory distress syndrome of the newborn. These retractions are usually thought to reflect the effects of a compliant chest wall attempting to expand a noncompliant lung. It is also conceivable that a chest wall without support would behave as a flail chest and aggravate respiratory distress. This hypothesis is supported by the fact that some infants who recover from the respiratory distress syndrome have true pectus excavatum in later life.

RIB

Minor abnormalities such as fusion or supernumerary ribs are frequent and are generally of no physiologic consequence. Supernumerary cervical ribs, however, can be troublesome in middle age and can cause pain through compression of brachial roots, requiring removal. Hypoplasia of ribs is a very infrequent occurrence; when present it appears to have little effect on respiration.

KYPHOSCOLIOSIS

The syndrome of scoliosis with or without kyphosis should be considered a reflection of disease affecting the supporting structures of the thorax, i.e., spine, ligaments, and muscle, permitting an imbalance between gravitational stress and mechanical support. Although its cause is frequently not determined, it should not be considered idiopathic until a careful search has been made for known causes. This is particularly true when the deformity is recognized before 10 years of age.

At some time all of the congenital diseases producing spinal deformity are undoubtedly metabolic in nature; in only a few is the metabolic defect defined. For purposes of arriving at a diagnosis by orderly examination of anatomic structure and function a classification based on anatomy is provided (Table 1). Nearly all of these diseases are likely to go unrecognized in the

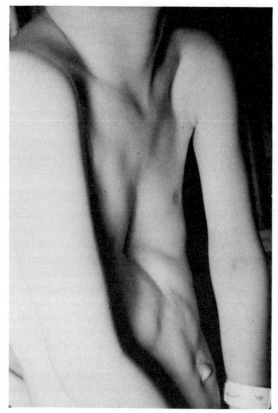

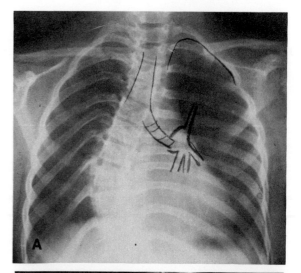

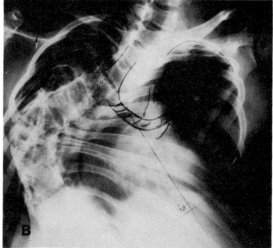

Fig. 1. A child of 8 years with severe pectus deformity and Marfan's syndrome. No deficit in ventilatory function or gas exchange was demonstrable in this child.

Fig. 2. Thoracic spine radiographs of a girl with neurofibromatosis and a scoliosis at age 12 years (A) (primary curve 65°) and when next examined at 18 years (B) (primary curve 110°).

newborn nursery except for vertebral anomalies found incidentally on chest radiography. In many of these diseases the resulting deformity of spine and thoracic structures contributes substantially to the pathophysiology of the disease.

Of all the thoracic deformities, scoliosis with or without kyphosis produces the most significant impairment of physiology. Kyphosis alone seems to have little effect on respiratory function, since patients with Scheuerman's disease, rheumatoid spondylitis, and mucopolysaccharidoses have normal lung volume and gas exchange for their size.

Based on the frequency of referral to an orthopedic surgeon, it is estimated that scoliosis affects 1 of 600 live births. This incidence among female family members is also increased, suggesting a common genetic or environmental factor. Idiopathic curves tend to begin and others tend to worsen with puberty to a degree that can be devastating to the child (Fig. 2). Whether this relates solely to greater mechanical imbalance during a period of rapid linear growth or to associated chemical, perhaps hormonal, changes is not known. Generally a child is not referred until the curve becomes quite obvious, on the average about 65 deg. This is fortunate since the child is asymptomatic and there is no demonstrable functional loss at this time. Causal factors must explain why 90 per-

cent of children with idiopathic curves are female and 90 percent of the curves are convex to the right.

PATHOPHYSIOLOGY

The degree of impairment of respiratory and cardiac function in these patients is directly related to the measured degree of the scoliotic curve. Those whose curves are due to neuromuscular disease tend to have even greater malfunction than those whose curves are idiopathic. In part this can be explained by the fact that lack of neuromuscular support permits the spine to sag under gravitational stress and in part by the fact that the intercostal component of inspiration may be deficient.

Scoliosis produces a progressive restriction of lung volume, a loss that is linear with the degree of primary curvature over 65 deg and affects vital capacity and total lung capacity to an equal degree (Figs. 3 and 4). Air-flow rates are generally normal. The gas-exchanging function of the whole lung and its distribution within the lung is impaired early. The alveolar–arterial oxygen gradient on

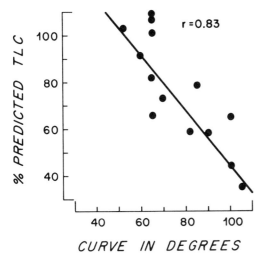

Fig. 3. The percentage predicted total lung capacity is related to the primary curve in degrees (Cobb's method) in 15 children. The relationship tends to be linear with a correlation coefficient of 0.83. Those with curves less than about 65° have total lung capacity within the normal range of $100 \pm 20\%$.

room air is increased to 35 mm Hg with no clear relationship to the degree of curvature. Since increased shunting is not a major abnormality in kyphoscoliosis, the increased O_2 gradient on room-air breathing reflects ventilation/perfusion inequality. The loss of diffusing capacity is linear with the loss of lung volume. Pulmonary blood flow is redistributed away from the lung base in those curves exceeding 70 deg and particularly in the lung on the convex side of the curve, generally the right lung. Thus the functional changes during adolescence are characterized by loss of functioning lung volume, ventilation/perfusion inequality, and increased pulmonary vascular resistance. These changes set the stage for the onset of respiratory failure and cor pulmonale during the

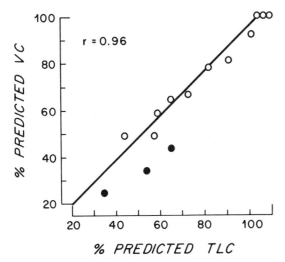

Fig. 4. The percentage predicted vital capacity versus the percentage predicted total lung capacity in the same 15 children has a correlation coefficient of 0.96. Thus there is a pure restrictive defect.

third to fourth decade, particularly in those with curves exceeding 90 deg.

THERAPY

Just as prevention of poliomyelitis has virtually eliminated that disease as a cause of scoliosis, so prevention of idiopathic scoliosis will be possible when its cause is known. Until then treatment should be instituted early so that the later irreversible pathophysiologic effects can be prevented. From available physiologic data the appropriate time for treatment is defined not by age but by the degree of curvature and should be effected before the curve exceeds 65 deg, since the loss of functioning lung volume associated with greater curves is irreparable. A variety of orthopedic techniques are successful in bracing, distracting, and fusing the spine with excellent cosmetic effect. In addition to this cosmetic improvement and its attendant psychologic benefit, there is a modest improvement in ventilation/perfusion inequality.

Children with scoliosis due to pleural disease following empyema should generally be treated with nonoperative methods. They will have abnormal lung function for several months but will gradually return to normal with time and with physical therapy. Therefore there should be no attempt to correct their deformity, e.g., by pleural decortication, for at least 6 months after the acute illness.

REFERENCES

Bartlett D: Postnatal growth of the mammalian lung: Influence of excess growth hormone. Respir Physiol 12:297, 1971

Bergofsky EH, Turino GM, Fishman AP: Cardiorespiratory failure in kyphoscoliosis. Medicine 38:263, 1959

Dwyer EM, Troncale F: Spontaneous pneumothorax and pulmonary disease in the Marfan syndrome. Ann Intern Med 62:1285, 1965

Maroteaux P, Savart P: La Dystrophie Thoracique Asphyiante: Etude radiologique et rapports avec le syndrome d'Ellis van Creveld. Ann Radiol 7:332, 1964

Orzalesi MM, Reynolds EOR, Cook CD: Lung function in scoliosis and pectus excavatum. Cesk Pediatr 20:404, 1965

Shannon DC, Riseborough EJ, Kazemi H: Ventilation perfusion relationships following correction of kyphoscoliosis. JAMA 217:579, 1969

PULMONARY NEOPLASMS

Gerald Nash

EPIDEMIOLOGY

During the past four decades the incidence of carcinoma of the lung has risen steadily (Fig. 1). From 1950–1952 to 1965–1967 the age-adjusted death rate for cancer of the lung per 100,000 population increased 106 percent in males and 70 percent in females. This increase was far greater than that of any other malignant tumor. Cancer of the pancreas showed the second highest increase, 32 percent in males and 24 percent in females. Carcinoma of the lung is currently second only to skin cancer as the most common malignancy in U.S. males, and for the two

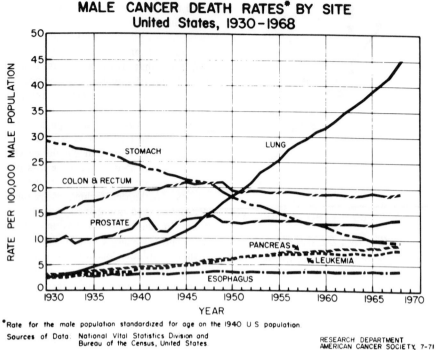

MALE CANCER DEATH RATES* BY SITE
United States, 1930-1968

Fig. 1. Male cancer death rates by site. (Courtesy of Research Department, American Cancer Society.)

sexes combined no tumor has a higher mortality rate. The peak age incidence is about 60 years in males and 70 years in females. The disease is four to six times as frequent in men as in women.

Epidemiologic evidence suggests that contamination of the air we breathe is a major cause of lung cancer. Carcinogenic compounds are found in large quantities in the contaminated atmospheres of industrialized cities, and urban populations have a higher risk of developing lung cancer than rural ones. Many individuals also produce their own private air pollution by inhaling cigarette smoke. Both tobacco and tobacco smoke have been found to contain a number of carcinogenic materials, and numerous studies have demonstrated an increasing risk of developing lung cancer as the quantity of cigarettes consumed goes up and the duration of the smoking habit lengthens. Recent investigations have also determined that a smoker may reduce his risk if he stops smoking. In a similar vein, morphologic studies have shown that the incidence of precancerous changes in bronchial epithelium increases with the level of cigarette consumption and decreases after the smoking habit is discontinued. The weight of evidence accumulated thus far demands that cigarette smoking be considered a major factor in the etiology of lung cancer.

Industrial workers exposed to certain chemicals have a higher than expected incidence of pulmonary malignancy. Substances that have been incriminated include asbestos, arsenic, chromium, nickel, iron, coal-tar fumes, petroleum mists, and uranium. Asbestos is perhaps the best known example. Asbestos workers face a risk of developing lung cancer that is seven to eight times that of

the general population. Asbestos may be even more notorious for its striking association with mesotheliomas, malignant tumors of the pleura and peritoneum. Given the ubiquity of asbestos fibers in the urban environment, it is possible that this substance may influence the chances of development of lung cancer by people who have no direct industrial exposure. It is known, for example, that individuals living in the vicinity of an asbestos industry have an increased risk of developing lung cancer.

CLASSIFICATION

Lung cancers may be classified on the basis of site of origin into three broad groups: bronchogenic, alveolar cell, and "scar" carcinomas. The bronchogenic carcinomas, which arise in the bronchial tree, are by far the most common and clinically important pulmonary malignancies and are of several histologic types. Seventy-five percent have their origin in major bronchi. These are usually squamous cell or undifferentiated carcinomas, the two types that are most frequently associated with cigarette smoking. The other 25 percent arise in peripheral bronchi and are usually adenocarcinomas. Squamous cell carcinoma accounts for approximately 60 percent of lung carcinoma in males and about 25 percent in females. These tumors are usually bulky and may occlude the bronchus and invade surrounding pulmonary tissue (Figs. 2 and 3). Necrosis with subsequent cavity formation occurs in 10 to 30 percent of all lung cancers, but the tumor that most frequently cavitates is the squamous cell type. Undifferentiated carcinomas make up to 30 to 40 percent of lung cancers. They, too, tend to be bulky and to occlude the bronchus of origin. The two histologic types included under this heading are the small

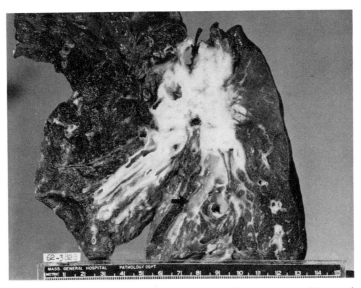

Fig. 2. Squamous cell carcinoma of the right main bronchus (curved arrow) with extensive invasion of the right middle and lower lobes. Note bronchiectasis (straight arrow) distal to tumor mass.

cell or oat cell carcinoma and the large cell undifferentiated carcinoma (Fig. 4). The third major type of bronchogenic carcinoma is the adenocarcinoma (Fig. 5). This tumor accounts for only about 10 percent of lung cancers in males, but makes up 25 to 30 percent of lung cancers in females. Adenocarcinomas are not associated with cigarette smoking. They tend to arise more peripherally in the bronchial tree and are usually smaller than other bronchogenic carcinomas. Bronchial adenomas are included under the heading of bronchogenic carcinomas because unlike most "adenomas" they act more like low-grade carcinomas than benign neoplasms. Although about 25 percent of these tumors are truly endobronchial, most extend beyond the confines of the bronchus, and some metastasize to regional lymph nodes and distant organs. The carcinoid type accounts for approximately 85 percent of these lesions. Cylindromas, also known as adenoidcystic carcinomas, account for

most of the remaining 15 percent and are the most malignant of the bronchial adenomas.

As their name implies, bronchiolar-alveolar cell carcinomas are thought to arise from bronchiolar or alveolar lining epithelium. They have a distinctive microscopic pattern consisting of cuboid to columnar cells lining alveolar walls (Fig. 6). These tumors make up only 3 to 4 percent of lung cancers, are not related to smoking, and occur with equal frequency in both sexes. Like adenocarcinomas, these tumors arise in the periphery of the lung.

Occasionally a lung cancer appears to have arisen in a pulmonary scar. Most so-called scar carcinomas are adenocarcinomas or bronchiolar-alveolar cell tumors; a minority are squamous cell carcinomas. Malignancy may develop in focal peripheral scars such as those resulting from pulmonary infarcts or healed granulomas, or it may occur in a setting of diffuse interstitial fibrosis.

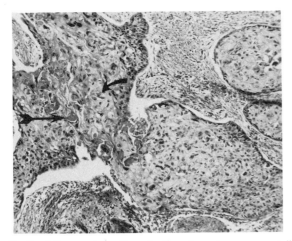

Fig. 3. Microscopic section of a bronchogenic squamous cell carcinoma showing individual cell keratinization (curved arrow) and poorly formed horn pearls (straight arrow) (H&E, ×130).

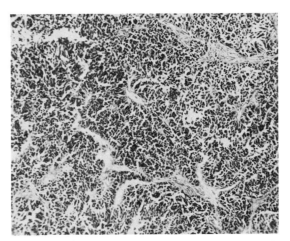

Fig. 4. Microscopic section of an oat cell carcinoma. This is a highly malignant undifferentiated tumor composed of uniform small oat-shaped cells (H&E, ×130).

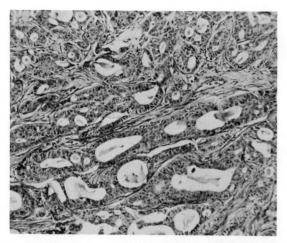

Fig. 5. Microscopic section of a bronchogenic adenocarcinoma. Well-formed malignant glands are readily apparent (H&E, ×130).

BEHAVIOR

The local growth characteristics and metastatic potential of lung cancers differ somewhat according to histologic type. In general, squamous cell carcinomas grow slowly and become very large; they often extend directly to the thoracic wall and may invade regional lymph nodes directly rather than by lymphatic metastasis. Only about 35 percent have extrathoracic metastases. In contrast, adenocarcinomas tend to have small primary growths and metastasize early, usually via the bloodstream. Approximately 85 percent are associated with extrathoracic metastases. Oat cell carcinomas grow very rapidly and metastasize widely via the lymphatics. Approximately 90 percent develop extrathoracic metatases, and half of the patients with this neoplasm have bone-marrow involvement at the time of initial evaluation. Bronchiolar-alveolar cell carcinomas begin as a small focus in the periphery of the lung and spread diffusely through both lungs, eventually causing

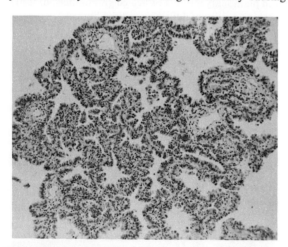

Fig. 6. Microscopic section of a bronchiolar-alveolar cell carcinoma. In this type of lung cancer the tumor cells line alveolar spaces; they are thought to be derived from bronchiolar or alveolar epithelium. (H&E, ×130).

respiratory insufficiency. Many observers believe that these tumors spread by exfoliation and endobronchial dissemination. Others think that they are of multicenteric origin. Approximately 80 percent are bilateral when the patient is first seen. Metastasis to hilar lymph nodes may occur, but spread to distant sites is rare.

In general, regional lymph nodes are the most common site of metastasis for lung cancer, with involvement in about three-fourths of cases. The liver is involved in one-third of cases, and the bones, adrenals, kidneys, and brain in about one-fifth of cases. It is not uncommon for the presenting complaint to be related to an extrathoracic metastasis rather than to the primary tumor. In one series of men who died of lung cancer, for example, approximately 10 percent presented with symptoms and signs referable to central nervous system involvement.

SYMPTOMS AND SIGNS

As a general rule localized lung cancers are seldom associated with respiratory symptoms, and patients who are symptomatic usually have extensive tumor. The symptoms of carcinoma of the lung may be caused by mechanical effects of the main tumor mass, extension to involve other thoracic structures, and distant metastases. In addition, many lung cancers are associated with a number of interesting nonmetastatic extrapulmonary manifestations.

The initial symptoms are usually those that are caused by partial bronchial obstruction and commonly consist of persistent cough, "asthmatic" breathing, and increased sputum production. The sputum often has a mucoid character. Patients with bronchiolar-alveolar cell tumors may produce voluminous amounts of frothy, clear sputum. Hemoptysis is frequent and may occur at any time in the course of the disease. Eventually complete bronchial obstruction results in distal atelectasis, which is followed by recurrent pneumonitis, bronchiectasis, or lung abscess. Symptoms and signs of obstructive pneumonitis usually persist following antibiotic therapy. However, on occasion they may disappear with treatment. It is therefore best to have follow-up chest roentgenograms on male patients over the age of 45 a few weeks following recovery from pneumonia, in order to avoid missing an underlying tumor.

Tumors arising in the apices of the upper lobes may invade the cervical sympathetic plexus, subclavian vessels, and brachial plexus, causing Horner's syndrome, vasomotor symptoms, and dysesthesias of the arm; this symptom complex is known as the superior sulcus tumor (or Pancoast) syndrome. Involvement of the superior mediastinum or lymph nodes beneath the aortic arch at the hilum of the left lung may damage the left recurrent laryngeal nerve, resulting in vocal cord paralysis and hoarseness. A phrenic nerve may become involved by tumor in the lateral superior mediastinum, causing paralysis of the homolateral hemidiaphragm. This can be diagnosed on fluoroscopy by the observation of paradoxical motion of the paralyzed hemidiaphragm. Tumor in the mediastinum may compress the esophagus, causing dysphagia. It may also compress the superior vena cava, producing edema and venous congestion of the face, neck, and arms, a condition known as the superior vena cava syndrome.

Carcinomas of the lung are associated with a variety of manifestations that are related to neither the primary organ nor the sites of metastatic spread. These extrapulmonary complications may dominate the clinical picture and on occasion may alert the physician to the existence of an otherwise occult tumor. Lung cancers can produce polypeptide hormones capable of causing a variety of endocrine syndromes. There is an association of specific histologic tumor types with specific hormonal dysfunction. Cushing's syndrome is probably the most common endocrine disorder associated with carcinoma of the lung. In most cases the tumor is an oat-cell carcinoma of the lung, but less often the carcinoid type of bronchial adenoma is implicated. Analysis of tumor tissue in such cases demonstrates a significant ACTH content; the hormone cannot be distinguished from normal ACTH by physiologic, physicochemical, or immunochemical methods. Oat cell carcinomas and carcinoid bronchial adenomas have also been associated with the carcinoid syndrome, with urinary excretion of excessive amounts of 5-hydroxyindole acetic acid or 5-hydroxytryptophan. Recent evidence suggests that both tumors may have their origin in the Kulchitsky (argentaffine) cells, which occur normally in the bronchial epithelium and mucus glands. Oat cell carcinoma is also associated with a syndrome of inappropriate ADH production, and immunoassays of tumor tissue in such cases have demonstrated the presence of ADH-like material within it. A hyperparathyroidlike syndrome, with symptoms secondary to hypercalcemia, is related to pulmonary cancer, almost always of the squamous cell type. Removal of all or part of the tumor has been followed by complete disappearance of symptoms, and the serum calcium and phosphorous levels have returned to normal within 48 hr after surgery. Some men with lung cancer develop tender gynecomastia and are found to have high blood and urine titers of gonadotropin, which is also contained in the tumor. Most gonadotropin-producing pulmonary tumors have been large cell undifferentiated carcinomas, but some have been squamous, oat cell, or bronchiolar-alveolar cell varieties.

Probably the most frequent nonmetastatic extrapulmonary manifestations of lung carcinomas are the so-called carcinomatous neuromyopathies. In approximately 60 percent of these cases the tumor type is an oat-cell carcinoma, and in about one-third the neuromuscular disorder precedes the appearance of other symptoms by a year or more. The neurologic syndromes that may occur include subacute cerebellar degeneration, dementia, psychosis, peripheral neuropathy, myasthenia, and polymyositis. The etiology and pathogenesis of these neuromyopathies are unknown. One hypothesis is that the tumors produce a substance that is directly toxic to the nervous system; another is that the tumor produces an organ-specific antigen to which the patient becomes sensitized as part of an autoimmune mechanism.

Hypertrophic osteoarthropathy is another nonmetastatic complication of lung cancer. It causes considerable discomfort and may be responsible for the patient's initial complaint. It involves the long bones, particularly near the wrists or ankles, and is characterized by swelling and edema of periarticular areas and marked subperiosteal bone formation. The condition may regress promptly following removal of the tumor. Digital clubbing, dermatomyositis, acanthosis nigricans, and nonbacterial thrombotic endocarditis are other nonmetastatic manifestations that may be associated with lung cancer, as well as with a variety of other diseases.

DIAGNOSIS

Almost all patients with symptomatic carcinoma of the lung have some abnormality on chest x-ray. Roentgenologic findings in lung cancer include one or more of the following: (1) a density in the lung field that represents tumor alone or tumor plus atelectasis and pneumonitis distal to an obstructed bronchus; (2) widening of the hilar shadow from tumor in a main bronchus, metastases to hilar lymph nodes, or vascular enlargement; (3) widening of the mediastinum; (4) pleural effusion. Rarely, a symptomatic bronchogenic carcinoma is not large enough to produce radiologic signs. Partial bronchial obstruction by such tumors may be detected on roentgenograms taken during forced expiration. During this procedure, air trapped distal to the partially obstructed airway shows up as an area of increased translucency. Routine chest x-ray may detect some occult lung cancers. Asymptomatic patients seem to have a better prognosis, since their tumors are usually smaller and are more often resectable. In addition to multiple projections and fluoroscopy, special roentgenographic techniques such as laminography, stereography, bronchography, and pulmonary arteriography may aid in the detection and differential diagnosis of lung masses. The extent of tumor spread beyond the confines of the lung can be evaluated when necessary by angiocardiography, superior vena cavography, and azygography.

A radiologic diagnosis of lung cancer is only presumptive; it is desirable to have morphologic confirmation prior to treatment. This may be obtained by biopsy or by cytologic examination of tracheobronchial secretions of pleural fluid. Bronchoscopy, mediastinoscopy, scalene lymph node biopsy, and biopsy of palpable cervical lymph nodes and other accessible sites of presumed metastases may yield a tissue diagnosis and provide valuable information on resectability. These procedures have been discussed in an earlier section. Needle biopsy of a peripheral pulmonary lesion may be performed in order to obtain a histologic diagnosis of tumor. This procedure, however, is usually performed only to confirm the diagnosis of carcinoma when the tumor is obviously inoperable, and it is not recommended when surgery for an attempted cure is anticipated.

Cytologic examination of sputum and bronchial aspirates has become a very accurate and valuable laboratory procedure and will often supply a morphologic diagnosis when biopsy has failed. If three satisfactory sputum samples are examined, an accurate preoperative diagnosis can be established in approximately 80 percent of all cases of carcinoma of the lung. False positive results in most centers occur in less than 1 percent of cases. Morning sputum specimens, representing the overnight accumulation of secretions, provide the best results. Some peripheral tumors may not contribute enough cells to the pool of sputum to permit a positive cytologic diagnosis. In such instances bronchial aspirates or washings obtained during bronchoscopy and the use of aerosols to promote sputum production may yield a positive diagnosis. The technique of bronchial brushing, in which small brushes are guided by x-ray television visualization to selected peripheral bronchi and cells are scraped from the bronchial mucosa, may also be helpful. These ancillary methods may increase the yield of cytologic diagnosis of lung cancer to almost 90 percent of cases.

Despite the variety of diagnostic procedures available, many patients who are evaluated for carcinoma of the lung must still undergo exploratory thoracotomy in order to confirm the diagnosis or to assess resectability.

TREATMENT AND PROGNOSIS

Surgery remains the treatment of choice for attempted cure of lung cancer. Unfortunately, in many patients the tumor has spread beyond the confines of the lung and is inoperable by the time medical attention is sought. Only 25 to 40 percent of patients who are evaluated for lung cancer have resectable tumors. Surgery is contraindicated not only in patients with unresectable lung tumors but also in individuals who have frank pulmonary insufficiency or who on the basis of their pulmonary function and overall clinical status might be expected to develop significant respiratory insufficiency following thoracotomy and removal of functioning lung tissue.

Resection consists of either a pneumonectomy or a lobectomy. Wherever possible lobectomy is performed, since its operative mortality is less and it leaves the patient with more functioning lung tissue. Pneumonectomy is performed only when involvement of the main bronchus or a major pulmonary vessel precludes a lobectomy. In cases in which resection for cure is not possible, palliative surgery is not recommended because it has been shown not to improve the quality of life or the survival time. The present role of radiotherapy in lung cancer is palliative; it may increase the length and quality of survival time in patients with inoperable tumors. In the treatment of oat cell carcinoma radiotherapy has been shown to be as good as or better than surgery. For this reason radiotherapy is the treatment of choice in most patients who have this highly malignant tumor. Preoperative radiotherapy of lung cancer has been evaluated in numerous studies and has not been shown to improve the survival rate as compared to surgery alone. It may, moreover, cause increased postoperative morbidity. Mediastinal lymph node involvement is considered by most authorities to be a contraindication to pulmonary resection. A recent study suggests, however, that in certain selected patients with mediastinal lymph node metastases (e.g., those with squamous cell carcinoma) an increase in survival may be obtained with mediastinal irradiation following pulmonary resection and mediastinal lymph node dissection. Chemotherapy currently plays a minor role in the treatment or palliation of lung cancer, since there is no convincing evidence that any drug is particularly helpful. Combination drug therapy however, has shown promise, increasing the survival time of patients with oat cell carcinoma.

In general the prognosis for patients with carcinoma of the lung is poor. The 5-year survival for all cases is between 5 and 10 percent. For patients who undergo pulmonary resection and have no lymphatic involvement, the 5-year survival is between 25 and 40 percent. The 5-year survival drops to between 15 and 20 percent if hilar nodes are involved, and it is less than 10 percent if there are mediastinal metastases. Patients treated with radiotherapy alone have a 5-year survival of approximately 10 percent. Tumor type alters the prognosis to some degree. Median survival is longest for patients with adenocarcinoma and shortest for those with oat cell carcinoma. Squamous cell and undifferentiated large cell tumors occupy an intermediate position.

This discussion has been concerned almost entirely with malignant pulmonary neoplasms, since they are by far the most common and important tumors of the lung. The only significant benign lung tumor is the pulmonary hamartoma. Typically this lesion occurs as a small well-circumscribed nodule that consists of proliferated bronchial elements, including epithelium and cartilage. Pulmonary hamartomas are usually peripheral and asymptomatic. They are commonly discovered on routine chest x-rays, in which they appear as rounded or lobulated densities ("coin lesions"). Foci of calcification are often visualized within them and are helpful in differentiating them from malignant neoplasms. Nevertheless, a patient with the typical roentgenographic picture of hamartomas should undergo thoracotomy and resection of the lesion, since malignancy cannot be ruled out in any other way.

REFERENCES

Ackerman LV, del Regato JA: Cancer: Diagnosis, Treatment and Prognosis (ed 4). St Louis, CV Mosby, 1970, p 329

Auerbach O, Gere JB, Forman JB, et al: Changes in the bronchial epithelium in relation smoking and cancer of the lung. N Engl J Med 256:97, 1957

Collaborative study: Preoperative irradiation of cancer of the lung. Cancer 23:419, 1969

Hinshaw HC: Diseases of the Chest. Philadelphia, WB Saunders, 1969, p 374

Kirsch MM, Kahn DR, Gago O, et al: Treatment of bronchogenic carcinoma with mediastinal metastases. Ann Thorac Surg 12:11, 1971

Liebow AA: Tumors of the Lower Respiratory Tract, Atlas of Tumor Pathology, Section V, Fascicle 17. Washington, Armed Forces Institute of Pathology, 1952

Morton DL, Itabashi HH, Grimes OF: Nonmetastatic neurological complications of bronchogenic carcinoma: The carcinomatous neuromyopathies. J Thorac Cardiovasc Surg 51:14, 1966

Omenn GS, Wilkins EW: Hormone syndromes associated with bronchogenic carcinoma. J Thorac Cardiovasc Surg 59:877, 1970

INDEX

Page numbers in italics refer to illustrations. Page numbers followed by *t* refer to tables.